Mosby's
Rapid
Review
Series

NURSING
PHARMACOLOGY

Mosby's Rapid Review Series

NURSING PHARMACOLOGY

Series Editor

Paulette D. Rollant, PhD, RN

President, Multi-Resources, Inc.
Newnan, Georgia

Karen Hill, PhD, MSN, RN

Assistant Professor
Southeastern Louisiana University
Hammond, Louisiana

second edition

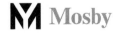

An Affiliate of Elsevier Science

St. Louis   London   Philadelphia   Sydney   Toronto

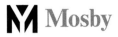

An Affiliate of Elsevier Science

Vice President, Nursing Editorial Director: Sally Schrefer
Senior Editor: Loren Wilson
Sr. Developmental Editors: Brian Dennison, Nancy L. O'Brien
Project Manager: Deborah L. Vogel
Design Manager: Bill Drone

SECOND EDITION

NOTICE
Pharmacology is an ever-changing field. Standard safety precautions must be followed, but as new research and clinical experience broaden our knowledge, changes in treatment and drug therapy may become necessary or appropriate. Readers are advised to check the most current product information provided by the manufacturer of each drug to be administered to verify the recommended dose, the method and duration of administration, and contraindications. It is the responsibility of the licensed health care provider, relying on experience and knowledge of the patient, to determine dosages and the best treatment for each individual patient. Neither the Publisher nor the editor assumes any liability for any injury and/or damage to persons or property arising from this publication.

Mosby, Inc.
An Affiliate of Elsevier Science
11830 Westline Industrial Drive
St. Louis, Missouri 63146

Printed in United States of America

Library of Congress Cataloging-in-Publication Data

Rollant, Paulette D.
    Nursing pharmacology/Paulette D. Rollant, Karen Hill.—2nd ed.
        p. cm—(Mosby's rapid review series)
    Includes bibliographical references and index.
    ISBN 0-323-01167-5
        1. Pharmacology—Outlines, syllabi, etc. 2. Pharmacology—Examinations, questions, etc. 3. Nursing—Outlines, syllabi, etc. 4. Nursing—Examinations, questions, etc. I. Hill, Karen, Ph.D. II. Title. III. Mosby's review series.
    RM301.14.R65 2001
    615'.1—dc21   00-062483

02   03   04   CL/MVY   9   8   7   6   5   4   3   2

To Dan, Mom, Dad, and my sisters and brothers:
Joanne, Joe, Alan, and Amy

Paulette Rollant

To Bobby, B.J., Kristopher, and Lindsey

Karen Hill

Preface

HOW TO USE *MOSBY'S RAPID REVIEW SERIES*

Mosby's Rapid Review Series is designed to help you get the most from your prep, study, and review time for nursing exams. These books can be used to review essential concepts, theory, and content prior to nursing courses and challenge, certification, or licensing examinations. The rapid review series can also be used to prepare for clinical experiences and as a quick reference while in the clinical setting. *Mosby's Rapid Review Series* consists of three books:

Maternal-Child Nursing
Medical-Surgical Nursing
Nursing Pharmacology

The series is designed to highlight and prioritize important information about the specific content as indicated in each title. It is not meant to provide comprehensive, in-depth coverage of the selected area of nursing.

In the revised editions, the new features, "Fast Facts," "Warning," "Essential Odds and Ends" chapter, "WEB Resources," the updated bibliography, the glossary, and the revised questions, answers, and test tips give you the added advantage for test prep. The CD-ROM disk of 265 new higher level questions, which include management and home care content, provides an opportunity to practice for the real test.

Keep in mind that this series, in combination with other texts, should be consulted when a more comprehensive discussion of a particular topic is desired. Use these books to jog your memory, to reinforce what you know, to guide you to identify what you don't know, and to lead you to appropriate sources for more details. If you are in a formal education setting, these books are not intended as a substitute for class attendance or the completion of any required reading assignments.

Used consistently and correctly, *Mosby's Rapid Review Series* can help you to:

1. Enhance your skills to prioritize in clinical situations, especially management and home care situations, by applying the nursing process.
2. Increase your ability to easily remember essential content.

3. Increase the productivity of your review and study time to leave time for you and your family.
4. Apply new behaviors for the improvement of your test-taking skills.
5. Evaluate your strengths and weaknesses for specific content areas or testing situations.

WHAT IS UNIQUE ABOUT *MOSBY'S RAPID REVIEW SERIES?*

1. The 265-question test on an accompanying CD-ROM
2. Comprehensive rationales for each answer option
3. Test-taking tips to eliminate test-taking errors
4. Chapter format of the nursing process with prioritized content
5. Web sites and traditional bibliography for further exploration of content areas
6. Odds and Ends chapter for the unfamiliar
7. Glossary of key terms

Test questions on CD-ROM

Each book in the series is accompanied by a comprehensive exam of 265 questions. The comprehensive exam questions, like the end-of-chapter questions, include the answers, comprehensive rationales, and test-taking tips. The disk has a tutorial and a test mode. Both allow you to repeat the test as many times as you wish. The level of the questions varies from knowledge, recall, application, and analysis. In many of the questions, all the options are correct; the task of the test taker is to select the highest priority.

Comprehensive rationales

The rationales include the answers and the rationales for each option. In questions where all options are correct but they must be prioritized, rationales state why or how each option is correct and why only one option is the best answer.

Test-taking tips

These tips build your decision-making skills to set nursing priorities and for managing and delivering home care wisely. The tips help to further develop your logical thinking skills to narrow the options to two and then select the correct answer based on what you know. After working with the questions in these books or on the CD-ROM, you will more often select the correct answer on those harder questions. You will have increased confidence from new learning methods and actions to think "how can I answer this question" rather than "if I only knew. . . ." You will learn how to get the correct answer on those questions about content you don't know.

Chapter format

Each chapter contains an easy-to-follow format divided into five sections:

1. "Fast Facts" are placed at the beginning of each chapter. These items are the "must know" information in that chapter.

2. "Content Review" is organized and structured by the nursing process to help you identify what is most important. Within each chapter the highlights include:
   - Prioritized information within each heading
   - The "Warning" feature is used throughout and focuses on critical and life-threatening issues
   - Client education is focused for the settings of hospital, clinics, and home
   - Management and home care content are included where applicable
   - You are alerted to issues regarding older adults where applicable
   - Evaluation criteria include decision-making tools about which actions to take when the client's clinical status shows improvement or deterioration
   - Tables, charts, and figures contrast, cluster, and simplify information for ease of grasp, recall, and review
3. "Review Questions" are stand-alone, four-option multiple choice questions. The test questions are of all difficulty levels and include management and home care situations for decision-making. The stems vary from being brief to lengthy to provide a realistic drill that mimics the NCLEX exam.
4. "Answers, Rationales, and Test-Taking Tips" focus on:
   - Comprehensive rationales, which are given for each option to explain why or how it is correct or incorrect. Additional information is given for less common facts or entities in the options. Other pertinent advice is also included to help you recall or review unfamiliar content or issues.
   - Test-taking tips give actions and strategies to use. For the more difficult questions, such as when options are narrowed to two; when you have no idea of a correct answer; when the content or issue is unfamiliar; or when all of the options are correct answers, specific approaches are given for each type of situation. The explanations include ways to prevent test-taking errors and ways to change your reading of the stem and options to get results—more correct answers. Specific prescriptions are given to raise your test scores.

"WEB resources" and bibliography

Web site resources for a particular condition, disorder, or topic are found throughout each book. A bibliography, including some books used in the development of the series, suggests areas for further study if more in-depth facts are needed.

Glossary

This list of key terms is provided to save you time in looking up unfamiliar terms or words.

WHAT'S IN *MOSBY'S RAPID REVIEW SERIES: NURSING PHARMACOLOGY?*

This book describes basic principles of pharmacology and practice. Within the initial four chapters, essential information, such as the fundamentals and principles of pharmacology and drug therapy, provides a basis for the remainder of the chapters, which are organized by major systems. The most common drug classifications act as the building blocks within each chapter. The development of content is by prioritization. The most common elements are written to include what is essential for study, review, and finding information in an expedient manner.

ABOUT THE AUTHORS

The original idea, the design, and the development of the *Rapid Review Series* were by Dr. Rollant. The original co-authors were the content experts for their respective books. They provided their expertise and hard work to develop the specific content and the questions. In the first edition, Dr. Rollant expanded the rationales for the question answers and then added the test-taking tips for each question.

In this revised second edition, each book has an author who is expert in the field, and Dr. Rollant is the series editor. Dr. Rollant has directed, coordinated, and managed the consistency of the revision as well as provided additional test questions, rationales, and test-taking tips. Dr. Rollant, with the expertise of test-taking skills development, expanded the discussion in the rationales for the correct answer and the discussion of each option for the questions written by the authors.

As a team, the series editor and the authors have worked diligently to provide the best test preparation and review format available to nursing students and graduates. We wish you the best in your nursing career. We encourage you to let us know what you have found the most or least helpful and what other needs you may have for test preparation. You can contact Dr. Rollant at rollant@bellsouth.net or 22 Village Lane, Newnan, GA 30265.

ACKNOWLEDGMENTS

I express my heartfelt gratitude to those who have endured with me throughout this publication of a nursing review series: an adventure from idea to reality.

I especially want to thank the following people who were involved in the first edition of the review series:

Beverly Copland, who thought that I had the potential to complete this project and who eagerly gave me tons of strong support in the initial and ongoing book development phases.

Laurie Muench, who picked up the ball in the middle of manuscript preparation and persisted with me through the process to completion of book publication. The response "OK . . . when can I expect it?" provided silent encouragement and sometimes comic relief when my mental and physical energies ran quite low. Laurie's thoughtfulness and guidance to help me set priorities were invaluable! I am very grateful and fortunate to have worked with Laurie.

Suzi Epstein, who was full of enthusiasm and total support from the birth of the idea to the final publication of the books. Suzi's creativity and suggestions provided essential building blocks in the overall development of the series.

My *coauthors*, for their enormous efforts to produce manuscript in a short time. Their nursing expertise was helpful for the development of the unique aspects of each book.

I also want to thank the following people who were involved in this second edition of the series:

Brian Dennison, who headed up the meeting of the authors for the revisions, coordinated the manuscript schedule and provided guidance up to the production of the changes. Brian's creativity, framed with his organizational skills, allowed for the process to be quite enjoyable. Brian's patience and steadiness were of great strength to me.

Nancy O'Brien, who entered at the production phase and carried the task to completion; however, not without a lot of bumps along the way. Nancy left no stone unturned as she strongly supported my colleagues and me. I appreciate her talent, skills, and patience to enter a project midway and complete it with ease and detail.

My wonderful husband, *Dan*, for his patience, humor, support, and love. His faith in my abilities has sustained my energies and maintained my sense of self. He has been my sounding board throughout both editions of the review series and through the publication of the *Soar to Success: Do Your Best on Nursing Tests* book.

My parents, *Joseph* (deceased March 7, 2000) and *Mildred Demaske*, for their love, encouragement, and prayers.

Paulette Demaske Rollant

I would like to thank the following people for helping me through the writing and revisions of this text:

Brian Dennison, Loren Wilson, and Mosby, for allowing all the authors to meet with Paulette Rollant to conceptualize the second edition.

Paulette Rollant, for her continued support in making this text a wonderful tool for students to use in preparing for NCLEX. She has given me support from the beginning and her input is always valued. I feel very grateful and fortunate to work with her and I value her expertise.

My wonderful *husband* for his support, love, and dedication in helping me to do the work when other things needed to be done. He has always supported me in my work and I am grateful for his faithfulness.

My three wonderful children, *B.J., Kristopher,* and *Lindsey,* for eating hotdogs and listening to their mom say she had to work all the time. Thanks for understanding.

Karen Y. Hill

Contents

INTRODUCTION
How to Use This Book
for Rapid Review
& Study

This book is designed to work for you at your convenience to save you time and energy. Read the following guidelines first. They will help save you additional time and energy for test preparation. These guidelines are divided into three areas of concern: the NCLEX–RN test plan structure, rapid study steps, and rapid review tips.

The chapters in this book are designed for short, quick intervals of review. Carry this book with you to catch those times when you are stuck and have nothing to do for that 5 to 15 minutes. Talk yourself into a brief rapid review and study period.

The directions for rapid review and study will give you the edge to:

- Maximize your individual performance on test prep and test questions
- Identify your personal priorities for test prep
- Sharpen your thinking and discrimination skills on multiple choice tests

NCLEX–RN test plan structure
The framework of *client needs* is the universal structure used on the NCLEX-RN. This framework of client needs defines the nursing actions and expected competencies across all settings for all clients. An integration of concepts and processes with nursing practice will be tested on the NCLEX-RN throughout the following four major categories of client needs. These categories, their subcategories, and related content, which includes, but is not limited to this list, are:

1. Safe, effective care environment
    - Management of care: advanced directives, advocacy, case management, client rights, concepts of management, confidentiality, continuity of care,

delegation, ethical practice, continuous quality improvement, incident/irregular occurrence/variance reports, informed consent, legal responsibilities, organ donation, consultation and referrals, resource management, supervision
- Safety and infection control: accident prevention, disaster planning, error prevention, handling hazardous and infectious materials, medical and surgical asepsis, standard (universal) precautions, use of restraints

2. Health promotion and maintenance
- Growth and development through the life span: the aging process, ante/intra/postpartum and newborn stages, developmental stages and transitions, expected body image changes, family planning, family systems, human sexuality
- Prevention and early detection of disease: disease prevention, health and wellness, health promotion programs, health screening, immunizations, lifestyle choices, techniques of physical assessment

3. Psychosocial integrity
- Coping and adaptation: coping mechanisms, counseling techniques, grief and loss, mental health concepts, religious and spiritual influences on health, sensory/perceptual alterations, situational role changes, stress management, support systems, unexpected body image changes
- Psychosocial adaptation: behavioral interventions, chemical dependency, child abuse/neglect, crisis intervention, domestic violence, elder abuse/neglect, psychopathology, sexual abuse, and therapeutic milieu

4. Physiological integrity
- Basic care and comfort: assistive devices, elimination, mobility/immobility, non-pharmacologic comfort interventions, nutrition and oral hygiene, personal hygiene, rest and sleep
- Pharmacological and parenteral therapies: administration of blood and blood products, central venous access devices, chemotherapy, expected effects, intravenous therapy, medication administration, parenteral fluids, pharmacologic actions and agents, side effects, total parenteral nutrition, untoward effects
- Reduction of risk potential: alterations in body systems, diagnostic tests, laboratory values, pathophysiology, therapeutic procedures, potential complications after tests, procedures, surgery, and health alterations
- Physiological adaptation: alterations in body systems, fluid and electrolyte imbalances, hemodynamics, infectious diseases, medical emergencies, pathophysiology, radiation therapy, respiratory care, unexpected response to therapies

Website: http://www.ncsbn.org/dxp.html
Other helpful sites:
National Student Nurses Association
   http://www.NSNA.org/index.htm
American Nurses Association
   http://www.ANA.org/index.htm

Rapid study steps

Step 1. Identify a study routine—What can be changed for efficiency and effectiveness?

a. What are your best days to study? First, list or think about all weekly activities that are set, such as work time, your children's school obligations, or attendance at church.

b. Write these activities on the days of your personal calendar and the calendar at home – yes, the big one that everyone uses to coordinate family activities; it is usually in the kitchen on the refrigerator. Be sure to include the time needed for each activity, including travel time to and from the activity.

c. Oh! You don't use one. Maybe it is time to get one and get writing! This communicates the weekly needs to your family or support systems. It highlights the time you will be available or unavailable to them.

d. Now write in your study times. What are the best times to study? Just look at "the time left" on each day. Decide if you desire to schedule in study, relaxation, or catch-up activities at these times. Then stick to it.

e. To have designated study time written on a readily accessible calendar is a nice reminder every day to yourself that study is important to you. Be sure to cross off completed tasks! You will feel great as you cross off the completed daily or weekly study times. These actions give you a sense of accomplishment.

  1) Does the designated study time have to be blocked for at least a few hours? No. Set aside your designated study time in 15- to 30-minute increments. These times might be set when you know that others in the family will be involved in their own activities.

  2) Remember the nursing process: assessment of the immediate situation is the first step in any given client situation. Get started with the application of the nursing process to your own life. The more you use these steps in your daily life, the more skilled you become in answering those test questions based on the nursing process. Weekly, assess what time you have and what content is weak and needs attention.

Step 2. Launch a rapid textbook study routine for each given class

a. Scan the table of contents in your textbook, noting assigned required reading

  1) Put a check mark in front of the content for 10 items with which you are comfortably strong.

  2) Circle 10 content areas with which you are shaky or which you dislike.

  3) Prioritize the shaky content, then the comfortable content.

    i. Put numbers from 1 to 10 in front of your shaky content, and then in front of the comfortable content.

    ii. Number 1 should be the weakest content area and number 10 should be the strongest area within each category of shaky or comfortable content.

b. When you are feeling a high-energy day, go to the number 1 chapter of the shaky content area and read.

c. When you are having a low-energy day, go to the number 1 chapter of the comfort content area and read.

d. Continue to work your way through all 10 areas of each category. Once you have completed all areas, start again with this process for the remainder of the content.

Step 3. Resort to rapid chapter reading

a. Read the summary at the end of the chapter or the introduction if no summary is provided.
b. Read the major and minor headings in the chapter in an attempt to put together a picture of the importance and the sequence of the content.
   1) If you are at this point and it is before class, make a brief list of what you don't understand. Use this list as the basis of the questions that you ask during class.
   2) If you are doing this after you have attended the class, more in-depth reading of the selected subject matter may be needed.
c. Next, read each chapter. Start by first reading the sections of the unfamiliar subject matter. Use this process to read the paragraphs: Read the first and the last sentence of each paragraph. Then, if you need to read the entire paragraph, do so. Recall from English class that paragraphs are formed with the key sentences at the first and last position. Apply this "process of writing" to your "process of reading."
d. Continue to use this process for assigned readings, such as journal articles, as well as for your enjoyment in reading books, newspapers or magazines.

Step 4. Achieve actions for accurate and retentive rapid study

a. Develop a system of study that meets the needs of your schedule.
   1) Select time when you are least tired or stressed, both mentally and physically.
   2) Limit your study time to a maximum of 90 minutes. This time frame results in the most effective, efficient retention of content.
b. If possible, relax and take a nap after the study period to cement the information into your long-term memory. Some research reveals that sleeping for 2 to 3 hours after studying results in a 70% to 80% retention rate of content in long-term memory. In contrast only a 30% to 40% retention rate is achieved when you are active after the study session.
c. Breathe deeply and slowly three times at the onset and at the end of your study time. S-L-O-W, deep breathing with concentration on the air going in and out is one of the best ways to get relaxed, both physically and mentally.
d. Use one other relaxation technique at the halfway mark of your study session.
e. If your time is limited, use 10- to 15-minute intervals to study small pieces of the content. For example, you may want to review the different aspects of hypertension in one study session.

Step 5. Select a theme for the day

a. When you plan at the beginning of the semester, use the approach of selecting a theme or topic for the day. For example, if there is enough time between

your test and when you begin to study, review something every Monday on sodium from the book. Then, at work, find clients with sodium imbalances, review their charts, and discuss their situations with colleagues or with the clients' physicians. Continue with themes for each day such as:
1) Tuesdays: potassium.
2) Wednesdays: calcium.
3) Thursdays: magnesium.
4) Fridays: acidosis situations.
5) Saturdays: alkalosis situations.
6) Sundays: fun days. Don't forget to keep one day to relax and have fun. This allows your mind to work; your mind will automatically reorganize the retained content for better recall.
b. Weekly themes also might be of help. Do one system per week, such as pulmonary, endocrine, and so forth. Think of a way to associate the theme with meaning. For example, during the first week, study the pulmonary system since this is the first system with basic cardiac life support (BCLS). Then during the second week, study the cardiovascular system.

Step 6. Set up a study place
a. Designate a place to sit and study. Have all of your schoolbooks, references, computer, and so forth, at this location for ease of access.
b. A designated study place eliminates the "set up" time if all of your stuff is centralized and not scattered throughout the house. You can get more done in less time.
c. On days you aren't motivated to study, simply sit at this location for a minimum of 5 minutes. Within that time frame, tell yourself you might "flip through" a book. Before you know it, you will be into a productive study session.

Rapid review tips
1. Are there a few basic essential actions I can use for recall? Yes! Yes! Yes!
   a. Use yellow or lime green notebook paper or index cards. These colors enhance recall in long-term memory.
   b. Underline single words instead of phrases. The mind becomes more alert and attentive.
   c. Use a lime green or yellow highlighter.
   d. PRINT with CAPS when you make notes. Recall is enhanced. Avoid cursive writing of notes.
   e. Talk out loud to whomever will listen—even talk to your pets—cat, dog or fish.
   f. Review for 15 to 30 minutes before you go to sleep.
   g. Repeat items at least 3 times.
2. How can I use this review book for a rapid review before my class?
   a. Complete the review questions at the end of each chapter for a specified content area.
   b. Review the answers, rationales, and test-taking tips.

   c. Review content for the missed areas.

   d. Refer to your textbook, which has more details, if you still do not understand the information.

3. How should I use my notes from class?

   a. Read over your notes from class—every day! Yes, every day! Three repetitions enhance recall: You hear the instructor. You take notes. You reread your notes.

   b. Every day before going to sleep, take 10 minutes for a quick read-over of your class notes.

   c. Read over the notes for each class in the same sequence as the classes were attended that day.

4. What is an easy way to know key terms or content?

   a. Card them.

   b. Use a 3- x 5-inch index card to write the terms or condition on one side and the definitions of the key terms or the content information on the opposite side.

   c. Use the nursing process format to outline critical content.

   d. Look at the term and state your definition out loud.

   e. Uncover the definition and read the given definition out loud.

   f. Speaking the content as well as seeing the content will enhance your retention. If you have a few related terms that you can't remember, make a story out of the terms.

   g. Carry the card with you for a few days to review this content again. Suggestion: put these cards on your sunvisor in the car and review them at the stoplight or if stopped in traffic.

5. How can I prepare for the end of the semester comprehensive exam?

   a. Complete the comprehensive exam on the CD-ROM. Use it in the test mode.

   b. Review which questions were missed. Be sure to read the rationales and test-taking tips.

   c. Note if the test item was missed because of a lack of content knowledge or because you simply misread the question or some of the options.

   d. If a content problem is identified, list the specific content missed. Then cluster these under umbrellas of similar content. Use index cards for this activity.

     1) Prioritize these clusters, with number 1 being the least familiar content.

     2) Review additional content as indicated by the questions that you missed.

     3) Review the most familiar content last, or on low-energy days. Review the weakest content first, or on high-energy days.

   e. If your problem was identified as misreading, make a list of where the misreading occurred—in the question? In an option? If in an option, which one? Is there a pattern to the misread options? Was the misread option a series of items or a two-part option? Did you misread the second part of the option? Identify the pattern of errors you made in reading. Most test takers have 3 to 5 consistent errors that they repeat over and over again.

Think of actions that you can take to eliminate or minimize these types of testing errors.

6. Should I repeat the same practice test questions?
   a. Yes. However, do practice questions at different times of the day than when the comprehensive test was initially done. Repeat the comprehensive exam on the CD-ROM in the test mode, and then in the tutorial mode, and then again in the test mode.
   b. Note whether the test item was missed because of a lack of content knowledge or because of simply misreading the question or some of the options.
   c. Note that even though the questions are repeated, you should evaluate how your reading of the questions and options differed.
   d. Do you have a pattern in perception and consistent ability to identify key words, terms, age, and developmental needs?
   e. Did the fatigue factor or tenseness influence your thinking skills? And what did you do or could you have done to minimize these factors to improve your abilities?
   f. Did anticipatory thinking of the correct answer enhance or hinder your selection of the correct answer?
   g. Doing the same test questions over can be helpful to reinforce content, fine tune test skills, and establish better reading habits.
7. How do I evaluate my performance for testing?
   a. For any practice test questions, read all of the rationales and test-taking tips. Do this for the questions you got correct and those that you missed. The rationales and test-taking tips often contain pearls of wisdom on how to remember or get a better understanding of the content.
   b. Remember to do a relaxation exercise before you begin your questions, during the examination, and as you review the results. Do at least one mental and one physical relaxation exercise at least every 30 minutes or every 30 questions.
   c. When you miss a question ask yourself:
      1) Did I not know the content?
      2) Did I misread the question or options?
   d. If you miss questions because of a knowledge deficit:
      1) Make a list on a 3- x 5-inch card for 3 to 4 days.
      2) Group or cluster the content according to the steps in the nursing process, the content area, or a system.
      3) Look up that content.
      4) Do not look up content after every practice test. A better approach is to cluster the content and look it all up every 3 to 4 days. With this approach you will have better retention in long-term memory and the best recall at a later time.
   e. If you misread the question or the option(s):
      1) Try to identify new ways to approach reading questions and their options.
      2) Try to identify what key words, time frames, ages, and developmental stages that you may have overlooked.

8. How can I improve my test scores?
   a. Practice, practice, and practice doing questions.
   b. Practice, practice, and practice doing relaxation before you begin the practice exam, after every 10 to 20 questions, and then at the end of the examination to refresh your thinking and diminish your tenseness or tiredness.
   c. Look for a pattern or cluster of wrong answers.
      1) Where did you miss questions?
      2) Are there clusters of missed questions? If so, did this happen after what type of question? One related to the nursing process? One that asks for a priority and where all of the options are correct? One that had terms of "all but the following"? One that asked for the most or the least important item? One that had information you had never seen?
      3) Did you miss clusters of questions at the beginning of the test?
         i. If so, you have a tension or anxiety problem.
         ii. Simply do at least one mental and physical relaxation exercise before the test and at question 25 to control your thinking.
      4) Did you miss clusters of questions at the middle or the end of the test?
         i. If so, you have a fatigue or tiredness problem.
         ii. First be alert to the event of "feeling tired" or fatigued.
         iii. When you feel this way, get up and leave the room for 2 to 4 minutes. While you are out of the room, MOVE and be active. Touch your toes 10 times. Swing your arms from side to side. Mentally tell yourself: "I know something. I'll figure it out."
         iv. Return to the test in a more sharp, attentive state.
9. What is most essential to preparation for the NCLEX? What are the most essential actions to prepare for "the big test"?
   a. Be sure to do a practice exam with the exact number of questions as the NCLEX or your "big test."
   b. Write down on a note card when you were the most tired, anxious, or nervous during this examination. List the question number you were at when you were feeling this way.
   c. Do a relaxation exercise at these tense or fatigued times during the exam. Note which actions helped the most.
   d. Avoid the thought, "I am tired and just want to get done with the test."
   e. Your success is directly correlated to your degree of effort to review content as well as to deal with any tension and fatigue during the review and exam processes.

Summary

We would be pleased if you use this book as a major tool to supplement your textbooks, clinical, and classroom activities. We hope that after you have used this book you will have learned to take actions to:

- Maximize your individual performance in study, review, and testing situations.
- Identify personal actions to help you set priorities for test preparation.
- Sharpen your thinking and reading skills during tests.

We hope that this book makes it easy, enjoyable, and effective to study and review at convenient times. The short, condensed, and prioritized chapter content may spark new ways to develop your skills in critical thinking and recall of content.

It is feedback from students, graduates, and practitioners in nursing that prompted the development and publication of this rapid review series. We welcome your comments. Please contact Dr. Rollant at rollant@bellsouth.net or 22 Village Lane, Newnan, GA 30265. We wish you a successful career in the nursing profession and hope that *Mosby's Rapid Review Series* has made that success a little easier to obtain!

The material on rapid study steps and rapid review tips was taken from Rollant PD: Soar to Success: Do Your Best on Nursing Tests, St. Louis, 1999, Mosby.

1

Fundamentals of Pharmacology

FAST FACTS

The nursing process applied to drug therapy:

1. Assessment actions for drugs include the five rights, use of over-the-counter (OTC) medications, drug allergies, cultural characteristics, life span considerations, and how the four factors of pharmacokinetics (i.e., absorption, distribution, metabolism, and excretion) might be altered in clients.
2. Nursing diagnoses for medication therapy are as follows: knowledge deficit, noncompliance, and any diagnosis related to side effects of the medicines.
3. Planning action includes the time at which medications are administered in relation to their desired effects.
4. Implementation is the accuracy and safety precautions necessary to administer medications.
5. Evaluation involves documentation of the therapeutic or subtherapeutic effects and any side effects of drugs.
6. Administration of medications within legal and ethical considerations for drug therapy involves five areas: (1) drug legislation affecting drug administration, (2) Food and Drug Administration (FDA) classifications of new and approved drugs, (3) use of controlled substances, (4) use of investigational drugs, and (5) the Nursing Code of Ethics.
7. The common forms of preparations are as follows: oral (solids and liquids), topical, injected, vaginal, rectal, ophthalmic, otic, and other nonspecific methods such as implants, insulin pumps, venous access devices, etc.
8. Routes of administration include enteral, parenteral, topical, inhalation, and absorption through mucous membranes.

CONTENT REVIEW

I. Nursing process

A. Assessment

1. Obtain a drug history. Include each of the following:
   a. Prescription drugs
   b. OTC drugs
   c. Herbal or other similar substances
   d. Drug specifics
      (1) Name
      (2) Amount of dose
      (3) Route of administration
      (4) Frequency: how often administered; time of last dose
   e. Allergies to drugs—Ask client: What exactly does the medicine do?
2. Identify diseases in the body system that may affect the following:
   a. Drug absorption through the gastrointestinal (GI) tract, lungs, mucous membranes
   b. Distribution by the circulatory system
   c. Metabolism by the hepatic system
   d. Excretion by the renal system
3. Assess the use of illegal drugs
4. Identify special considerations for the older adult, pediatric, and pregnant client
5. Know the FDA pregnancy categories of the drugs
6. Identify client's ability to explain why each medication prescribed or unprescribed is being taken
7. Identify cultural considerations related to drug therapy (Box 1-1)

B. Diagnosis

1. Identify nursing diagnoses related to the medications currently in use
2. Begin a plan of care related to the client's drug regimen; consider side effects, dietary factors, and compliance level
3. Apply nursing diagnoses taken from the North American Nursing Diagnoses Association (NANDA, 1996) specific to drug therapy. Consider the following:
   a. Knowledge deficit related to drug treatment regimen
   b. Noncompliance related to side effects of medication or financial difficulty
   c. Risk for injury related to side effects of medication
   d. Constipation related to slowing of peristalsis due to narcotic use for pain management
   e. Diarrhea related to side effects of medication (name specific drug)
   f. Risk for infection related to specific drug's effect of compromising immune system (name drug)

Box 1-1
Cultural Considerations

A knowledge deficit may make client education about drug therapy a high priority before a client is discharged.

Language barriers and cultural customs may present a barrier to communicating how to safely administer medications.

Belief Systems

Belief systems vary according to the culture of the client.
Western cultures: Demonstrate considerable participation in health care; demand more explanation about disease, treatment, and prevention of diseases.
Asian: Believe in traditional medicine and use physicians and herbalists in their health care.
African: Practice folk medicine and also employ "root workers" as healers.
European: Hold traditional health beliefs; may still practice folk medicine.
Response to medications can vary according to cultural beliefs.
Chinese: More sensitive to sedative effects; require lower doses of antidepressants; more sensitive to cardiovascular and respiratory effects of analgesics; and more sensitive to beta-blocking agents.
Hispanic: Have more side effects to antidepressants.
Asian: Require lower doses of neuroleptics; more sensitive to side effects of alcohol.
Indian: Have a greater clearance rate for analgesics.
Native Americans: Have a faster metabolism; less tolerant to alcohol.
African Americans: Respond better to diuretic agents than to beta-blocking agents.

From Lilly, LL, Aucker RS: *Pharmacology and the nursing process,* ed 2, St. Louis, 1999, Mosby; McKenry, L, Salerno, E: *Mosby's Pharmacology in nursing,* ed 20, St. Louis, 1998, Mosby.

Box 1-2
Additional Nursing Diagnoses for Drug Treatment

Ineffective individual coping
Impaired home maintenance management
Risk for poisoning
Sexual dysfunction
Altered sexuality patterns
Disturbance in sleep pattern
Altered thought processes
Urinary retention

    g. Ineffective management of individual therapeutic regimen related to limited financial resources

    h. Health-seeking behaviors, such as help for physical dependence related to chronic and abusive use of cocaine

    i. Other common diagnoses related to medication administration (Box 1-2)

C. **Planning**
1. Identify outcome criteria for documenting client responses to drug therapy
2. Determine the best schedule for administering the prescribed drugs
   a. Consider drugs to be administered with and without meals
   b. Plan diuretics and laxatives early in the morning to avoid unnecessary interruptions in sleep during the night for elimination
   c. Identify potential drug interactions and schedule accordingly
3. Establish nursing observations and interventions needed for safe drug therapy
   a. Recognize safety factors for drugs that interfere with level of consciousness
   b. Develop guidelines for reporting abnormal side effects
4. Identify necessary client teaching for safe drug administration at home

D. **Implementation**
1. Provide drug therapy as directed on the plan of care
2. Prepare the medication with consideration to the proper technique for the ordered route and correct drug calculation
3. Consider the five rights of drug administration: right drug, dose, route, time, and client
4. Monitor for the effectiveness of the drug and for adverse side effects
5. Teach appropriate information for home drug therapy
6. Accurately document the medication prescribed

E. **Evaluation**
1. Document the effectiveness of the drug
2. Document any side effects and the actions taken to relieve them
3. Determine the client's knowledge of the drug regimen
4. Evaluate laboratory work necessary for safe drug administration

II. Drug legislation within the United States (Table 1-1)

A. FDA classifies investigational new drug applications and new drug approvals to benefit the reviewer of those drugs (Table 1-2, p. 7).
B. Maintaining updates of new drugs is a responsibility of the nurse. The Center for Disease Control and Prevention (CDC) offers free updates and provides access to new drug developments through the World Wide Web.

⚠ Warning!

Nurses must know the new drugs being approved through the FDA and therefore must keep up with the literature through brochures, advertisements, the Internet, inserts, and workshops.

III. Controlled substances (Table 1-3, p. 8)

A. Controlled substances are drugs that have the potential for causing physical or psychological dependence

TABLE 1-1 Federal Drug Legislation in the U.S.

Date	Title of Law	Major Provisions
1906	Pure Food and Drug Act	Established USP and NP as official standards. Set standards for proper drug labeling.
1912	Shirley Amendment	Prohibited fraudulent claims for therapeutic effects of drugs.
1914	Harrison Narcotic Act	Legally defined term "narcotic." Regulated and restricted importation, manufacture, sale, and use of opium, cocaine, marijuana, and other drugs likely to produce dependence.
1938	Food, Drug, and Cosmetic Act	Maintained major provisions of previous laws. Required that a drug be demonstrated to be safe before it was marketed. Added *Homeopathic Pharmacopoeia of the United States* as a third standard for drugs.
1941-1945	Amendments to Pure Food and Drug Act	Required that biologic products that are used as drugs (i.e., insulin or antibiotics) be certified on a batch-by-batch basis by a government agency.
1952	Durham-Humphrey Amendment	Designated certain drugs as "legend" drugs that must be marked "Caution: Federal Law prohibits dispensing without prescription." Restricted right of pharmacist to distribute legend drugs.
1962	Kefauver-Harris Amendment	Required proof of efficacy for a drug to remain on market. Authorized FDA to establish official names for drugs.
1970	Comprehensive Drug Abuse Prevention and Control Act (or Controlled Substances Act)	Defined drug dependency and drug addiction. Classified drugs according to abuse potential and medical usefulness. Established methods for regulating the manufacture, distribution, and sale of controlled substances. Established education and treatment programs for drug abusers.
1978	Drug Regulation Reform Act	Shortened the drug investigation process to release drugs sooner to the public.
1982	AAPA Model Practice Act	American Academy of Physicians Assistants introduced the Model Practice Act.
1983	Orphan Drug Act	Offered tax relief to companies marketing orphan drugs. Protected companies for 7 years against competition on nonpatentable orphan drugs.
1984	Drug Price Competition and Patent Term Restoration Act	Drugs first marketed after 1962 are eligible for abbreviated new drug application. Generic drugs are more easily introduced. Established guidelines for bioequivalence. Restored up to 5 years of patent protection for time used in drug development.

Data from Clark JB, Queener SF, Karb VB: *Pharmacologic basis of nursing practice,* ed 6, St. Louis, 2000, Mosby; McKenry LM, Salerno E: *Mosby's Pharmacology in nursing,* ed 20, St. Louis, 1998, Mosby

Continued

TABLE 1-1	Federal Drug Legislation in the U.S.—cont'd

Date	Title of Law	Major Provisions
1986, 1988	National Childhood Vaccine Injury Act	Private health care providers are required to keep records on adverse events after immunization; covers diphtheria, measles, mumps, pertussis, poliomyelitis, rubella, and tetanus toxoids or vaccines.
1987	Prescription Drug Marketing Act	Bans diversion of prescription drugs from legitimate channels. Restricts reimportation of drugs from other countries.
1988	Food and Drug Administration Act	Establishes the FDA within the Department of Health and Human Services. Sets mechanism for appointing the Commissioner of Food and Drugs.
1997	Nurses Prescriptive Authority	Gives authority to the nurse practitioner to write prescriptions according to established protocols or under physician supervision or collaboration

Data from Clark JB, Queener SF, Karb VB: *Pharmacologic basis of nursing practice,* ed 6, St. Louis, 2000, Mosby; McKenry LM, Salerno E: *Mosby's Pharmacology in nursing,* ed 20, St. Louis, 1998, Mosby

B. **The nurse's responsibility is to maintain accurate records of the use of controlled substances in health care agencies**

⚠ Warning!

The nurse must not
- sign for wasted narcotic agents if the disposal has not been witnessed
- sign for another nurse in relation to controlled substances
- leave the facility without an accurate count of the inventory of controlled substances

IV. Drug names
A. *Chemical name* is the chemical nomenclature. EXAMPLE: N-Acetyl-para-aminopenol
B. *Generic name* is the nonproprietary name assigned by the United States Adopted Names (USAN) council. EXAMPLE: acetaminophen
C. *Brand name* is the proprietary (or trade) name assigned by the manufacturing company. EXAMPLE: Tylenol

⚠ Warning!

Nurses should know both the generic and brand name of a drug in clinical practice (and for nursing examinations).

TABLE 1-2 FDA Classifications of New Drug Applications

The FDA classifies investigational new drug applications and other new drug applications by chemical type and potential benefit.

Chemical Type
1. New molecular entity: An active ingredient never marketed in this country before.
2. New derivative: A chemical that is from an active ingredient already on the market.
3. New formulation: A new form of dosing or using an active ingredient already on the market in a new form.
4. New combination: Combining two or more compounds that have never been marketed together.
5. Already marketed drug product, new manufacturer: A product with the same active ingredient, formulation, or a combination of the two.
6. Already marketed drug product, but new use: A new use for a drug currently marketed by another company.
7. Drug already legally marketed without FDA approval: Products marketed prior to 1938, DESI-related products marketed between 1938 and 1962, or those marketed without NDA's after 1962.

Effectiveness Codes
SE1	New indication or essential modification of an indication in existence
SE2	New dosage regimen
SE3	New route
SE4	Comparative efficacy claim
SE5	Change in sections that significantly change the population of clients to be treated
SE6	Switch from prescription to OTC

Treatment Potential
P (priority review drug): Offers advanced therapy over present therapy
S (standard review drug): Qualities of drug are similar to drugs currently on market
AA (AIDS drug): Treatment of AIDS or related diseases
E (subpart E drug): Developed under special circumstances to treat life-threatening or severely debilitating illnesses
V (orphan drugs): Sponsor eligible for tax credits and has exclusive rights for marketing the drug

Center for Drug Evaluation and Research: FDA Drug Approvals List, October 1999, U.S. Department of Health and Human Services. (From website: http://www.fda.gov)

V. Legal and ethical considerations
A. **Three conditions should be met before a nurse can legally administer a medication:**
   1. The medication order must be valid.
   2. The physician or prescriber and the nurse must be licensed. A nonphysician prescriber acts within the regulations of the state. A nurse should know the policies of the institution for the nonphysician to prescribe drugs.

TABLE 1-3	Controlled Substances	
Schedule	**Dispensing Restrictions**	**Information**
C-I	Only with approved protocol	No medical use, high abuse potential, severe dependency (examples: heroin, LSD, marijuana)
C-II	Written prescription only or written prescription within 24 hours for telephone order; no refills, must have warning label	Accepted medical use, high abuse potential, severe physical and/or psychological dependency (examples: codeine, meperidine, morphine, amphetamine, methadone, pentobarbital)
C-III	Written or oral prescription that expires in 6 months; 5 refills in 6-month period; must have warning label	Accepted medical use, less abuse potential than C-II, moderate to low physical or high psychological dependency (examples: codeine, paregoric, nonopioid preparations, combination products)
C-IV	Written or oral prescription that expires in 6 months; only 5 refills in 6 months; must have warning label	Accepted medical use, abuse potential less than C-III; limited physical or psychological dependency (examples: phenobarbital, benzodiazepines, chloral hydrate)
C-V	Written prescription or OTC; varies with each state law	Accepted medical use, potential for abuse less than C-IV, limited physical or psychological dependency (examples: medications for relief of coughs or diarrhea containing limited opioid-controlled substances)

From Lilley LL, Aucker RS: *Pharmacology and the nursing process,* ed 2, St. Louis, 1999, Mosby

   3. The nurse must know the purpose, actions, desired effects, major side effects and toxic effects of the drug and the teaching required to enable the client or caregiver to safely and accurately administer the drug.

B. Nurses are required to know the limitations of their own skills, expertise, knowledge, and experience and understand these limitations according to the Board of Nursing regulations for the state in which the nurse practices

⚠ Warning!

Nurses' actions will be judged by expert witnesses as well as what the literature documents (e.g., drug reference manuals, *Physician's Desk Reference*)

Box 1-3
Prescriptive Authority

Independent Authority*	Dependent Authority*	Dependent Authority†
Alaska	Arkansas	Alabama
Arizona	California	Florida
Colorado	Connecticut	Hawaii
Delaware	Georgia	Idaho
District of Columbia	Indiana	Kentucky
Iowa	Kansas	Michigan
Maine	Louisiana	Missouri
Montana	Maryland	New Jersey
Nebraska	Massachusetts	Nevada
New Hampshire	Minnesota	Ohio
New Mexico	Mississippi	Tennessee
Oklahoma	New York	Texas
Oregon	North Carolina	Virginia
South Carolina	North Dakota	
South Dakota	Pennsylvania	
Vermont	Rhode Island	
Washington	Utah	
Wisconsin	West Virginia	
Wyoming		

From McKenry LM, Salerno E: *Mosby's Pharmacology in nursing,* ed 20, St. Louis, 1998, Mosby
*Includes controlled substances.
†Excludes controlled substances.

   C. **Nurses practice under the Code of Ethics for Nurses when considering ethical issues about drug administration**

   D. **The nurse should question orders that are incomplete, incorrect, inappropriate, or invalid**

   E. Prescriptive Authority **for nurse practitioners within the United States can be** independent **or** dependent **(Box 1-3)**

   F. **Nurses should never give a medication that is unfamiliar to them**

   G. **Nurses may be involved in research projects concerning drug therapy. Informed consent is required of clients.**

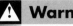 **Warning!**

Nurses do not hold the responsibility of *explaining* a research project or the drugs included in the project.

   H. **Nurses may administer placebo therapy, but they have an ethical responsibility to consider all aspects of the client's care and must have a direct order for the placebo therapy**

VI. Forms of medications

   A. **Preparations**
     1. Oral solids
       a. Tablets that are compressed (may be scored)
       b. Capsules with a dissolvable gelatin sheath
         (1) Timed-release or sustained-release tablets or capsules may include several types of specially coated medications that dissolve at different times. The suffixes SA and SR or the term "extentab" may be used (Box 1-4)
         (2) Enteric-coated tablets or capsules dissolve in the intestine instead of in the stomach
         (3) Timed-release and enteric-coated tablets should not be crushed (see Box 1-4)
       c. Lozenges or troches dissolve in the mouth on top of the tongue
       d. Powders must be dissolved in liquid before use
     2. Oral liquids
       a. Elixirs, spirits, and extracts contain alcohol
       b. Syrups contain large amounts of sugar

Box 1-4
Drug Formulations that Should
Not Be Crushed or Chewed

Enteric-coated tablets.
Sustained-release forms, which often have these suffixes added to the drug name:
- Dur (duration)
- SR (sustained-release)
- CR (controlled- or continuous-release)
- SA (sustained action)
- Contin (continuous-release)
- LA (long-acting)

Trade names that imply sustained-release, such as spansules, extentabs, or extencaps.
Trade names with the twice-daily abbreviation (bid) in the name, such as Theobid or Cardabid.
Liquid-containing capsules, although it may sometimes be acceptable to puncture the capsule and squeeze out the contents; consult the pharmacist or manufacturer.
The name alone may not provide enough information. Consult the pharmacist if in doubt. Some formulations that look like sustained forms are not, and vice versa. Some capsules containing small, slow-released pellets may be opened and the pellets sprinkled on applesauce or gently mixed into liquid or food, but they should not be crushed or dissolved.
Scored tablets may be broken along the scored line but should not be chewed or crushed.

From Clark JB, Queener SF, Karb VB: Pharmacologic basis of nursing practice, ed 6, St Louis, 2000, Mosby.

     c. Suspensions, such as emulsions, gels, and magmas, are mixtures that are not dissolved. These must be shaken well before use.

     d. Tinctures are portions of drugs mixed in a solution with alcohol

     e. Oral sprays

  3. Topical

     a. Creams, lotions, and ointments

     b. Topical sprays

     c. Transdermal disks are medicated and allow for slow absorption of the medication through the skin, usually over a period of 3 to 7 days

  4. Injectable

     a. Powders must be mixed with a diluent

     b. Single-dose and multidose vials

     c. Intravenous (IV) fluids

  5. Vaginal and rectal

     a. Creams and tablets

     b. Suppositories

     c. Vaginal douches

     d. Rectal enemas

  6. Ophthalmic and otic

     a. Drops: may be suspensions, etc.

     b. Ointments

  7. Other

     a. Nasal sprays

     b. Inhalants

     c. Implants (subcutaneous)

     d. Insulin pumps

B. Routes of administration

  1. **Enteral:** by way of the GI tract

     a. Oral (PO) preparations

     b. Nasogastric (NG) tubes

     c. Gastrostomy tubes

     d. Intestinal tubes

  2. **Parenteral:** by injection

     a. Intradermal (ID)

     b. Subcutaneous (SC) or (SQ)

     c. Intramuscular (IM)

     d. Intravenous (IV)

     e. **Intrathecal**

     f. **Epidural**

     g. Continuous portable infusion systems (patient-controlled analgesia (IV), insulin pumps (SQ), etc.)

     h. Other routes: **intraarticular, intraosseous, intraperitoneal, intrapleural,** access devices (medi-ports, port-a-caths, Hickmans, etc.)

   3. **Topical:** by way of a body surface part, such as through the skin, mucous membranes, or the cornea
     a. Through the skin
       (1) Transdermal drug delivery system (TDDS)
       (2) Skin ointments, creams, and gels
     b. Through mucous membranes and cornea (absorbed through the mucous membranes of various parts of the body)
       (1) Eye and ear ointments and drops
       (2) Vaginal applications: creams and tablets
       (3) Rectal suppositories
       (4) Buccal administration to the cheek or mouth
       (5) Inhalants: nasal drops
       (6) Sublingual (SL) medications absorbed under the tongue
   4. **Inhalants** are absorbed through the lungs
     a. Oxygen administered by nasal cannula (NC) or mask, in L/min or percentage of total gas
     b. Aerosols; inhalers

Web Resources

http://www.fda/gov/cder/whatsnew.htm
   Subscribe to new drug development information.

http://www.fda.gov/cder/da/da.htm
   New drugs approved by the month of the year.

http://www.fda.gov/cder/approval/index.htm
   Approvals lists by alphabet.

http://health.yahoo.com/health/drugs_tree/medication_or_drug
http://www.health-center.com/english/pharmacy/meds
   Other resources.

REVIEW QUESTIONS

1. A client with abdominal pain reports to the emergency department. A brief history reveals an allergy to the analgesic morphine sulfate. The nurse should follow through by first asking which of these questions?
   1. What other analgesics are you allergic to?
   2. Have you had this allergy long?
   3. Exactly what does the morphine do to you?
   4. Does the morphine make you nauseated?

2. A client reports to a cardiac rehabilitation session complaining of not feeling well. The nurse questions what is wrong and is told, "I've been having angina for several days." During further assessment, the client reports that no nitrate has been used because it causes a terrible headache. Which of these nursing diagnoses is most appropriate?
   1. Knowledge deficit related to the side effects of nitroglycerin
   2. Knowledge deficit related to the need for nitrates
   3. Alteration in comfort: headache related to the side effects of the vasodilator
   4. Noncompliance related to the side effects of nitroglycerin

3. A nurse's neighbor calls, concerned that the medicine prescribed for her daughter is too big to swallow. After a brief discussion, the nurse discovers that the capsule the child is having trouble swallowing is a sustained-release capsule. The nurse should:
   1. encourage the mother to open the capsule and mix it with ice cream.
   2. explain to the mother how to crush the medicine and then give it with plenty of liquid.
   3. explain that sustained-release capsules cannot be crushed; the mother should call her physician to report that the pills are too difficult for the child to swallow.
   4. explain that sustained-release capsules cannot be crushed; the mother should stop the medication and inform her physician at the child's follow-up visit.

4. The nurse is asked to give an investigational drug to a client. Upon entering the room, the nurse asked if the study and the use of the drug had been explained to the client. If the client answers "no", the nurse should:
   1. proceed to administer the drug anyway.
   2. give a brief explanation about the drug and proceed to administer it
   3. explain the study, secure a consent, and administer the drug.
   4. refuse to administer the drug and notify the investigational physician.

5. An appropriate example of the nurse's action in the planning stage of drug therapy would be which of the following:
   1. determine drug allergies and list the current medication regimen.
   2. calculate the correct dosage.

3. schedule the diuretic at 5:00 pm instead of 9:00 pm.
4. assess the international normalized ratio (INR) while the client is on Coumadin therapy.

6. In which of these clients would it be most important not to ingest elixirs?
1. A client in chronic renal failure on peritoneal dialysis
2. An alcoholic client who is on medication for the cessation of drinking
3. A client who had gastric surgery 2 weeks ago
4. A client with a new diagnosis of asthma

7. The nurse had a discussion with a group of clients. One of the questions from a client was to explain what the topical route means for medication delivery. The nurse should have responded based on the knowledge of which of these statements?
1. Topical means "only applied to the skin surface"
2. Topical administration of medication takes at least 2 hours to be effective
3. Topical drugs are not found in over the counter form
4. Topical route means "by way of a body surface part, such as the skin, mucous membranes, or cornea"

ANSWERS, RATIONALES, AND TEST-TAKING TIPS

Rationales	Test-Taking Tips

1. Correct answer: 3

Determining the exact nature of the allergic reaction will best help the nurse distinguish an allergy from a common side effect. A listing of all medications the client is allergic to would be an appropriate question after option 3. The length of time the client has had the allergy is irrelevant. Nausea is a common side effect, not an allergic reaction.

One strategy is to eliminate options that are false or not the best. Options 2 and 4 offer little information, since they are "yes or no" questions. The question in option 1 ignores the issue of the morphine allergy. It is a good question but is not the best answer for the "first" question, given the situation in the stem. Thus, select option 3.

2. Correct answer: 4

Headache is a common side effect of nitroglycerin and can lead to noncompliance. There is not enough information to determine if options 1 and 2 are true. Option 3 is an appropriate nursing diagnosis. However, it is not the best answer in this situation. The priority is the omission of the prescribed medication and not the discomfort of the headache.

Options 1 and 2 can be eliminated, since there is no information in the stem to support a knowledge problem. If you read option 3 too quickly, you may have had the headache on your mind instead of the more important fact that the client omitted the medication and had physical symptoms (angina) as a result. This error of reading too quickly is common for this type of question, especially if you are tired or tense. You may have had a knee-jerk reaction to select option 3 and not even read option 4. If you did this, make a pact with yourself to read each option.

3. Correct answer: 3

A different medication or a liquid form of the drug must be ordered by the physician. Opening the capsule can alter absorption and cause toxicity. Crushing alters the absorption and destroys the sustained-released action of the medication.

Key words in the question are "sustained-release capsule." Options 1 and 2 can be immediately eliminated because of the word clues "open the capsule" and "crush the medicine." These methods are never used for time-released or enteric-coated medications. If you have difficulty deciding between options 3 and 4, a clue exists in

Rationales	Test-Taking Tips

option 4: "inform physician at the follow-up visit." A medication should never be discontinued without notification of the physician. To notify the physician about the medication should be done the day the client decides to stop it and not later.

4. Correct answer: 4

Follow the basic principle that a client needs to be informed of any procedure. Investigational drug programs can be classified as procedures. Option 1 ignores the fact that the client has no knowledge of the therapy. Options 2 and 3 are similar except that option 3 has the consent obtained. In investigational drug programs the nurse is not the typical person to explain and to obtain the consent document.

If you have no idea of a correct answer, use the cluster or grouping technique. In options 1, 2, and 3 the medication is given. Select the odd option that is 4 where the medication is held. Be sure to read all parts of each option. With options that have a series of items, it is common to read the last option quickly and less intensely.

5. Correct answer: 3

Option 1 is an action in the assessment stage of drug therapy. Option 2 is an action in the intervention stage of drug therapy. Option 4 is an action in the evaluation stage of drug therapy.

The approach to read these options is to expect that they are all correct actions. The question asks which action falls into a certain stage. The question does not ask which action is correct. If you read the options for 3 incorrect actions and one correct action you have approached this question and these options in the wrong manner. Thus, you may have a tendency to misread the question or the options. The clue in the question is "the planning stage" which guides you to think of the nursing process steps as you read the options. To label the options with a step of the nursing process as you read is a good action to take on these types of questions.

6. Correct answer: 2

An elixir contains alcohol. It would result in severe reactions for a client who is on medication to help them stop drinking alcohol. Note that all of the options are correct answers. None of these clients should ingest alcohol for various reasons. The clients with renal failure or asthma may have interactions between their routine medications and the alcohol. The client who has had gastric surgery would have gastric irritation from the alcohol.

If you have no idea of a correct answer, use the match approach. Recall that elixirs have a biting taste from the alcohol content. Match this fact to the option with alcohol in it, option 2.

7. Correct answer: 4

Option 4 is the most comprehensive answer. Option 1 is too narrow with only the area of the skin. Option 2 is a false statement. The effect depends on if the preparation is drops, a cream, or ointment, and the site of application. Option 3 is a false statement.

Eliminate option 1 because of the absolute "only." Options with absolutes such "always, never, forever" or "every" are usually incorrect answers. Eliminate option 2 based on your knowledge that many factors influence the onset of drug effectiveness. Eliminate option 3 from your knowledge that OTC drugs include topical preparations. Remember to focus on what you know, then go with it. Refrain from second-guessing yourself.

2

Principles of Drug Therapy

FAST FACTS

1. Any ingested drugs go through a four-step process in the body: absorption, distribution, metabolism, and excretion.
2. Absorption can be affected by several factors: surface area available, drug formulation, route of administration, availability of circulating blood, circulation to a specific site, pain, stress, drug solubility, drug interactions, and pH level of the body.
3. Plasma protein-binding is one form of distribution that occurs in the circulatory system. Low albumin levels can lead to failure of the drug to be distributed properly or can result in competition between two highly protein-bound drugs.
4. The blood-brain barrier serves as a protective permeability process of the cerebral capillaries that determines which drugs are distributed within the brain.
5. Metabolism of all substances and drugs is primarily done in the liver, where they are broken down into either of two forms: harmless substances or substances that are capable of further drug activity.
6. Hepatic first-pass effect can interfere with the adequate absorption and metabolism of a drug. Enterohepatic recycling can hinder a drug from being properly eliminated.
7. Excretion of drugs is primarily by the kidneys. The pH of the urine and the presence of kidney disease affect excretion. The half-life of a drug is maintained by normal kidney function.
8. Drugs produce local or systemic effects, and some can produce both.
9. The therapeutic response obtained by the administration of a drug can be affected by the body size of the individual, age, presence of disease, immunologic state, psychological belief in the drug, environment, gender, and genetic factors.
10. All drugs have a primary effect, which is intended, and are capable of secondary effects, or side effects.

11. Drugs are often given in a loading dose to achieve a therapeutic level quickly and then followed by a maintenance dose. Plasma concentration levels of many drugs are measured to assess the need to increase the dosage in situations of subminimal blood levels or decrease the dosage in the event of toxic levels.

CONTENT REVIEW

I. Four reasons for medication administration
A. Treatment, examples: acetylsalicylic acid (aspirin) for fever, digoxin (Lanoxin) for heart failure
B. Cure, example: antibiotic for infection
C. Maintenance, example: insulin for diabetes
D. Support, examples: IV-administered fluids, potassium supplements

II. The study of pharmacology includes three areas
A. Pharmacokinetics: the study of how drugs are absorbed, distributed, metabolized, and excreted; think about transport
B. Pharmacodynamics: the study of how the medicine exerts an effect once it reaches the target cell; think about action
C. Pharmacotherapeutics: the study of how drugs are used to treat various illnesses and the client's responses; think about barriers that prevent drugs from meeting specific needs

III. Pharmacokinetics: transport of a drug
A. Four steps
1. Absorption
2. Distribution
3. Metabolism
4. Excretion
B. Absorption: what happens to a drug from the time it enters the body until it enters the circulating fluid
1. Mechanisms of absorption
   a. Active transport: carriers plus an energy source
   b. Passive transport: without an energy source
   c. Pinocytosis: engulfing of the molecule to move it across the cell wall
2. Variables affecting absorption
   a. Absorption surface: irritation to the lining of the stomach, abrasion to the skin
   b. Drug formulation: enteric-coated, timed-release, liquid vs solid
   c. Route of administration: linked to blood flow; IV route usually absorbed quicker than IM route
   d. Circulation: more blood flow increases absorption; less blood flow decreases absorption
   e. Pain and stress: can decrease absorption; may be linked to blood flow

    f. Effects of the pH in the stomach and in the small intestines: may increase or decrease absorption rate

    g. Drug solubility: drug must become liquid to be absorbed

    h. Motility of the GI tract: may increase or decrease absorption rate

    i. Drug interactions: drug to drug and drug to food

  3. Absorption can be affected by the different routes for administering medications (Table 2-1)

TABLE 2-1 Comparison of Drug Administration Routes and their Effects on Absorption

Enteral

Absorption is rapid in small intestine.
Presence of food often diminishes absorption.
Absence of food may increase absorption.
Liquids absorb more rapidly than solids.
Absorption occurs within 3 to 5 min. with sublingual or buccal administration.
Increased intestinal motility decreases available time for absorption.
Absorption through the GI tract may be undependable.

Parenteral

IM injection has effects within 10 to 15 min.
SC injection can have effects within 10 to 15 min.
IV route requires no absorption and has immediate effects.
Poor circulation may hinder IM or SC absorption.
Shock, edema, trauma, and coolness of tissue slow absorption.
Massage and heat to tissue increase absorption.

Topical

Local application of drugs can have a systemic effect; for example, lidocaine (Xylocaine) + epinephrine (Adrenalin).
Some medications may be applied locally for a systemic effect; for example, nitrol paste or patch (nitroglycerin).
Scarred or burned skin can hinder absorption.
Damaged or irritated skin can enhance absorption systemically.

Inhalation

May be absorbed systemically; for example, anesthetic agents.
May be absorbed locally; for example, corticosteroids.
Absorption is enhanced because of the large surface area of the lungs. Expect results within 2-3 minutes.

Mucous Membranes

May produce either local or systemic effect.
Rectal route may result in incomplete absorption if feces is present in sigmoid colon or there are numerous internal hemorrhoids.
Absorption is rapid through the rectal route because of the large vascular surface; for example, acetylsalicylic acid (aspirin). Expect results in 10 to 15 minutes.
Absorption by the vaginal route is usually enhanced because of the dense vascularity.

C. **Distribution: ways in which drugs are transported by body fluids to their sites of action**
 1. Factors affecting distribution
    a. Drugs may have an affinity for certain areas, such as fatty tissue, bone, or other body tissues. The drug may be stored in these areas, only to be released at a later time and possibly result in toxicity.
    b. Amount of blood flow to specific organs
 2. Factors related to plasma protein–binding
    a. Certain drugs must be bound to a protein to be distributed. The drug book will specify "highly protein-bound" followed by a percentage. For example, warfarin sodium (Coumadin) is 99% protein-bound. Most references consider high protein-binding to be more than 65%, moderate to be 35% to 64%, and low to be less than 34%. Other common drugs that are protein-bound are: aspirin, Tylenol, oxycodone hydrochloride and acetaminophen (Percocet, Tylox), nonnarcotic analgesics, and the selective serotonin reuptake inhibitors (SSRI) antidepressants. Drugs bound to the protein albumin are transported by the protein and cannot be used until unbound or free from the protein.
    b. Situations that alter protein-binding
       (1) Hypoalbuminemia: decreased albumin level in the blood; in this situation, more of a drug may be available than there is albumin to bind it, which may result in toxic effects
       (2) Competition for protein can occur between two highly protein-bound drugs; example: aspirin and warfarin sodium (Coumadin)
 3. Blood-brain barrier: a special property of the permeability of the cerebral capillaries that protects brain by preventing many medications from penetrating. Agents that can penetrate the blood-brain barrier include:
    a. Anesthetics
    b. Barbiturates
    c. Penicillin G
    d. Atropine sulfate (Atropair)
    e. Scopolamine hydrobromide (Hyoscine)
D. **Metabolism: the breaking down or detoxification of medications**
 1. Occurs primarily in the liver
 2. Other sites of metabolism: kidneys, lungs, blood, and intestinal mucosa
 3. Results of metabolism on a drug
    a. Converted into a harmless substance
    b. Converted into metabolites that are capable of exerting a therapeutic effect
    c. Unchanged
    d. Competition resulting in toxicity
 4. Hepatic first-pass effect: inactivation of drug by enzymes in the liver before the drug reaches the systemic circulation for distribution

E. Excretion: process of elimination from the body
1. Occurs primarily in the kidneys
2. Other excretory sites: sweat glands, feces, salivary glands, bile duct, lactating breasts, lungs
3. Steady state: obtained when absorption equals elimination
4. **Half-life:** the amount of time necessary to reduce the plasma concentration of a drug by half; usually takes five half-lives to completely eliminate a drug
5. Factors affecting elimination are as follows:
   a. Urine pH can enhance or delay excretion
   b. Kidney diseases may interfere with drug clearance from the body
   c. Enterohepatic recycling can occur, in which a drug is reabsorbed from the small intestines into the bile and then into the circulatory system. These drugs remain in the system much longer than normal.

> ⚠ **Warning!**
>
> Laboratory tests that help to determine kidney problems include blood urea nitrogen (BUN), serum creatinine level, which is the most specific for abnormal kidney function (both will rise in the presence of kidney disease) and the urine creatinine clearance (which will decrease in the event of kidney disease). If clearance through the kidneys is hindered, drugs will stay in the system longer.

IV. Pharmacodynamics: therapeutic effect or action

A. Alteration in the cell environment by drugs occurs as follows:
1. Physical modification of the cell environment by alteration of the surface tension (stool softeners) or by osmosis (osmotic diuretics)
2. Chemical modification of the cell environment, such as changing the pH of stomach contents (antacids)

B. Alteration in the cell function may occur when drugs interact to alter the cellular process; for example, insulin facilitates transfer of glucose into cells

C. Drug-receptor theory is the most commonly accepted theory about the action of drugs. Receptors attract drug molecules that attach and fit into the receptor (lock and key effect).
1. **Agonist:** a drug with a certain affinity for a receptor. Example: morphine sulfate (Astramorph).
2. **Antagonists:** drugs that form a complex with the receptor, prohibiting a pharmacologic action or counteracting the effect of other drugs. Example: naloxone hydrochloride (Narcan).

D. Effects of drugs
1. Local: usually affecting one body part; effect occurs at the site of application. Example: acyclovir (Zovirax) cream for herpes simplex viral infection

2. Systemic: may affect more than one body part; effect may not occur at the site of administration. Example: promethazine hydrochloride (Phenergan) given IM for nausea.
3. Local and systemic: an agent may be given for its local effect but produce a systemic effect also. Example: lidocaine hydrochloride (Xylocaine) with adrenalin chloride (epinephrine) SC.

⚠️ Warning!

A drug is often given for a local effect and is absorbed systemically to produce undesirable systemic effects.

V. Pharmacotherapeutic phase: target of medications and response by clients

A. **Factors influencing therapeutic response**
   1. Percentage of muscle mass, fat, and total body weight (20% below or above ideal weight) can affect the dosage.

⚠️ Warning!

The adult dose is calculated on the basis of the average person weighing 150 pounds between the ages of 16 and 65. Therefore, smaller or larger individuals may need dosage adjustments.

   2. Age: some clients are more prone to drug effects (Table 2-2).
      a. Neonates and infants because of immature organs
      b. Older adults because of decreased function of organs
   3. Disease states or dysfunction of the following systems:
      a. Circulatory, example: congestive heart failure (CHF)
      b. Hepatic, example: cirrhosis
      c. Renal, example: acute or chronic renal failure
      d. GI, example: bowel inflammation or resection
   4. Immunologic state: body's ability to form antibodies against medications can result in adverse effects
   5. Psychological factors: a client's belief in the effects of the drug (such as a placebo)
   6. Environmental factors: temperature and climate can affect dosage. High altitudes can affect individuals, especially elders, who may require dosage adjustments.
   7. Time of administration: normal human biorhythms can alter the response of a drug
   8. Gender: females contain proportionately less water, owing to a greater percentage of body fat, and absorption can vary according to water or fat solubility of the drug. Women are also usually smaller than men.
   9. Genetics: enzymes and acetylation rates are determined genetically, and alterations can cause toxicity
B. **Drug effects and interactions**
   1. Primary effect: that which is intended

TABLE 2-2	**Drug Therapy Across the Life Span**		
	Older Adult	**Pediatric**	**Pregnant**
Absorption	Delayed, but more complete	Exaggerated as a result of lack of gastric acidity and shorter intestines Impeded somewhat from a larger body surface *IM delayed Enteral route unpredictable	Delayed because of decreased motility and prolonged gastric emptying or may not be affected at all
Distribution	Low albumin level could create problem with plasma protein-binding; could cause toxicity Altered because of less lean mass, less body water, greater body fat	Protein binding may be a problem; greater chance of toxicity because of low albumin levels	Decreased protein binding because of decreased protein level can increase drug transfer across placenta
Metabolism	Decreased because of diseases; changes due to age, higher blood concentration, and less excretion cause greater chances of toxicity	Immature liver; metabolism may be altered; best to give drugs based on body weight to avoid toxicity	Decreased because of less blood flow to liver
Excretion	Less excretion from decreased glomerular filtration rate	Delayed as a result of immature kidneys Repeat dosing may cause problems	Increased excretion from increased renal perfusion

Continued

*IM, intramuscular.

TABLE 2-2	**Drug Therapy Across the Life Span—cont'd**				
	Older Adult		**Pediatric**		**Pregnant**

Considerations

Older Adult
- Polypharmacy: the use of a number of different drugs by a patient who may have one or several health problems
- Multiple medications can cause many problems in absorption, distribution, metabolism, and excretion
- Higher chance of drug-to-drug interactions
- Compliance may be a problem due to forgetfulness, cost, or ability to manipulate lids of medication bottles or equipment, such as syringes and aerosols and inability to see clearly
- Toxicity is the main concern

Pediatric
- Calculate dosage by *BSA or mg/kg
- Nursing implications
  1. Be honest about pain
  2. Allow choice of bandage
  3. Assure that crying is all right
  4. Offer comfort (pacifier, bottle, favorite toy)
  5. Tell how long procedure should last or if it will hurt
  6. Use age-appropriate words and a brief explanation
  7. Prepare all medication in advance
  8. Keep needle out of sight
  9. Solicit parents' help
  10. Act quickly; do not be nervous
  11. Position child correctly

Pregnant
- FDA rating of drugs for effects on pregnancy
  A–No risk
  B–No risk evident in human studies or animal studies
  C–Risk cannot be ruled out
  D–Positive evidence of risk exists
  X–Contraindicated in pregnancy
- Many drugs pass to infants through maternal milk
- Teratogenesis is the major concern first trimester
- Placental barrier is not a protective mechanism
- Common ingestants, such as alcohol, caffeine, and illegal drugs, can cause serious complications
- †FAS can be a side effect of alcohol consumption; FAS is a set of congenital psychological, behavioral, cognitive, and physical abnormalities: typical are limb and cardiovascular defects, retarded development, and craniofacial defects

*BSA, body surface area; †FAS, fetal alcohol syndrome.

2. Secondary effect: any effects other than those intended:
   a. Drug allergy
      (1) Unique tissue response, example: dermatitis.
      (2) Anaphylactic shock: systemic reaction within minutes that requires immediate attention
      (3) Serum sickness: reaction 1 week after administration of a drug
   b. **Idiosyncrasy:** an individual sensitivity to the effects of a drug caused by an inherited or other bodily constitution factor; example: malignant hyperthermia after receiving general anesthetics
   c. **Side effect** (also called adverse effect): an undesirable or unintended effect of a drug, examples: nausea or insomnia
   d. **Iatrogenic effect:** unintentional adverse effects that are physician- or health care-induced or treatment-induced, including renal damage, hepatic toxicity, and blood dyscrasias: anemias, leukopenia, thrombocytopenia
   e. Photosensitivity: an abnormal reaction to light, particularly sunlight, example: sunburn or pruritus after a short time in the sun
   f. **Extrapyramidal effect:** exhibiting movement disorders similar to Parkinson's disease, examples: dystonia, akathisia, and akinesia
   g. **Toxicity:** blood level above the **therapeutic level,** example: digoxin (Lanoxin) toxicity.
   h. **Teratogenicity:** causing harm to the fetus, example: alcohol ingestion by pregnant woman causing fetal alcohol syndrome (FAS)
3. Drug and food interactions occur, example: penicillin G potassium (Pentids) is destroyed by food in the stomach
4. Drugs may interact with other drugs:
   a. *Synergistic effect:* a substance that augments or adds to the activity of another substance or agent. Example: ethanol (alcohol) and diazepam (Valium). Synergistic effect is symbolized by the formula $1 + 1 = 3$.
   b. *Additive effect:* the combined effect of drugs that produces an enhanced effect greater than the sum of the separately measured individual effects. Example: acetaminophen + codeine (Tylenol #3) Additive effect is symbolized by the formula $1 + 1 = 2$.
5. Placebo effect: a physical or emotional change occurring after a substance is taken or administered that is not the result of any special property of the substance. Example: sodium chloride (normal saline solution) administered in place of a narcotic and produces the same pain relief.
6. Dependency:
   a. Physical: the need for continued use of a substance to avoid abstinence symptoms. Example: ethanol (alcohol) used to avoid delirium tremens (DTs).

    b. Psychological: the craving or desire to continue use of a substance to meet the demands of everyday life, example: continual, excessive or compulsive use of diazepam (Valium) to avoid or handle anxiety.
7. Tolerance: the need for increasing amounts of a substance to produce the same effect, example: caffeine
8. Cross-tolerance: tolerance between related chemicals, example: alcohol and anesthetics
9. Tachyphylaxis: a quickly developing tolerance after repeated administration of a drug

VI. Monitoring drug therapy

A. **The goal of drug therapy is to maintain a therapeutic serum drug level. Examples:**
  1. Digoxin (Lanoxin) level of 0.8 to 2.0 μg/ml
  2. Aminophylline level of 10 to 20 μg/ml

B. **A *loading dose* may be required to obtain a therapeutic blood level or to relieve symptoms quickly by inducing a therapeutic response. Most commonly used with the following:**
  1. Initial digitalization
  2. Urinary antiseptics
  3. Anticonvulsants
  4. Antidysrhythmics
  5. Antibiotics
  6. Bronchodilators, especially aminophylline

C. *Maintenance dose* **is the daily dose necessary to maintain a therapeutic blood level**

D. **Toxicity occurs at a dose greater than that needed to maintain a therapeutic blood level. Low plasma protein levels, hepatic or renal dysfunction may contribute to drug toxicity. Clients usually exhibit specific *toxic effects.***
  1. For theophylline, the toxic effects are initially nausea and then tremors
  2. For digoxin, toxic effects are initially anorexia, nausea, and vomiting

E. **The smallest drug dose needed to produce an effect is measured as the minimal concentration level (MCL)**

F. **A blood test may be ordered to measure the following:**
  1. Plasma concentration (also called blood or serum level)
    a. Digoxin (Lanoxin)
    b. Theophylline (Theo-DUR) or aminophylline
    c. Lithium carbonate
    d. Gentamicin sulfate (Garamycin) or any aminoglycoside
    e. Phenytoin (Dilantin)
  2. **Peak level:** the drug's greatest concentration in blood or plasma; usually obtained for IV antibiotics 1 hr after dose is completely infused; insulin depends on the specific type: fast-acting reaches peak level in 2 to 4 hr, intermediate-acting in 6 to 12 hr

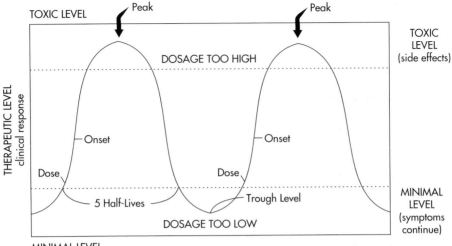

Figure 2-1   Onset, peak, and trough levels in relation to minimal, therapeutic, and toxic blood levels. (Adapted from Baer C, Williams B: *Clinical pharmacology and nursing,* ed 2, St. Louis, 1992, Mosby.)

3. **Trough level:** drug's lowest concentration before next dose; usually obtained immediately prior to antibiotic administration of a next dose

G. **The relationship of various concentration levels is demonstrated in Figure 2-1.**

Web Resources

http://www.fda.gov/cder/whatsnew.htm
   Subscribe to new drug development information.

http://www.fda.gov/cder/da/da.htm
   New drugs approved by the month of the year.

http://www.fda.gov/cder/approval/index.htm
   Approvals lists by alphabet.

http://www.health-center.com/english/pharmacy/med/index.htm
http://health.yahoo.com/health/drugs_tree/medication_or_drugs
   Other resources.

REVIEW QUESTIONS

1. A nurse applies a medication in the form of an ointment to a client's rash. Shortly after applying the ointment, the nurse begins to feel a burning sensation on the hand and notices that it has reddened. The nurse then sees some ointment next to the reddened area and realizes that this drug reaction is a (an):
   1. Systemic effect
   2. Local effect
   3. Idiosyncratic effect
   4. Synergistic effect

2. The nurse must monitor factors affecting drug action. Which of these clients has physiologic factors that would most significantly determine and modify drug activity?
   1. Mr. Carver, age 45, an alcoholic with an ulcer
   2. John, age 18, a large boy who fractured his leg and wrist in an accident
   3. Mr. Cannon, age 89, who is a frail, underweight man with high blood pressure and heart disease
   4. Susie, age 12, who has just been diagnosed with leukemia

3. A client who has received an initial dose of an antibiotic has severe wheezing within minutes. Which is the most appropriate documentation to describe the situation?
   1. Idiosyncratic reaction
   2. Anaphylactic reaction
   3. Serum sickness
   4. Cumulative effect

4. The normal therapeutic range for the drug theophylline is 10 to 20 μg/dl. A client has a serum level of 24 μg/dl. This level would be considered:
   1. Tolerance
   2. A high trough level
   3. Exaggerated peak
   4. Toxic

5. The nurse is caring for a client who has hypoalbuminemia. The nurse is concerned for which of these reasons?
   1. There may be difficulty with the elimination of a drug
   2. Excess free drug may result in toxicity
   3. A reduction in a drug effect may occur
   4. Excess bound drug may result in toxicity

6. A client has had most of the small intestine removed. The nurse would be most concerned about drug:
   1. Excretion
   2. Absorption

   3. Metabolism

   4. Distribution

7. A client is currently being maintained on a medication that is protein-bound. A second drug that is more highly protein-bound has been prescribed. What is likely to be the effect if both of these medications are administered?

   1. The second drug will produce a greater effect than the first

   2. The first medication will be inactivated

   3. Toxic effects may occur from the first drug

   4. The second drug will have a synergistic effect on the first

8. Which variable will decrease the absorption of an oral drug?

   1. Increased surface area of the small intestine

   2. Reduced surface area of the small intestine

   3. Reduced stress

   4. Increased splanchnic blood flow

ANSWERS, RATIONALES, AND TEST-TAKING TIPS

Rationales	Test-Taking Tips

1. Correct answer: 2

The burning sensation indicates a reaction from contact with the skin and a local reaction. In option 1 a systemic effect would require absorption through the circulatory system and may be exhibited by a headache or nausea. Option 3, an idiosyncrasy, is an unusual response, usually more an individual reaction rather than a common finding such as nausea or vomiting. Option 4, the synergistic effect, involves the combination of two drugs where one substance augments the activity of another agent.

Use a common sense approach: "ointment next to the reddened site" is a local effect. Do not select options 3 or 4 if you can't recall such terms. Go with what you know!

2. Correct answer: 3

Hypertension, heart disease, and weight greatly influence drug activity. In option 1, the alcohol and ulcer can affect absorption, but more information is needed. In option 2, the client has no significant factors that will modify drug activity. Leukemia could lower the resistance, but more information is needed to choose option 4.

A common sense approach would also work here. Look at the youngest given age, 12, and the oldest, 89. Look at these clients' diagnoses first, since the young and the very old are more at risk for complications. Then list the number of variables given for each: the young person has one and the older client has four. Thus, option c is the best choice. Avoid the error of forgetting what the question is as you read through the options. To maintain focus on complex questions such as this one, use this reading process: select an option, then read the question followed by your option to see if it flows for the correct answer.

3. Correct answer: 2

The descriptors "severe" and "within minutes" signals that the answer is anaphylactic reaction.

Be cautious to avoid an emotional reaction that may block your thinking process. Since you might

Respiratory distress as an anaphylactic response is common to antibiotics, especially the penicillins or the cephalosporins. The anaphylactic response may occur with an initial dose or with later doses. Option 1, idiosyncratic reaction, means unusual and specific to an individual. Option 3, serum sickness, usually manifests within a week after a medication administration. Option 4, a cumulative effect, occurs after multiple doses of a medication. The clue "initial" dose indicates that the medication is being given for the first time.

not document the situation with these types of terms, you may become angry that this is a ridiculous question. Remember to get focused on the question. Answer the question to the best of your ability. Then move on to the next question without question hangover of anger or other emotions.

4. Correct answer: 4

Toxicity occurs when the level is greater than the highest number indicated (Figure 2-1). In option 1 tolerance is the need for increasing amounts of a drug to produce the same effect. An increased dose of a medication is not indicated from the information in the stem. In option 2 a high trough level would be a higher amount than expected in the circulatory system before the next dose. No peak time is given from which to determine if it is exaggerated, so option 3 cannot be correct.

Remember that toxic levels top the therapeutic maximum serum level of a substance. With theophylline specifically, the clinical findings would first be nausea, and later, tremors or twitching. Another approach is that if you have no idea of the correct answer, cluster the first three options under the umbrella of "normal or less harmful." In option 4, "toxic" indicates abnormal and harmful, so select it.

5. Correct answer: 2

A low albumin level allows more unbound drug to circulate in the body and results in toxicity. A low albumin level has no association with elimination problems. An increase in the drug effect would be seen and lead to a toxic situation. In

Eliminate options 1 and 3 because of the clue from the key words "elimination" and "effect." Note that options 2 and 4 have the similar words "excess . . . result in toxicity." To decide between these two options, use common sense: if a free amount of a drug is available,

Rationales	Test-Taking Tips

option 4 the event of excess bound drug would result in a reduction in the drug effect since less would be available to work.

more action is possible than with the bound drug. Thus, option 2 is the best choice.

6. Correct answer: 2

Many drugs are absorbed through the small intestine. The kidney is the main organ that is involved in drug elimination. For option 3, the liver is the main organ for metabolism. For option 4, plasma protein and the circulatory system are the main elements of concern for drug distribution.

Recall the normal process that ingested medication goes through in the body after administration: (1) absorption, (2) distribution, (3) metabolism, and (4) excretion. Now look at the situation given in the question. The client had part of the GI tract removed. Oral medication would be affected by this change. Oral medications must be absorbed from the GI tract before they can complete the three remaining steps. Therefore, this first step, absorption, is of greatest concern. Note an easy recall tip to remember the sequence for this normal process after drug ingestion: The first three steps can be remembered in alphabetical order, with common sense dictating that excretion occurs last.

7. Correct answer: 3

More of the first drug will remain free, or unbound, since more of the second drug will be bound to the protein. Therefore, the first drug, being at higher serum levels, can produce toxic effects. The second drug is more bound with the protein and will have a lesser or subtherapeutic effect. Competition does not necessarily cause inactivation. There is not enough information in the question to select a synergistic effect, which would require a substance that augments or adds to the activity of another substance or agent.

An approach to use when you have no idea of the correct answer is to select the most severe or detrimental situation. The situations are: in option 1, a greater effect; in option 2, inactivated; in option 3, toxic effects; and in option 4, synergistic effect. Select option 3 because toxic effects are the most detrimental of the given choices.

8. Correct answer: 2

Less intestinal surface area or time in the small intestine will decrease absorption (e.g., diarrhea). Increased surface area will increase absorption. Reduced stress allows for more absorption. In contrast, increased stress will most likely decrease absorption. Increased splanchnic blood flow increases absorption. Splanchnic blood flow is the visceral circulation, which is the circulation to internal organs in the abdominal cavity.

Read carefully to focus on the specific direction asked in the question: decreases the absorption. As you read the options, keep common sense in mind. A decreased surface area results in decreased absorption, option 2. If you have no idea of the correct option, match the direction of the concern in the question "decreased absorption" with the same direction in the options to narrow it to options 2 and 3. Then make an educated guess. Think in a logical manner: reduced stress means the body is relaxed and more absorption would occur. Thus, select option 2.

3

Administration of Medications

FAST FACTS

1. Medications should always be checked for the "five rights" ("5R's"): right drug, right dose, right route, right time, and right client.
2. When hurried, and especially with clients who have multiple medications ordered (such as elders), checking the 5R's is essential (none should be omitted).
3. Nurses are legally accountable for the proper signing out, use, and waste, if any, of controlled substances.
4. Nurses have an ethical responsibility to report improper use of any medications, especially controlled substances.
5. Nurses may delegate certain responsibilities for IV medications and fluids to a licensed practical nurse (LPN) if proper training has been provided to the LPN and the agency policy allows this delegation.
6. Handwashing before the preparation of drugs and between clients is essential
7. Z-track injection prevents leaking of the drug into the subcutaneous (SC) tissue and is used for irritating or oil-based medications and large quantities (more than 2 ml) of medication.
8. An air lock is not used with intradermal (ID) injections, is not required in SC injections, and should be 0.5 ml with Z-track injections and 0.2 ml with other injections

CONTENT REVIEW

I. General principles for medication administration
  A. **Remember the 5R's of medication administration**
    1. Right drug
    2. Right dose
    3. Right route

  4. Right time

  5. Right client

B. **Always check for client's allergies**

C. **Check all medications three times, as follows:**

  1. When locating in the cart or on the shelf

  2. When pouring or preparing

  3. Before returning to cart or shelf (or before giving a unit dose)

D. **Check all medications listed on the medication administration record (MAR) against the chart orders at least once per shift**

E. **Never administer medication another staff member has prepared**

F. **Sign only for controlled substance waste that you have witnessed**

G. **Give medications within 60 min before or after the time scheduled, if unable to give at the scheduled time**

H. **Identify clients by checking their identification band, and if possible, ask them to speak their names; ask parents to state children's names**

I. **Always double-check medications questioned by clients. (They are often right!)**

J. **Wash your hands before medication preparation and between clients**

K. **Use gloves to protect self from contamination and to avoid absorbing the medication through the skin**

L. **Assess the client according to the medication administered; example: check BP in a lying or sitting, then a standing position before an antihypertensive; check breath sounds before a bronchodilator; or assess pain type, location, and intensity prior to an analgesic**

M. **Never give an unfamiliar medication; be sure to question any unusual route, dosage, or combination of medications**

N. **Sign out all controlled substances**

O. **In the narrative charting, document all stat, one-time, and prn drugs; any necessary assessments or unusual findings; the evaluation of the drug's effectiveness; and the degree of desired effect**

P. **Discard needles, gloves, and alcohol swabs in containers clearly marked "hazardous waste"**

Q. **Check expiration dates of medications and IV fluids prior to giving**

II. Administration by injection

 A. **Three possible routes or sites**

  1. IM: into a muscle

  2. SC: into the subcutaneous or fatty tissue

  3. ID: into the dermis

 B. **Locating sites** (Figures 3-1 to 3-5)

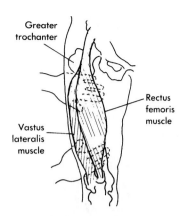

Figure 3-1 To define vastus lateralis (great lateral muscle) and rectus femoris muscle sites, place one hand below patient's greater trochanter and one hand above knee. Space between two hands defines the middle third of underlying muscle. Rectus femoris is on anterior thigh; vastus lateralis is on lateral thigh. (From Clark J et al: *Pharmacologic basis of nursing practice,* ed 6, St Louis, 2000, Mosby.)

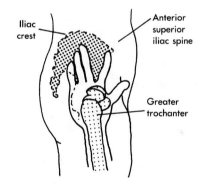

Figure 3-2 To locate ventrogluteal muscle injection site, place palm of hand on greater trochanter of femur. Make V with fingers, with one side running from greater trochanter to anterosuperior iliac spine and other side running from greater trochanter to iliac crest. (From Clark J et al: *Pharmacologic basis of nursing practice,* ed 6, St Louis, 2000, Mosby.)

    C. Angles of injections
       1. ID: 15 degrees
       2. SC: 45 or 90 degrees
       3. IM: 90 degrees

III. Key principles
    A. Oral route
       1. Avoid touching tablets when transferring into a cup
       2. Do not crush sustained-release or enteric-coated tablets
       3. Assess the client's ability to swallow and the presence of a gag reflex

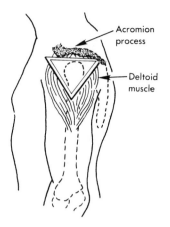

Figure 3-3 Deltoid muscle injection site roughly forms an inverted triangle, with acromion process as base. Muscle may be visible in muscular patients. (From Clark J et al: *Pharmacologic basis of nursing practice,* ed 6, St Louis, 2000, Mosby.)

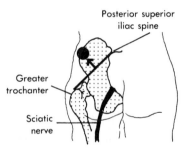

Figure 3-4 Accepted method for defining dorsogluteal injection site. Locate by palpation posterior superior iliac spine and greater trochanter, then draw imaginary line between them. Injection site up and out from that line should be used. (From Clark J et al: *Pharmacologic basis of nursing practice,* ed 6, St Louis, 2000, Mosby.)

    4. Assess whether the client has swallowed the tablet
    5. Elevate the head of the bed at least 60 degrees to administer oral medications
    6. Medications can be crushed or can be mixed with ice cream, applesauce, water, or juice to allow easier swallowing
 B. Injections
    1. Know which medications should be given **Z-track;** these are usually oil-based, irritating, or large doses. Z-track is a technique to prevent medication from leaking into the SC tissue (Figure 3-6)
      a. Use a 0.5-ml air lock: a small amount of air added to the syringe after the medication is accurately measured to clear all of the drug from the injecting needle
      b. Change the needle after drawing up the medication

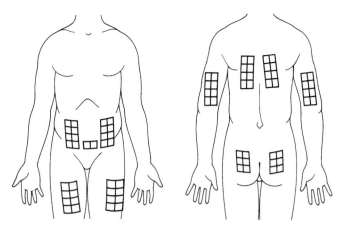

Figure 3-5   Commonly used subcutaneous injection sites. (From Clark J et al: *Pharmacologic basis of nursing practice,* ed 6, St Louis, 2000, Mosby.)

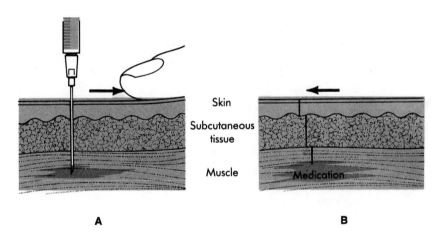

Figure 3-6   **A,** In Z-track intramuscular injection, skin is pulled laterally, then injection is administered. **B,** After needle is withdrawn, skin is released. Technique helps prevent medication from leaking into SC tissue. (From Clark J et al: *Pharmacologic basis of nursing practice,* ed 6, St Louis, 2000, Mosby.)

2. In children who are not yet walking, the lateral great muscle (vastus lateralis) is the injection site that is recommended
3. Always aspirate by pulling back on the plunger before injecting medications to check for a blood return. If blood returns, remove the needle and discard the medication. This blood return means the needle is in a large vessel rather than in the muscle. For medications administered subcutaneously, such as heparin sodium

or insulin, aspiration technique is not recommended since large vessels are not in the subcutaneous tissue.

4. Use an **air lock** of 0.2 ml for injections that are not Z-track. No air lock is needed for ID injections. The use of an air lock of 0.2 ml for SC injections is the decision of the nurse. However, consistency must be maintained so that the dosage given to the client is not altered. Examples: insulin, heparin sodium

5. Must produce a bleb for ID injections

6. Use the deltoid muscle for 1 ml or less. The dorsal gluteal muscle can tolerate a maximum of 5 ml per site.

7. Massage increases the absorption of medication. Avoid massaging heparin sodium SC injections to prevent bruising at the site.

8. Know which medications (usually oil-based) cannot be mixed with other medications for IM injections; example: diazepam (Valium)

9. Change the needle after withdrawing the desired dose for irritating medications; example: iron dextran (Imferon)

10. Penicillin injected IM is given Z-track, measured in millions of units, and given with 16-gauge or 18-gauge needles, 2 to 3 in long

C. **NG (route): medications administered through a tube passed through the nose into the stomach; gastrostomy tube (G-tube): tube inserted into the stomach through the upper abdominal wall for long-term feedings**

1. Wear gloves

2. Be sure medication can be crushed to mix with water for instillation into an NG tube. Liquid forms are available for some medications.

3. Check placement of the tube before instillation of any medications; withdrawal of green gastric fluid is most reliable

4. Follow the medication with 30 to 60 ml of tap water to flush the tube

D. **IV (into a vein)**

1. Know how fast an intravenous push (IVP) should be given or an intravenous piggyback (IVPB) should be run. The literature identifies certain limits for some IVP medications. Most IVP medications should be given over at least 1 to 3 minutes, IVPB over 30 minutes.

2. Use sterile technique for all forms of IV administration

3. Wear gloves during administration to protect self from bloodborne diseases

4. Monitor for signs and symptoms of the following:
   a. **Phlebitis:** inflammation of a vein; redness, warmth, pain
   b. **Infiltration:** fluid passes into the tissue: pallor, edema, coolness, decreased IV flow, usually no blood return

5. Do not rely on an IV pump alone; check the accuracy of the flow rate

6. Cleanse the ports on the IV tubing with a disinfectant before use of the port for an IVP or IVPB
7. Never push medicines through a difficult or clogged IV line
8. Know which medications can and cannot be mixed together. If medications do not mix, flush with sterile water or normal saline (NS) before administering, or use another site. Example: diazepam (Valium) cannot be mixed with any other medications or diluted with NS.
9. Know the hospital protocol for the rotation of IV peripheral sites; usual recommendation is every 72 hr
10. Prime the IV line before beginning an infusion and prime all the ports
11. Know which medications need a filter. IV substances usually *not* filtered (think of the word "LATIN"):
    a. Lipids
    b. Amphotericin B
    c. Alteplase recombinant (Activase)
    d. TPN—total parenteral nutrition
    e. Insulin
    f. Nitroglycerin (NTG)
12. Monitor for common complications of IV therapy, including:
    a. Infiltration or **extravasation:** the process whereby a fluid or drug passes into the tissues
    b. **Thrombophlebitis:** inflammation of a vein, often accompanied by a clot
    c. Pain at the insertion site
    d. Fluid overload: excess accumulation of intravascular fluid; may be manifested by tachycardia, tachypnea, pulmonary edema
    e. Infusion-related infection: contamination of the IV system, site, or solution; manifested by purulent drainage, cellulitis, erythema, pain, thrombophlebitis
    f. **Tissue necrosis:** localized tissue death that occurs in groups of cells in response to disease or injury
13. Avoid taping over the IV cannula or needle insertion site, must be easily viewed at all times
14. Know care differences for IV central lines; major action is to prevent air embolism with tubing change by closing clamp near insertion site, have client bear down or hold breath (Valsalva's maneuver), and then change tubing

E. Other routes
1. Vaginal
    a. Wear gloves
    b. Offer the client a sanitary pad for comfort after application
    c. Wash the applicator with warm water and soap. Applicators can be reused.

2. Rectal
   a. Wear gloves
   b. Use a water-soluble lubricant, such as K-Y Jelly
   c. Instruct the client not to expel the suppository immediately after application and to try to retain it for at least 30 minutes
3. Otic drops
   a. Pull pinna back and down for children under age 5; pull pinna back and up for adults; remember "grow-up" and "pull-up"
   b. Keep the dropper aseptic; avoid touching the ear
   c. Allow the drop to slide down the wall of the ear canal to decrease a sudden discomfort of medication falling on the eardrum
   d. Instruct clients to lie on their sides or keep their heads tilted to the side for 5 to 10 min
   e. Cotton may or may not be recommended after instillation of the drops
4. Ophthalmic drops and ointments
   a. Instill in the everted lower lid while client looks up and slightly tilts head backwards with hyperextension of the neck (Figure 3-7)
   b. Avoid touching the dropper on the eyelid
   c. Hold pressure on the lacrimal sac for 1 to 3 min after instillation to decrease risk of sinus and systemic absorption
   d. Wait 2 to 3 min before instilling another drop or ointment
5. Topical
   a. Use gloves for application of creams
   b. Date the outside of transdermal patches

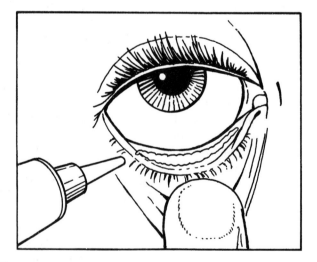

Figure 3-7   Administering ophthalmic ointment. To instill ointment, gently pull lower lid down as patient looks upward. Squeeze ophthalmic ointment into lower sac. Avoid touching tube to eyelid. (From Clark J et al: *Pharmacologic basis of nursing practice,* ed 6, St Louis, 2000, Mosby.)

    c. Apply a clear plastic wrap over nitroglycerin (NTG) ointment paper, which will increase the absorption

    d. Rotate sites to prevent irritation to the skin; cleanse old site after patch removal

    e. Do not shave hairy areas, because shaving may inflame the skin, which then increases absorption; avoid hairy areas if possible

F. Venous access device or port (VAP): internal surgically implanted infusion device placed in the chest wall, abdomen, or antecubital area of the arm designed for continuous access to the venous system. Examples: Port-a-Cath, Infuse-a-Port, Mediport, Chemo-Port.

    1. Secure the implanted device with two fingers before injecting (Figure 3-8)

    2. Cleanse site with povidone iodine (Betadine) before puncture

    3. Aspirate for a blood return

    4. Irrigate with sterile water or saline before and after administering the medication

    5. Recommended needle size is 20- to 22-gauge; commonly, a Hubor point, straight or at a 90-degree angle, is used with a 22-gauge needle

G. Venous access device (VAD): external central VAD; most common are Hickman, Broviac, and Groshong. Care is similar to care of an IV central line.

IV. Needles

    A. ID: 26-gauge, ¼ or ⅜ in. long

    B. IM: 22-gauge, 1 to 1 ½ in. long; 16- to 18-gauge, 2 to 3 in. long for penicillin injections

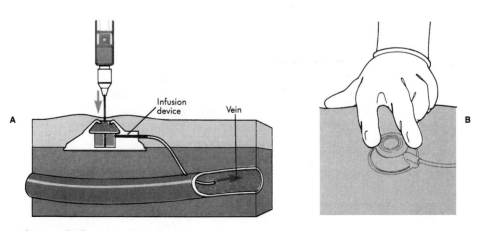

Figure 3-8 Inplanted infusion device. **A,** Side view, illustrating needle inserted through skin and top of infusion device. Distal end of device is in vein. **B,** Use one hand to secure device before inserting needle. (From Clark J et al: *Pharmacologic basis of nursing practice,* ed 6, St Louis, 2000, Mosby.)

C. **SC: 25- or 26-gauge, ½ to ⅝ in long**
D. **IV: 18- to 22-gauge for general IV; 14- to 20-gauge for blood transfusion**
E. **Hubor needle is especially designed with a sharp-angle bevel and is used only for implanted venous infusion or access ports (VAP): can be either 22-gauge straight or 90-degree angled (right-angled)**

V. Calculation of dosages can be accomplished by three formulas

A. **Desired/have: 50 mg ordered, have on hand 100 mg/2 ml**
   1. Formula:

$$\frac{\text{Desired dose}}{\text{Have on hand}} \times \text{Quantity} = \text{Dose to give}$$

   2. Example:

$$\frac{50 \text{ mg}}{100 \text{ mg}} \times 2 \text{ ml} = 1 \text{ ml}$$

B. **Ratio/proportion (RP): 50 mg ordered, have on hand 100 mg/2 ml**
   1. Formula:

$$\frac{\text{Dosage on hand (units)}}{\text{Dosage on hand (ml)}} : \frac{\text{Desired dose (units)}}{\text{Unknown} \times \text{(ml)}} = \text{Dose to give}$$

   2. Example:

$$\frac{100 \text{ mg}}{2 \text{ ml}} : \frac{50 \text{ mg}}{\text{x}}$$

(Note: Cross-multiply 50 mg with 2 ml and 100 mg with x)

$$100 \text{ mg x} = 100 \text{ mg/ml}$$

$$\text{x} = \frac{100 \text{ mg/ml}}{100 \text{ mg}}$$

$$\text{x} = 1 \text{ ml}$$

(Note: milligrams cancel out)

C. **Dimensional analysis (DA): 50 mg ordered, have on hand 1 gr/2 ml**
   1. Formula

Dose ordered $\times$ Conversion factor $\times$ Dose on hand $=$
                                        Dose to give (or dose needed)

(Note: all units should cancel except the desired dose)
   2. Example:

$$50 \text{ mg} \times \frac{1 \text{ g}}{1,000 \text{ mg}} \times \frac{15 \text{ gr}}{1 \text{ g}} \times \frac{2 \text{ ml}}{1 \text{ gr}} = 1.5 \text{ ml}$$

REVIEW QUESTIONS

1. Which client response below should make a nurse double-check the tablets, dose, and timing of the medication that has been prepared by the nurse?
   1. "I don't know what these are for"
   2. "I've never taken a yellow one before"
   3. "Can you tell me what these do?"
   4. "The blue tablet always makes me sleepy"

2. An injection of iron dextran (Imferon) should be given Z-track on an adult client in which location?
   1. Dorsogluteal muscle
   2. Ventrogluteal muscle
   3. Deltoid muscle
   4. Lateral great muscle (vastus lateralis)

3. Medications given by the nasogastric (NG) route require that:
   1. The medications are followed with formula
   2. Heart sounds are assessed
   3. Instillation of 30 to 60 ml of water is done after medication instillation
   4. All medications are crushed, or liquid forms are used

4. Which of these IV complications would be manifested by pallor, coolness of the skin, and edema at the site?
   1. Tissue necrosis
   2. Thrombophlebitis
   3. Infiltration
   4. Infection

5. A client complains of nausea and has been given hydroxyzine hydrochloride (Vistaril), 50 mg IM q4h prn. The nurse knows the medication must be given Z-track with a 0.5-ml air lock. The purpose of an air lock is so that the medication:
   1. Will completely clear the hub
   2. Cannot leak out
   3. Is accurately measured
   4. Will not irritate the muscle

6. A client has received an antipyretic medication via rectal suppository at 8:00 AM. When should the nurse recheck the client's vital signs?
   1. 8:30 AM
   2. 10:00 AM
   3. 12:00 PM
   4. 4:00 PM

7. A nurse administers a buccal antihypertensive drug. Within how many minutes should the client's blood pressure be rechecked?

    1. 60 min

    2. 30 min

    3. 15 min

    4. 5 min

ANSWERS, RATIONALES, AND TEST-TAKING TIPS

Rationales	Test-Taking Tips

1. Correct answer: 2

Clients often know the shape, color, and number of tablets they take every day. Unless a new medication has been added, the nurse could have made a drug error. Clients may not know what every medication is for, especially if new medications were ordered. Clients often want to know what actions drugs have. Drowsiness is a common side effect and does not require rechecking the medications.

Use what you know to think logically to figure out the answer if you have no idea of the correct one. Look at each option to establish a theme. Options 1 and 3 are knowledge-deficit. Option 2 is questioning a new pill. Option 4 is familiarity. Go back to get refocused on the question: "which causes the nurse to doublecheck?" By looking at the themes, it is obvious the question about the new pill is the best answer.

2. Correct answer: 1

The dorsogluteal muscle is a large muscle used for the injection of irritating drugs. The ventrogluteal muscle is used for IM injections but is not the preferred location for Z-track injections. The deltoid muscle is too small and is typically used for vaccine administration and less than 1 ml injections. The great lateral muscle (vastus lateralis) is used for IM injections but is not the preferred site for the injection of irritating medications.

Remember that the ventrogluteal and the great lateral muscles are both chosen on the lateral aspect of the body for IM injections, and only as a second choice for deep IM and Z-track injections. An easy way to remember the difference between deltoid and dorsogluteal muscles is that deltoid comes first alphabetically and also is the first site at the top of the body on the upper arm. Dorsogluteal is next alphabetically and is positioned lower on the body. Recall tip—the dorsogluteal muscle is for "down-deep" injections.

3. Correct answer: 3

Water flushes the tube, clears all the medication, and prevents the clogging of the tube. Clients often need additional water administered separately from the formula. To flush the tube with water before and after is correct. This is also important because

Option 1 is somewhat vague, since after you give medications you do continue with the formula. Option 2 introduces new information that is unrelated to the focus of the question. These types of options can usually be eliminated. Option 4 has the absolute "all" in it; options that

Rationales	Test-Taking Tips

some of the medications may not mix with the ingredients of the formula. Heart sound assessment is not necessary for administration of NG administration of medications. Time-released or enteric-coated tablets should never be crushed.

contain absolutes are often misleading and an incorrect choice.

4. Correct answer: 3

Infiltration is manifested by pallor, edema, and coolness, because the fluid escapes into the tissue around the site. Tissue necrosis is manifested by warm, irritated, and usually red or purplish-red skin. Warmth, redness, and various degrees of swelling are findings consistent with thrombophlebitis. Infection is indicated by findings of redness, warmth, pain, and possibly exudate or pus.

Use this action if you have no idea of the correct option. Cluster options 1, 2, and 3 under "inflammatory response," which is characteristically red. Eliminate these three answers, since they conflict with the given data of "pallor."

5. Correct answer: 1

An air lock clears all medication from the hub and needle, since the air clears after the medication is injected. The Z-track method prevents medication from leaking back into the SC tissue. Accurate measurement should occur before you draw up an air lock. The Z-track method is used to prevent irritation by injection of oil-based or caustic drugs or large amounts of IM medications.

Read the question carefully. If you read too fast, you may have focused on the Z-track and selected option 2 or 3. Z-track is a distracter in the question. The question is asking for the reason for the use of an air lock in the syringe.

6. Correct answer: 1

The absorption of rectal medications is fast via the mucous membranes. This is

Focus on the absorption route rather than the type of medication. Another approach, if you had no similar to absorption by the mucous membranes in the mouth. If changes do not appear in the client within 15 to 30 min after a rectal suppository is given, the nurse should check for insertion of the suppository into fecal matter instead of next to the mucous membranes or for excessive internal hemorrhoids. The other times are too long.

idea of the time, is to look at the type of medication: antipyretics are given for a fever. Clients with high fevers who require medication have their temperatures checked every 30 minutes until the preferred body temperature is achieved. One way to remember antipyretics is to think of a pyromaniac, a person who likes to set fires and watch them burn. A fire is hot. Therefore an antipyretic fights the fever (or fire) in a sick client.

7. Correct answer: 4

The buccal route, absorption through the mucous membranes in the mouth, is effective within 5 min. To refresh your memory, the buccal route is the placement of a medication between the gums and the cheeks.

Associate the buccal route with the sublingual route, by which nitroglycerin is given. Recall that nitroglycerin can be repeated after 5 minutes. Both are absorbed through the mucous membranes.

4

Drugs Affecting the Autonomic Nervous System

FAST FACTS

1. The four drug classifications in the autonomic nervous system (ANS) are: adrenergic or sympathetic (sympathomimetic), cholinergic or parasympathetic (parasympathomimetic), adrenergic blockers, and cholinergic blockers.
2. Cardiac terms: **chronotropic** means heart rate (think "chronologic" or "numbers"); **dromotropic** means conduction of impulse (think of how fast the drive is through the heart of the impulse); and **inotropic** means contractility of muscle.
3. Sympathetic receptor sites include alpha (vascular smooth muscles or the blood vessel walls); beta$_1$ (heart, think "one heart"); and beta$_2$ (lung, think "two lungs").
4. Adrenergic blocking agents may result in findings consistent with parasympathetic stimulation.
5. Cholinergic blocking agents may result in findings consistent with sympathetic stimulation.
6. Evaluation of the effectiveness of ANS drugs is completed by clinical assessment for changes in (listed in order of priority):
   - Increase or decrease in heart rate (HR) or BP, irregular heart rhythm
   - Respiratory rate (RR) and lung sounds: clear, wheezes
   - Level of consciousness (LOC): excitement or dullness
   - GI: bowel sounds, increased or decreased; mucous membranes, dry or moist
   - Laboratory test results, increased or decreased serum glucose level
   - Pupils, constricted or dilated
7. Sympathetic (adrenergic) response is stimulated by stress and can cause mydriasis, increased HR, dilated bronchioles, release of renin in kidneys,

constricted arteries and veins (increased BP), decreased motility of the bowel and relaxation of bladder muscle, dilated uterus in non-pregancy and contraction of uterus in pregnancy, ejaculation.

8. Parasympathetic (cholinergic) response is stimulated by common daily needs for body functions. If overstimulated, it can cause miosis, decreased HR, constricted bronchioles, vasodilation of arteries and veins, increased voiding, increased gastric secretions and motility, erection.

CONTENT REVIEW

ADRENERGIC AGENTS: SYMPATHOMIMETIC

Sympathetic—

I. Adrenergic agonists

"High ddny"

A. Division by types (Table 4-1)

1. Includes alpha$_1$, alpha$_2$, beta$_1$, beta$_2$, and dopamine agonists. The drugs are selective for either alpha or beta-adrenergic receptors, or both.

TABLE 4-1	Classification of Autonomic Nervous System Drugs	
Sympathetic		**Parasympathetic**
Adrenergic Response		**Cholinergic Response**
Catecholamines: norepinephrine epinephrine dopamine	**Neurotransmitters**	Acetylcholine ACh
Beta$_1$ Beta$_2$ Alpha Dopaminergic	**Receptor Sites**	Nicotinic Muscarinic
	Agents	
Adrenergic Drugs (Sympathomimetic) • Catecholamines • Noncatecholamines		**Cholinergic Agents** (Parasympathomimetic) • Direct-Acting Cholinergic Agents • Anticholinesterase Agents
Adrenergic-Blocking (Sympatholytic) • Alpha-Adrenergic Blockers • Beta-Adrenergic Blockers • Ganglionic Blockers		**Cholinergic-Blocking** (Parasympatholytic) • Anticholinergic Agents

2. Divided into two groups as follows:
   a. Catecholamines: a group of sympathomimetic compounds that cannot cross the blood-brain barrier or be taken orally and act directly:
     (1) Endogenous: norepinephrine, epinephrine, and dopamine
     (2) Synthetic (exogenous): dobutamine, isoproterenol
   b. Noncatecholamines: compounds that can cross the blood-brain barrier, act directly or indirectly, and be taken orally: ephedrine, albuterol, phenylephrine

B. Overall therapeutic uses
1. Anorexiants
2. Produce bronchodilation in respiratory system, uterine relaxation and increase force of contraction of the heart muscles
3. Reduce intraocular pressure and dilate pupils (mydriasis)
4. Decrease nasal and conjunctival congestion
5. Support the heart during cardiac failure or shock (cardioselective drugs)

C. Catecholamines
1. Actions (Table 4-2)
   a. Positive **inotropic action:** increases force or contractility of the heart
   b. Positive **chronotropic action:** increases HR
   c. Positive **dromotropic action:** increases conduction of electrical impulse through the heart
   d. Adrenergic neurotransmission
   e. Bronchodilation

TABLE 4-2   Autonomic Action of Cardiovascular Medications

Action	Refers To	To Increase	To Decrease
Contractility	Stretch	+ Inotropic	− Inotropic
Heart rate	Beats/min	+ Chronotropic	− Chronotropic
Conduction	Speed of electrical impulse transmission through heart	+ Dromotropic	− Dromotropic

Effects		Positive	Negative
Inotropic	Cardiac output	↑	↓
	Urinary output	↑	↓
	Cardiac workload	↑	↓
Chronotropic	+ Tachycardia, or increase in heart rate		
	− Bradycardia, or decrease in heart rate		
Dromotropic	+ Attribute to dysrhythmias		
	− Decrease in dysrhythmias		

+ = positive
− = negative

2. Uses
   a. Hypotension
   b. Anaphylactic shock
   c. Asthma
   d. Hypoglycemia
   e. Control local bleeding
   f. Local anesthetic
   g. CHF
   h. Mild renal failure
3. Major side effects
   a. Tachycardia
   b. Hypertension
   c. Myocardial ischemia
   d. Hyperglycemia
4. Nursing implications
   a. Monitor vital signs (VS) and the cardiac function by means of an electrocardiogram (ECG)
   b. Assess respiratory effort and lung sounds
   c. Monitor blood glucose levels
   d. Monitor intake and output (I&O)
   e. Avoid extravasation

⚠ Warning!

Check IV patency at least every 15 to 30 min, especially when using norepinephrine bitartrate (Levophed), which can cause necrosis of tissue if infiltration occurs and result is need for the amputation of the affected extremity. Use with caution in children. Avoid use in pregnancy.

   f. Special considerations: Dopamine can be given in low, moderate, or high doses with varied results, as follows:
      (1) 1 to 5 μg/kg/min for renal perfusion
      (2) 5 to 10 μg/kg/min for cardiac effects
      (3) 10 to 20 μg/kg/min for cardiac effects but may produce adverse effects from generalized vasoconstriction; can result in decreased kidney function
5. Common drugs
   a. Epinephrine hydrochloride (Adrenalin Chloride)
   b. Dobutamine hydrochloride (Dobutrex)
   c. Dopamine hydrochloride (Intropin)
   d. Isoproterenol hydrochloride (Isuprel)
   e. Norepinephrine bitartrate (Levophed)
D. Noncatecholamines
   1. Action
      a. Selective catecholamine action because of the drugs' similarity
      b. Selective $beta_2$ action

2. Uses
   a. Asthma
   b. Nasal decongestion
   c. Prevent premature labor (Terbutaline sulfate [Brethine] only)
   d. Hypotension (especially orthostatic hypotension)
   e. Appetite suppression
3. Major side effects
   a. Central nervous system (CNS) reactions: nervousness, anxiety, headache, insomnia
   b. ECG changes: palpitations, tachycardia, dysrhythmias
   c. Musculoskeletal: weakness, mild tremors, cramps
4. Nursing implications
   a. Monitor vital signs and mental status
   b. Teach patient how to properly administer inhalants; the amount of drug in the canister can be assessed by placing it in a bowl of water: if it floats, it is empty; if it floats half out of the water it is half full; and if it sinks, it is full.

> ⚠️ **Warning!**
> Report any CNS changes immediately.

5. Common drugs
   a. Terbutaline sulfate (Brethine)
   b. Albuterol (Proventil, Ventolin)
   c. Metaproterenol sulfate (Alupent)
   d. Phenylephrine hydrochloride (Neo-Synephrine)
   e. Pseudoephedrine hydrochloride (Sudafed)
   f. Tetrahydrozoline (Murine, Visine)
   g. Midodrine (ProAmatine)
   h. Amphetamines, benzphetamine (Didrex), dextroamphetamine (Dexedrine)

ADRENERGIC BLOCKING AGENTS

I. Divided into three groups (see Table 4-1, p. 54)
A. Alpha-adrenergic blockers
B. Beta-adrenergic blockers
C. Ganglionic blockers

II. Alpha-adrenergic blockers (antiadrenergic)
A. Actions
   1. Interrupt or antagonize the sympathomimetic agents
   2. Dilate vessels in smooth muscle
   3. Lower peripheral vascular resistance
B. Uses
   1. Peripheral vascular disease
   2. **Raynaud's disease**

3. **Pheochromocytoma**
4. Hypertension
5. Vascular headaches (especially migraine)

C. **Major side effects**
1. Nasal congestion
2. GI irritation, nausea, vomiting
3. Ergotism: an acute or chronic disease caused by excessive dosages of medications containing ergotamine, an ergot alkaloid; symptoms may include circulatory impairment from various degrees of vasoconstriction, such as spasms, cramps, weakness, cyanosis, muscle pains, or dry gangrene of the upper or lower extremities

> ⚠️ **Warning!**
>
> To avoid ergotism, patient should not exceed recommended dose. Dry gangrene of the upper or lower extremities, acute or chronic, can occur if these drugs are improperly used.

4. Rebound tachycardia: sudden return of the heart rate to more than 100 beats/min
5. Postural hypotension: drop in blood pressure of more than 20 mm Hg when patient changes from a lying to a standing or sitting position

D. **Nursing implications**
1. Monitor vital signs; measure lying, sitting, and standing BP
2. Instruct the patient to change positions slowly
3. Direct the patient to take the medication at the first sign of severe headaches
4. Assess for signs of ergotism: numbness, weakness, tingling of fingers and toes
5. Instruct the patient how to take ergotamine products and follow the dosing instructions until the headache is gone; products vary as to the time for repeat dosing and the maximum dose within a 24 hour period
6. Instruct patient to limit caffeine intake, since caffeine causes vasoconstriction

E. **Common drugs**
1. Ergotamine tartrate (Ergostat)
2. Ergotamine tartrate and caffeine (Cafergot)
3. Phentolamine mesylate (Regitine)
4. Prazosin hydrochloride (Minipress)
5. Terazosin (Hytrin)

III. **Beta-adrenergic blockers (antiadrenergic)**

A. **Actions: block sympathetic response by competing for beta receptors; also block the stimulation of the heart and have the potential to block bronchodilation**

B. Uses
  1. Hypertension
  2. Angina
  3. Tachyarrhythmias
  4. Migraine headaches
  5. Myocardial infarction
  6. Anxiety

C. Major side effects
  1. Bradycardia
  2. Hypoglycemia
  3. Orthostatic hypotension
  4. Impotence
  5. Bronchospasm, especially in patients with asthma or other COPD
  6. Depression ("beta blocker blues")

> ⚠ **Warning!**
>
> These drugs interact with alcohol and other central nervous system depressants; teach patient to avoid combining these agents with alcohol or other depressants. Avoid some OTC drugs, such as decongestants. Do not abruptly discontinue the medication. Severe angina may result.

D. Nursing implications
  1. Monitor VS, especially for bradycardia and hypotension
  2. Monitor blood glucose level for hypoglycemia (less than 50 mg/dl)
  3. Instruct patient to self-monitor pulse and BP and to change positions slowly
  4. Tell the patient about the possibility of impotence
  5. Assess lung sounds for inspiratory and expiratory wheezing
  6. Advise patient to avoid extreme heat, hot tubs, hot showers
  7. Monitor for a need to increase dosage, because these drugs are subject to the hepatic first-pass effect

> ⚠ **Warning!**
>
> Careful evaluation for the desired effect is essential; the dosage may need to be increased or decreased.

E. Common drugs (tip: these drugs end in "-lol")
  1. Atenolol (Tenormin)
  2. Propranolol hydrochloride (Inderal)
  3. Metoprolol tartrate (Lopressor)
  4. Nadolol (Corgard)
  5. Pindolol (Visken)
  6. Timolol maleate (Timoptic)—eye drop medication

IV. Ganglionic blockers

A. Action: compete with acetylcholine and affect both the sympathetic and the parasympathetic systems

B. Uses
1. Hypertension, especially hypertensive crisis
2. Pulmonary edema resulting from pulmonary hypertension

C. Major side effects
1. Hypotension
2. Bradycardia
3. Anticholinergic effects, such as dry mouth, dilated pupils, tachycardia, decreased GI and urinary motility

D. Nursing implications
1. Monitor every 5 to 10 min for a decrease in BP of 20 mm Hg and decrease in HR of 20 beats/min from the initial readings
2. Provide comfort measures for anticholinergic side effects, such as saliva substitutes
3. Monitor I&O, assess elimination patterns

> ⚠ **Warnings!**
>
> Avoid these drugs in patients with glaucoma. Use cautiously in patients with cardiac disease. Monitor BP for a rapid decrease; expect a sudden drop in BP. Note the patient's symptoms and adjust the dosage as necessary.

E. Common drugs
1. Mecamylamine hydrochloride (Inversine)
2. Trimethaphan camsylate (Arfonad)

CHOLINERGIC AGENTS: PARASYMPATHOMIMETIC

(like Adrenergic blockers?)

I. These agents are divided into the following types (see Table 4-1, p. 54):
A. Direct-acting cholinergic agonists
B. Anticholinesterase agents

"low + slow + moist"

II. Direct-acting cholinergic agonists
A. Action: mimics acetylcholine to produce parasympathetic stimulation

B. Uses
1. Glaucoma
2. Bladder atony
3. Constricted pupils (miosis) (see Chapter 19)
4. Gastroesophageal reflux disease; delayed gastric emptying
5. Nausea and vomiting before chemotherapy

C. Major side effects
1. Bronchoconstriction, wheezing, shortness of breath
2. Bradycardia, hypotension
3. Headache, flushing
4. Increased salivation, sweating
5. Nausea, vomiting, diarrhea, cramping
6. Impaired vision, impaired night vision

> ## ⚠ Warnings!
>
> Interactions: expect a decrease in action when given with adrenergic drugs. Have atropine sulfate, an anticholinergic, available for emergency reactions.

D. Nursing implications
  1. Assess respiratory and cardiac status
  2. Instruct patient to take before or after meals to limit GI symptoms
  3. Instruct patient how to instill eye drops, if ordered. Eye drops for glaucoma have a miotic effect (constrict the pupil). Caution the patient about driving at night.

E. Common drugs
  1. Bethanechol chloride (Urecholine) for bladder atony
  2. Pilocarpine hydrochloride (Pilocar) for glaucoma
  3. Carbachol intraocular (Miostat) for glaucoma
  4. Metochlopramide hydrochloride (Reglan) for gastric reflux, delayed gastric emptying, and nausea and vomiting

III. Anticholinesterase agents

A. Action: inhibit the enzyme acetylcholinesterase, which breaks down acetylcholine

B. Used to treat the following:
  1. Myasthenia gravis
  2. Glaucoma
  3. Postoperative complications of bladder distention or paralytic ileus

C. Major side effects
  1. GI distress, such as nausea, vomiting, diarrhea
  2. Bradycardia, hypotension
  3. Diaphoresis, increased salivation
  4. Muscle cramps, fatigue, weakness, paralysis
  5. Respiratory depression

> ## ⚠ Warnings!
>
> Keep atropine sulfate handy to counteract drug effects in case of an emergency. Edrophonium chloride (Tensilon), which is used as a diagnostic agent for myasthenia gravis, is the antidote for the neuromuscular blocker pancuronium (Pavulon).

D. Nursing implications
  1. Assess neuromuscular status; provide safety measures if side effects occur
  2. Assess respiratory rate, depth, and rhythm; assess for diminished lung sounds
  3. Assess for change in bowel function and elimination pattern; offer antiemetic as needed
  4. Assess VS for changes in HR and BP
  5. Monitor I&O

E. **Common drugs**
1. Edrophonium chloride (Tensilon) for diagnostic testing
2. Neostigmine bromide (Prostigmin) for maintenance
3. Pyridostigmine bromide (Regonol) for maintenance

CHOLINERGIC BLOCKING AGENTS

I. Anticholinergic agents

High + dry likde sympathetic adrenj

A. **Action: compete with acetylcholine at muscarinic receptors**
B. **Uses:**
1. Preoperatively, to reduce salivation and gastric secretions and increase peristalsis during surgery
2. Symptoms of Parkinson's disease
3. Motion sickness
4. GI spasms, urinary spasms
5. Reverse heart blocks
6. Induce dilatation of the eye (mydriasis) and paralyze accommodation (cycloplegia) during eye examinations and surgery (see Chapter 19)
C. **Major side effects**
1. Dry mouth
2. Blurred vision due to dilated pupils
3. Flushed skin color, decreased sweating, intolerance to heat
4. Constipation, urinary retention
5. Confusion, delusional status

⚠ Warnings!

These drug groups interact with CNS depressants, antidysrhythmics, and antihistamines. Carefully monitor elderly patients to prevent *severe* complications from the expected side effects. Use with caution in patients with decreased renal function and avoid in patients with myasthenia gravis.

D. **Nursing implications**
1. Provide comfort measures if side effects occur
2. Encourage the use of ice chips and good oral care to relieve dry mouth
3. Encourage fluid consumption to decrease risk of constipation
4. Direct the patient to use the agent 30 minutes to 1 hour before traveling to relieve motion sickness
5. Monitor vital signs routinely and if side effects occur
E. **Common drugs**
1. Atropine sulfate (Isopto Atropine)
2. Scopolamine hydrobromide (Hyoscine)
3. Hyoscyamine sulfate (Levsin)
4. Propantheline bromide (Pro-Banthine)
5. Benztropine mesylate (Cogentin) for symptoms of Parkinson's disease; to treat extrapyramidal symptoms associated with neuroleptic or antipsychotic drugs
6. Oxybutynin chloride (Ditropan) for bladder spasms

REVIEW QUESTIONS

1. While being admitted to the emergency department for signs of CHF, a patient experiences extreme hypotension, a BP of 78/50 mm Hg. The patient is stabilized on dopamine hydrochloride (Intropin) IV drip. The nurse would assess which of the following items initially?
   1. Glucose level
   2. Heart sounds
   3. Neuromuscular status
   4. Mental status

2. Which one of these drugs is indicated for a patient who is in respiratory distress from an anaphylactic reaction to a first dose of cephalexin (Keflex)?
   1. Atropine sulfate
   2. Albuterol (Ventolin)
   3. Ergotamine tartrate and caffeine (Cafergot)
   4. Epinephrine hydrochloride (Adrenalin)

3. A child, age 5, enters the clinic with wheezing, shortness of breath, and a history of severe asthma. The physician orders epinephrine hydrochloride (Adrenalin) SC stat. After the epinephrine is given, which result should cause concern?
   1. HR of 140, BP 90/50
   2. Severe tremors, HR of 99
   3. HR of 160, BP 130/94
   4. Blood glucose level of 32 mg/dl, severe twitching

4. A child, age 3, was sent home on twice daily albuterol (Ventolin) treatments for severe allergic bronchitis. The mother phones complaining of the child's inability to sleep at night. The mother should be instructed to do what?
   1. Skip the evening treatment unless absolutely necessary
   2. Give the second treatment at noon instead of in the afternoon
   3. Give the second treatment around 4 PM instead of 8 PM
   4. Divide the evening dose; give half at 4 PM and the other half at 8 PM

5. A young adult, age 22, with migraine headaches, should be given which of these instructions for taking ergotamine tartrate (Cafergot)?
   1. Take one tablet when the headache is just beginning and another every 4 hr until the headache is gone
   2. Take one tablet at the first sign of the headache, then every hour until relieved, not to exceed five tablets
   3. Take one tablet at the first sign of the headache, then every hour until relieved, not to exceed 10 tablets
   4. Take one tablet once the headache occurs in full force, then every hour thereafter

6. Important information from a nursing history for the patient taking metoprolol tartrate (Lopressor) would be a history of which of these medical diagnoses?
1. Hypertension
2. Asthma
3. Myasthenia gravis
4. Myocardial infarction

7. Atropine sulfate is more commonly used for which of these side effects?
1. Cardiovascular complications
2. Glaucoma
3. Hypertension
4. Hypersalivation

8. Hyoscyamine sulfate (Levsin) is ordered for a 4-month-old infant who is experiencing extreme episodes of colic during the early morning hours. The infant's parent should be instructed to monitor for which of the following?
1. Diarrhea
2. Constipation
3. Polyuria
4. Hypothermia

ANSWERS, RATIONALES, AND TEST-TAKING TIPS

Rationales	Test-Taking Tips

1. Correct answer: 1

Adrenergic agonists can cause hyperglycemia. These agents cause tachycardia; therefore the vital signs, not the heart sounds, should be monitored. These agents do not affect neuromuscular status. These agents do not directly affect mental status.

Think of what you know from the given information. The patient has a low BP, so common sense dictates to raise it. Natural situations that raise blood pressure are stress situations. Think of what hormones are released during stress and what fuel is needed. One of the catecholamines released during events of stress is epinephrine, which constricts peripheral blood vessels, to raise BP and results in cool appendages. This catecholamine also stimulates the increase of serum glucose levels, which is needed for stressful situations. Since this stressed patient has low BP, he or she has been unable to produce the natural response. Thus, external substances are required, such as dopamine, a catecholamine and the serum glucose levels will most likely rise. A last approach to use, if you have no idea of the correct answer, is to cluster options 2, 3, and 4 under "bedside assessments." Option 1 is a serum test. Select the unique or different option, option 1.

2. Correct answer: 4

Epinephrine, a catecholamine, is used in anaphylactic reactions and shock. It results in overall clinical improvement during an emergency because of the positive inotropic, chronotropic, and dromotropic effects. It is given IV or SC in situations in which the patient is experiencing anaphylactic shock. Atropine, an

Remember that epinephrine is for emergencies. Avoid focusing on the wrong information. It is not important what caused the reaction. The patient is in respiratory distress. Think of the ABCs of resuscitation, even though the patient has not stopped breathing. Epinephrine is the drug of choice in resuscitation.

Rationales	Test-Taking Tips

anticholinergic, increases the heart rate and dilates the pupils. Albuterol (Ventolin, Proventil), a bronchodilator, is used to treat asthma and hypotension. Cafergot, an alpha-andrenergic blocker plus caffeine, is used for vascular headaches, usually migraines. Usually given orally (PO) or by suppository, it modulates the vessel tone to prevent extremes in vasoconstriction and dilatation.

3. Correct answer: 3

Side effects of epinephrine include both hypertension and tachycardia. Epinephrine causes hyperglycemia and, as seen in option 4, a blood glucose level of 32 mg/dl indicates hypoglycemia, which is defined as a serum glucose level of less than 50 mg/dl.

As you read the options, think of the focus of sympathetic response or the actions of epinephrine. Read the options with a vertical technique, which clarifies and helps to eliminate options without your having to read all of the information. Read down: HR 140 beats/min, yes, a concern; tremors, not typical (so eliminate option 2); HR 160 beats/min, yes, a concern; glucose 32 mg/dl, not a concern (so eliminate option 4). Then read the second series down for the options that are left: option 1 is BP of 90/50 mm Hg, of no concern; option 3 is BP of 130/94 mm Hg, yes, a concern—hypertension. The correct option is 3.

4. Correct answer: 3

Taking the drug earlier may decrease the irritability and insomnia and still allow the child to sleep. Option 1, skipping the dose, could cause increased symptoms of bronchitis. Option 2, a dose at noon, would be too soon after a

The clues are the key words in the stem question: the twice daily frequency and the severe allergies. The medication is needed. Thus, eliminate options 1 and 4. Use common sense to choose between options 2 and 3, since 4 PM is later in the day for a second dose than noon. Select option 3.

morning dose and too long before the next morning dose. Giving half the dose could lower the agent's therapeutic bronchodilatory effects.

5. Correct answer: 2

Taking the drug every hour until the headache is relieved should prevent it from developing to maximum severity. The recommended dose should not exceed five tablets per headache episode. Cafergot is to be taken to prevent a full-blown, severe headache. Cafergot taken every 4 hr after an initial dose would have a minimal effect. Ten tablets would exceed the recommended dose for an attack. Cafergot is to be taken before the full attack of a migraine headache. Benefits of the drug cannot be experienced if the patient waits until the headache has reached maximum pain.

The major action in management of migraine headaches is prophylactic rather than therapeutic. Usually, these options are narrowed to either 2 or 3, since they are both the same except for the number of tablets taken. Be conservative and make an educated guess. Select option 2, with the lesser number of tablets. Also note that, in option 4, there is no end point for stopping the medication; this is usually an inappropriate action.

6. Correct answer: 2

Lopressor, a bronchodilator, can cause bronchospasm with the result of respiratory difficulties for a patient with asthma. Option 1, hypertension, would indicate that the medication had a subtherapeutic effect, since Lopressor is used to decrease BP. This is a secondary concern and not the best answer to the question. Beta blockers should not interfere with myasthenia gravis. These agents may be recommended for patients after myocardial infarction and for those with hypertension.

If you have no idea of the correct option, use what you know, go with the ABCs (airway, breathing, circulation), and select option 2. Also, use the great recall tip to remember that with beta blockers "bb" the major complications are "bb": bronchospasm and bradycardia.

Rationales	Test-Taking Tips

7. Correct answer: 4

Atropine has an antisecretory action that decreases salivation, mucosal secretions, and peristalsis of the GI and genitourinary (GU) tracts. This action helps prevent intraoperative complications. Atropine is used preoperatively to limit potential side effects of aspiration during surgery. Atropine is contraindicated in glaucoma because of the effects of the agent: the mydriasis, pupillary dilatation, and cycloplegia (paralysis of the cilary muscle). Atropine increases heart rate but not the blood pressure.

Recall that atropine is an anticholinergic and therefore acts against (anti-) the normal day-to-day processes of the body, which encourage moist mucous membranes, peristalsis, pupillary response to light and visual gaze, and a HR within normal limits of 60 to 100 beats/min. Thus, these specific areas will change after the administration of atropine.

8. Correct answer: 2

Constipation is common with hyoscyamine from the anticholinergic effect. Fluids should be encouraged. Urinary retention, not polyuria, is a side effect of the drug. A late side effect of this drug is intolerance to heat (not hypothermia), since the drug causes flushing of the skin.

Read the options, remembering that colic causes spasms of the GI tract. Treatment would be to decrease the GI spasms or motility. Option 2 is the only answer that suggests a slowing down of motility or peristalsis (the opposite of spasms). Thus, constipation is most likely to occur as a side effect.

5

Drugs Affecting the Neuromuscular System

FAST FACTS

1. Evaluation for the effectiveness of neuromuscular drugs is completed by clinical assessment for changes in the following (listed in order of priority):
   - Respiratory: RR, pattern of respiration
   - LOC: excitement or dullness
   - Cardiac: HR, heart rhythm, and BP
   - Musculoskeletal (MS): extremity strength, skin condition, seizures, movement: tremors, rigidity, flaccidity
   - GI: swallowing, gag reflex, gums, mucous membranes: moist or dry, excessive saliva
   - Laboratory test results: serum creatinine level, complete blood cell (CBC) count, aspartate aminotransferase (AST) and alanine aminotransferase (ALT) levels, blood levels of drugs
2. The elderly, who tend to metabolize anticonvulsant medications more readily, should be carefully monitored for signs of toxicity.
3. Acetazolamide (Diamox) has been used effectively in combination with anticonvulsants for treatment of absence seizures, generalized tonic-clonic seizures, mixed seizures, and myoclonic seizure patterns.
4. As a carbonic anhydrase inhibitor, acetazolamide (Diamox) is thought to increase carbon dioxide that retards neuronal activity.
5. Acetazolamide (Diamox) has other therapeutic classifications: diuretic (of weaker action), antiglaucoma agent (decreases intraocular pressure), and antiepileptic.
6. A ketogenic diet, which consists of high-fat foods, has been used, especially in children, to decrease the amount of anticonvulsant medication needed. The diet is recommended in children who have disabling seizures or side effects

from conventional drug therapy. The diet is thought to mimic the effect of starvation on seizure activity.
7. Newer anticonvulsants are being used as a preventive treatment for migraine headaches.

CONTENT REVIEW

ANTICONVULSANTS

I. Agents used to prevent or treat the severity of epilepsy or other convulsive seizures

II. General information
   A. There is no ideal drug to control seizures; therefore, a trial period of evaluating the effects of a drug is needed
   B. Abrupt withdrawal of these agents may precipitate seizures
   C. Close supervision is needed to monitor the effects and serum levels of the drug
   D. The therapeutic goal is to control the seizure activity without hindering the client's ability to perform normal daily activities
   E. A baseline neurologic assessment should be made by the nurse before beginning the anticonvulsant therapy and then repeated every shift thereafter. More frequent assessments should be made before and during dosage changes.
   F. Several of these drugs are being used for "breakthrough" pain in clients with muscular conditions that cause chronic pain
   G. The most common anticonvulsants used for status epilepticus are diazepam (Valium), fosphenytoin (Cerebyx), and lorazepam (Ativan)
   H. *Fetal antiepileptic drug syndrome* is a side effect of several of the anticonvulsant drugs (phenobarbital {Luminal}, carbamazepine {Tegretol}, and valproate {Depakote}) and should be discussed with women who have seizures and are in the child-bearing years

> ⚠️ **Warning!**
>
> Because of the sedative effect of these agents, safety measures to prevent client injuries should be performed by the nurse and taught to clients. Dosage is highly individualized and commonly requires titration with several adjustments. Many drug interactions may occur when a client takes anticonvulsants and other medications. Clients are to eliminate all use of alcohol, which includes elixirs, mouthwash, and other OTC medications that contain alcohol. Alcohol may cause an additive effect and increase sedation if given with anticonvulsants. Compliance is a major factor for the control of this disease.

III. Hydantoin derivatives

A. **Actions: decrease the focal activity in the CNS, decrease the spread of the seizure process, and decrease abnormal hyperactivity**

B. **Use: first line drug therapy for all types of seizures except absence (petit mal) seizures**

C. **Major side effects: minimal at therapeutic levels. Common effects related to the dose prescribed include the following findings:**
   1. GI: Gingival hyperplasia: overgrowth of the gingival tissue; nausea, vomiting, anorexia
   2. Neurologic: sedation
   3. Dermatologic: hypersensitivity, rash
   4. Hematologic: agranulocytosis, leukopenia, aplastic anemia, thrombocytopenia
   5. Cardiovascular (CV): dysrhythmias and hypotension

   ### ⚠ Warning!

   Interaction may occur with enzyme inhibitors, folic acid, oral contraceptives, and other agents that are highly protein-bound. Withdraw or wean medication over a 1- to 2-week period; if done sooner, may precipitate seizure activity. Phenytoin (Dilantin) has an increased effect in clients with low serum albumin levels.

D. **Nursing implications**
   1. Monitor carefully for maintenance of the therapeutic serum level (10 to 20 μg/ml)
   2. Monitor carefully in pregnant or lactating client; teratogenicity is possible
   3. Give IV drugs slowly because hypotension and dysrhythmias may occur; give only through a saline IV line, at the most proximal port to the insertion site
   4. Do not mix with other agents when given IV; validate a good blood return; extravasation causes tissue death (purple glove syndrome)
   5. Assess oral cavity and degree of gum tenderness; no bleeding should occur
   6. Evaluate for oral intake of foods and fluids; record client's height and weight
   7. Implement and teach safety measures to the family
   8. Dosage is highly individualized and may require titration with several changes

E. **Common drugs**
   1. Phenytoin (Dilantin) is the primary drug within this group
   2. Fosphenytoin (Cerebyx) has fewer problems with IV administration
   3. Mephenytoin (Mesantoin) is less potent and has greater incidences of blood dyscrasias and dermatological side effects

IV. Barbiturates

A. **Action: limit the spread of seizures by increasing the seizure threshold**

B. **Uses**
1. All types of seizures, except absence seizures
2. **Status epilepticus** (newer drugs are used before barbiturates are used; consider barbiturates as secondary drugs)

C. **Major side effects**
1. Neurologic: sedation (most common), decreased LOC, agitation, confusion (especially in older adults)
2. Physical dependence or tolerance
3. Congenital abnormalities to the fetus: fetal antiepileptic drug syndrome
4. Toxicity

⚠ Warning!

Interactions may occur with other CNS depressants (additive effect) and oral contraceptives (decreased effect); avoid alcohol. A slow withdrawal or weaning should be used over a period of 1 to 2 weeks; never abruptly withdraw, as this may precipitate seizure activity.

D. **Nursing implications**
1. Teach the client considering pregnancy about the possibility of the effects to the fetus
2. Have knowledge that a loading dose may be required
3. Monitor for symptoms, since tolerance can develop and the dosage may have to be increased
4. Provide safety measures within an institution, such as bed in low position, side rails up, nightlight turned on, and teach client about these interventions

E. **Common drugs**
1. Phenobarbital sodium (Luminal Sodium)
2. Primidone (Mysoline)
3. Thiopental (Penthothal)
4. Phenobarbital (Luminal, Solfoton)

V. Succinimides

A. **Actions: inhibit spike and wave formation in absence seizures; decrease amplitude, frequency, duration, and spread of discharge in minor motor seizures**

B. **Used primarily for treatment of absence seizures**

C. **Major side effects: mostly GI, including epigastric pain and hiccups**

⚠ Warning!

Interactions: decreased effects of estrogens, oral contraceptives; antagonist effect with tricyclic antidepressants, resulting in unknown effects of both drugs.

D. **Nursing implications**
1. Teach clients to avoid alcohol ingestion and CNS depressants because combinations may result in increased sedation
2. Monitor blood studies: complete blood cell (CBC) count, hepatic and renal studies

E. **Common drugs**
1. Ethosuximide (Zarontin)
2. Methsuximide (Celontin)
3. Phensuximide (Milontin)

VI. Valproates

A. **Actions: similar to succinimides**
B. **Use:**
1. Primarily in absence seizures
2. Prevention of migraine headaches

C. **Major side effects**
1. CNS: tremors, drowsiness, confusion, sedation
2. GI: gastric distress, diarrhea, indigestion
3. Body changes: weight gain
4. Hormonal: irregular menses
5. Hematologic: prolonged bleeding time, thrombocytopenia, leukopenia

⚠ Warning!

Interactions: increased effects with CNS depressants; increased toxicity with salicylates, warfarin, and phenytoin.

D. **Nursing implications**
1. Give elixir alone; separate from other medications and do not dilute
2. Offer with food
3. Teach client that physical dependency may result if used over a long term
4. Monitor blood studies: CBC count, prothrombin time (PT), mean activated partial thromboplastin time (aPTT), and serum creatinine level
5. Teach and institute safety measures

E. **Common drugs**
1. Valproic acid (Depakene)
2. Valproate disodium (Depakote)

VII. Benzodiazepines

A. **Actions: facilitate *gamma-aminobutyric acid (GABA)* and inhibit nerve impulses**
B. **Use: as anticonvulsant especially in the event of status epilepticus (a medical emergency characterized by uninterrupted seizures)**

C. Major side effects
   1. CNS: drowsiness, fatigue, lethargy
   2. IV infiltration

> ⚠️ **Warning!**
>
> Tolerance and addiction are common with these drugs. They should be used as ordered and the amount monitored for frequency of refills, which may indicate that the client is taking more than prescribed. Refills are sometimes limited to 2-week quantities if there is a risk of suicide. Abrupt withdrawal is contraindicated, since there is a risk for precipitation of seizure activity. Advise clients not to take these drugs with alcohol; an additive effect and increased sedation could occur.

D. Nursing implications
   1. Administer IV slowly and in titrated dosages to most proximal site
   2. Drugs may precipitate if mixed with any other agents

E. Common drugs
   1. Diazepam (Valium)
   2. Clonazepam (Klonopin)
   3. Clorazepate (Tranxene)
   4. Lorazepam (Ativan)

VIII. Other anticonvulsants

A. Carbamazepine (Tegretol)
   1. Action: similar to phenytoin (Dilantin); used in cases refractory to first-line drugs because of side effects
   2. Uses: effective in tonic-clonic, simple partial, and complex partial seizures
   3. Major side effects
      a. CNS: vertigo, dizziness, drowsiness
      b. Hematologic: aplastic anemia, agranulocytosis, thrombocytopenia
      c. Skin: photosensitivity
      d. Systemic: toxicity
      e. GI: nausea or vomiting

> ⚠️ **Warning!**
>
> Interactions: decreased effects with phenobarbital, phenytoin; toxicity potential with cimetidine, isoniazid, lithium, erythromycin.

   4. Nursing implications
      a. Monitor CBC, hepatic and renal studies
      b. Instruct client that urine may turn pink or brown

      c. Monitor serum levels of the drug

      d. Implement safety measures and teach client and family to follow safety precautions

      e. Administer with food to decrease GI effects

      f. Teach clients to protect self with clothing when in the sun; sunscreens are ineffective

B. Gabapentin (Neurontin)

  1. Action: GABA neurotransmitter analog. Action is not fully understood. Thought to transport amino acids across neuronal membranes and possibly affect serotonin metabolism (related to phenytoin [Dilantin]).

  2. Uses

      a. Adjunctive therapy for partial seizures with and without secondary generalization

      b. Chronic pain management

  3. Side effects

      a. Neurologic: somnolence, dizziness, ataxia, fatigue, amnesia, nystagmus, and tremor

      b. Eye: diplopia, blurred vision

      c. Weight gain

      d. Mood: depression

      e. CV: hypertension

⚠ Warning!

Clients with reduced renal function (a serum creatinine level of more than 1.2 mg/dl) may require smaller doses because the drug is excreted unchanged in the urine. Should not be administered at the same time as an antacid.

  4. Nursing implications

      a. Monitor and teach about safety risks, especially to avoid driving

      b. Monitor VS, especially BP, and use cautiously in clients with cardiac disease

      c. Assess baseline renal function

ANTIPARKINSONISM DRUGS

  I. Parkinson's disease: a slowly progressive, degenerative, neurologic disorder characterized by nonintentional tremors, shuffling gait, masklike facial expression, muscle rigidity, and weakness

  II. Goal of these agents: to relieve the symptoms of the disease and to aid the client in carrying out normal daily activities. These agents do not cure; they only treat the symptoms.

III. Actions

A. Increase the dopaminergic system in three ways
   1. By increasing the release of dopamine in the brain
   2. By stimulating the dopamine receptor sites
   3. By enhancing conversion of levodopa (L-dopa) (Larodopa) to dopamine in the brain

B. Inhibit specific enzymes that interfere with dopamine. Monoamine oxidase B degrades dopamine in the brain and catechol *O*-methyltransferase (COMT) inactivates catecholamines, including dopamine.

C. Decrease the cholinergic system by blocking the acetylcholine receptors in the brain (anticholinergic agents). This action lessens the symptoms of the disease.

IV. Uses: decrease the rigidity, spasms, and tremors associated with Parkinson's disease. *These agents also control extrapyramidal effects caused by antipsychotic agents.*

V. Major side effects: *drug* effects are *dose-dependent*

A. GI: nausea, vomiting, anorexia, aversion to certain foods

B. CV: dysrhythmias, orthostatic hypotension

C. *Extrapyramidal effects:* tremors; tardive dyskinesia (rhythmic movements of the face manifested by active tongue movement, rocking, chewing, grimacing); dystonia (impaired muscle tone); and akathisia (pathologic condition consisting of restlessness, agitation, inability to sit still)

D. Behavioral symptoms: nervousness, agitation, anxiety

⚠ Warning!

Interactions: pyridoxine hydrochloride (hexa-Betalin) or vitamin B_6 can reverse or inhibit the effectiveness of levodopa.

VI. Nursing implications

A. Instruct the client to rise slowly if orthostatic hypotension occurs

B. Administer the medicine with food if GI symptoms occur

C. Assess the client's ability to carry out activities of daily living (ADLs)

D. Monitor for the following:
   1. *On-off phenomenon:* alteration in the control of symptoms from day to day or within each day
   2. *End-of-dose deterioration:* return of symptoms before the next dose

VII. Common drugs

    A. Dopaminergic agents: levodopa (L-dopa is the precursor of dopamine, which enters the brain). The problem with levodopa is that a majority of it is converted to dopamine in the periphery, so it cannot cross the blood-brain barrier. Carbidopa blocks the peripheral conversion of levodopa to dopamine and allows for more of the drug to enter the brain before it is converted to dopamine.

        1. Levodopa or L-dopa (Larodopa)

        2. Carbidopa-levodopa (Sinemet)

        3. Carbidopa (Lodosyn)

    B. Dopamine receptor agonists

        1. Amantadine hydrochloride (Symmetrel)

        2. Bromocriptine mesylate (Parlodel)

        3. Pergolide (Permax)

    C. Anticholinergic drugs (given to maximize side effects of the antipsychotics)

        1. Benztropine (Cogentin)

        2. Diphenhydramine (Benadryl)

        3. Trihexyphenidyl (Artane)

    D. Enzyme inhibitors

        1. Selegiline hydrochloride (L-Deprenyl), a monoamine oxidase (MAO) type B inhibitor

        2. Tolcapone (Tasmar), a COMT inhibitor

ANTIMYASTHENIC AGENTS

    I. Myasthenia gravis is an abnormal condition characterized by the chronic fatigue and weakness of voluntary muscles. The goal of therapy for clients with myasthenia gravis is to maintain a normal lifestyle. Drugs do not cure the disease.

    II. Action: these agents prevent the breakdown of acetylcholine at the neuromuscular junction, so that receptors are activated and the effects of the acetylcholine are prolonged; this improves the symptoms of the disease (Figure 5-1)

    III. Uses: to treat myasthenia gravis and to reverse the effects of neuromuscular blocking agents

    IV. Major side effects

    A. Muscle weakness, cramping, contractions

    B. Parasympathetic stimulation: excessive salivation, nausea, vomiting, sweating, bronchospasm

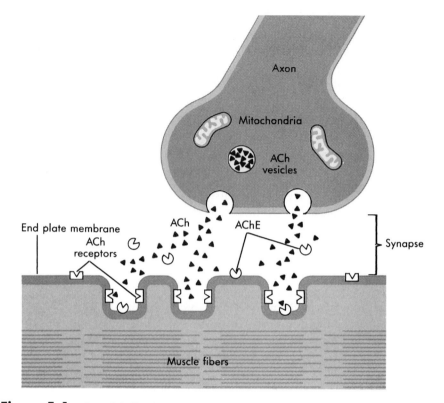

Figure 5-1   Acetylcholine is the neurotransmitter released by the nerve to occupy nicotinic receptors on the muscle, and thereby initiates biochemical events causing the muscle to contract. Acetylcholine is rapidly degraded by acetylcholinesterase, present throughout the synapse. In clients with myasthenia gravis, the number of receptors is greatly decreased. Acetylcholinesterase inhibitors prevent rapid breakdown of acetylcholine. With more acetylcholine present, fewer receptors are needed and loss of receptors is partially compensated. (From Clark JB, Queener SF, Karb VB: *Pharmacologic basis of nursing practice,* ed 6, St. Louis, 2000, Mosby.)

C. **Cholinergic crisis: a pronounced muscular weakness and respiratory paralysis caused by excessive acetylcholine or an overdose with anticholinesterase drugs, manifested by increased weakness, increased salivation, dyspnea, bradycardia, increased secretions, nausea, and vomiting**

D. **Myasthenic crisis: the sudden return of the original clinical findings after an insufficient (smaller) dose of the medicine**

⚠ Warning!

Interactions may occur when taken concurrently with other drugs having anticholinergic properties, resulting in increased side effects. Atropine sulfate is the antidote for these drugs. Periods of stress and infection may require an increased dose.

V. Nursing implications

A. Initiate a baseline neuromuscular assessment

B. Doses are highly individualized, because an insufficient dose can result in myasthenic crisis and an overdose may result in cholinergic crisis

C. Monitor for signs of lessening ptosis, increased ability to swallow, and increased muscle strength for evaluation of the drug's effectiveness

D. Teach the client the signs and symptoms of cholinergic crisis and to report them to physician immediately

E. Administer with food to decrease the GI side effects; administer 30 to 60 min before a meal to increase strength for chewing and swallowing

VI. Common drugs: acetylcholinesterase inhibitors are the drugs of choice for this disease

A. Ambenonium (Mytelase)

B. Pyridostigmine bromide (Mestinon)

C. Neostigmine methylsulfate (Prostigmin)

D. Edrophonium chloride (Tensilon) is used more in the initial diagnostic process and to differentiate between myasthenia crisis and cholinergic crises; it has a short duration of action. Tip: Edrophonium chloride (*T*ensilon) is the *T*est drug to *T*ell of or validate this diagnosis.

NEUROMUSCULAR BLOCKING AGENTS

I. Divided into two groups

A. Nondepolarizing agents

B. Depolarizing agents

II. General information about the classification

A. These drugs act to relax the skeletal muscles by disrupting the transmission of nerve impulses

B. These drugs do not cross the blood-brain barrier; therefore, the client remains conscious and aware of pain. The addition of narcotic analgesics or sedatives is required.

C. Three clinical indications for these drugs

1. Relaxation of smooth muscles during surgery

2. Decreasing the intensity of muscle spasms in drug-induced or electrically induced convulsions

3. Management of clients who need controlled mechanical ventilation

III. Nondepolarizing agents

A. **Actions: compete with acetylcholine for the receptor sites on the motor end plate or by blocking depolarization. Client remains conscious and experiences pain.**

B. **Uses**
   1. Facilitation of endotracheal intubation
   2. Decrease the amount of anesthetic used during surgery
   3. Relaxation of skeletal muscles of intubated clients on mechanical assistance to allow for total control of breathing

C. **Major side effects**
   1. CV: hypotension, tachycardia, dysrhythmias
   2. Respiratory: apnea, depression, bronchospasm, excess bronchial secretions
   3. Complications of paralysis

> ⚠ **Warning!**
>
> Antibiotics intensify the effect of the neuromuscular blocking agents. Some antidysrhythmic agents may potentiate the effects of these drugs. Administration of pain medication is essential with these drugs. Keep the antidotes (anticholinesterase drugs) available: usually edrophonium chloride (Tensilon) is given. These drugs do not cross the blood-brain barrier; therefore, the client remains conscious and aware of pain. The addition of narcotic analgesics or sedatives is required.

D. **Nursing implications**
   1. Implement and teach safety measures; eyes may need artificial tears and be patched during paralysis
   2. Use suction and intubation equipment as needed
   3. Offer pain medications if indicated
   4. Assess for signs of respiratory depression, if client is not ventilated
   5. Maintain a calm environment
   6. Monitor vital signs carefully
   7. If patient is on a ventilator, bring client out of paralysis once per shift to complete a neurologic check

E. **Common drugs**
   1. Pancuronium bromide (Pavulon)
   2. Gallamine triethiodide (Flaxedil)
   3. Pipecuronium bromide (Arduan)
   4. Vecuronium (Norcuron)

IV. Depolarizing agents

A. **Action: these agents mimic the action of acetylcholine and cause depolarization of the muscle fiber, which makes the muscle incapable of becoming stimulated by another impulse. These agents are not destroyed by cholinesterase and therefore have a prolonged action.**

B. **Uses**
   1. Short-term relaxation needed in orthopedic procedures
   2. Intubation
   3. Endoscopy
   4. Preanesthetic

C. **Major side effects**
   1. Hypertension
   2. Increased intraocular pressure
   3. Muscle pain

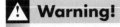 **Warning!**

Interactions: same as for nondepolarizing agents.

D. **Nursing implications: same as for nondepolarizing agents**
E. **Common drug: succinylcholine chloride (Anectine)**

WEB Resources

http://www.stanford.edu/group/ketodiet/
   Information about the ketogenic diet.

http://137.172.248.46/treatmen.htm
   Information on anticonvulsants.

http://pages.prodigy.net/stanley.way/myasthenia/causes.htm
   Information on treatment of myasthenia gravis.

REVIEW QUESTIONS

1. Nursing implications for care of the client who is taking an anticonvulsant medication include which of the the following items?
   1. A neurologic assessment is essential after the drug regimen begins
   2. Administration of the medicine around the clock may decrease sedation
   3. If toxicity occurs, the drug is abruptly discontinued
   4. Stress to the client that compliance is essential

2. A client with status epilepticus might be given which of these medications?
   1. Oxazolidones
   2. Iminostilbenes
   3. Valproates
   4. Benzodiazepines

3. A client is admitted to the hospital for the control of seizures. The physician prescribes a hydantoin derivative: phenytoin (Dilantin). This class of agents helps to treat seizures by which action?
   1. Limiting the spread of the seizure
   2. Facilitating GABA to inhibit nerve impulses
   3. Decreasing the focal activity in the CNS
   4. Inhibiting nerve impulses

4. While taking phenytoin (Dilantin), a female client should be advised to do which of these actions?
   1. Use alcohol conservatively
   2. Report for blood monitoring as ordered to avoid toxicity
   3. Continue to take oral contraceptives as ordered
   4. Hold one dose if the drug is too sedating

5. Which possible adverse reaction to phenytoin (Dilantin) should be reported to the physician?
   1. Cavities
   2. Hypertension
   3. Agitation, confusion
   4. Bleeding of gums

6. The drugs of choice in the treatment of Parkinson's disease are those that have which action?
   1. Block acetylcholine receptors in the brain
   2. Decrease dopamine
   3. Increase dopamine
   4. Increase cholinergic activity

7. The antiparkinsonism drug levodopa (L-dopa) has many side effects. The combination of levodopa and carbidopa (Sinemet) may work better because of which fact?
   1. The latter blocks all side effects of levodopa
   2. The levodopa is converted to dopamine more quickly after absorption
   3. The carbidopa blocks the conversion of the levodopa to dopamine before its entry into the brain
   4. The anticholinergic effects block the symptoms of the disease

8. A client is on an antiparkinsonism drug. The client receives the dose as scheduled (9:00 AM, 1:00 PM, 5:00 PM). The nurse notices that from 9:00 AM to 12:00 noon the client seems calm, is without tremors, and walks normally. Between 12:30 PM and 4:30 PM the symptoms worsen. The nurse should suspect which problem?
   1. End-of-dose deterioration
   2. On-off phenomenon
   3. Extrapyramidal effects
   4. Dawn phenomenon

9. Antimyasthenic agents exert their effects to diminish the findings of myasthenia gravis by which action?
   1. Deactivating receptors at the neuromuscular junction
   2. Decreasing the excitatory effects of the cholinergic system
   3. Inhibiting the breakdown of acetylcholine at the neuromuscular junction
   4. Increasing the destruction of acetylcholine

10. A client diagnosed with myasthenia gravis is placed on pyridostigmine bromide (Mestinon). The client calls the office and complains of severe diarrhea, drooling, and intestinal cramping. What is the best advice for this patient?
   1. Avoid the next dose and see the doctor tomorrow
   2. Report to the emergency room at once for treatment
   3. Increase the next dose and report back to the physician
   4. Come in to the office for an examination and perhaps an IV edrophonium chloride test

11. Which of these actions is appropriate for a client on a nondepolarizing blocking agent?
   1. Monitor VS once per shift
   2. Assess for the need to suction the client and for indications of pain
   3. Instruct the client to walk at least twice per shift unless contraindicated by the physician
   4. Allow frequent visitors to interact with the client during the therapy to make the time go faster

ANSWERS, RATIONALES, AND TEST-TAKING TIPS

Rationales	Test-Taking Tips

1. Correct answer: 4

Compliance is a major teaching topic for clients who are on these drugs for seizure control. A baseline neurologic assessment should be done before administering the agent, then used for comparison purposes later during the therapy or for complications of the therapy. Sedation is a major side effect. A bedtime (hs) dose is best for the elimination of the sedation effect. Abrupt discontinuation could cause the seizures to return. If toxicity occurs the dosage is usually decreased.

Clues in the form of key words in each option help you eliminate it as a choice. In option 1, the key word is "after;" in option 2, "decrease"; and in option 3, "abruptly."

2. Correct answer: 4

Diazepam (Valium), a benzodiazepine, is the drug of choice because of its effectiveness. Other drugs within this class can be used. Lorazepam (Ativan), an anticonvulsant agent, is also a drug of choice, since it has a longer duration with less respiratory depression for status epilepticus. A third drug for status epilepticus is fosphenytoin (Cerebyx), which causes fewer problems when administered IV. Barbiturates are used as second-line drugs for status epilepticus. Oxazolidones, which are extremely toxic, are rarely used for absence seizures and not used for status epilepticus. Iminostilbenes, such as

Go with what you know. If you cannot recall what the classifications of options 1, 2, and 3 are and you identified the classification in option 4, then select that with which you are familiar. Focus on facts you know!

carbamazepine (Tegretol), are used for cases refractory to phenytoin. Valproates are used in absence seizures.

3. Correct answer: 3

The action of hydantoin derivatives decreases the spread of the seizure by a decrease in abnormal hyperactivity. This action in option 1, to limit the spread of the seizure, is the action of barbiturates. Options 2 and 4 are the actions of benzodiazepines.

Go with what you know plus use common sense to match the need to "control" the seizure by "a decrease" in activity of the CNS. "Limit the spread" in option 1 would not control seizures. Avoid the selection of option 2 when you do not recall to what it pertains.

4. Correct answer: 2

Maintenance of a therapeutic level is absolutely necessary to control seizures. Alcohol should never be taken by a client while on an anticonvulsant drug because of the additive effect. Interactions can occur with this drug and oral contraceptives to decrease the effectiveness of the contraceptive. The client should have the physician reevaluate the dose of the oral contraceptive being taken or use other protective measures. The excess sedation should be reported to the physician. A client should never skip a dose without notification of the physician first.

When questions mention a specific drug, recall the classification for that drug. This action helps to stimulate your thinking skills so you can read the options in a more global sense of the classification. This drug is an anticonvulsant. Then, as you read the options add an additional step. Use a "true or false" approach as you read and think of the classifications. On the initial read, options 1 and 4 can be eliminated since alcohol is usually prohibited and doses are not to be skipped. Of the two options left, 2 and 3, go with what you know to select option 2, since monitoring serum levels may help avoid toxicity of any drug. Do not select option 3 if you are unsure of the connection between anticonvulsants and oral contraceptives.

5. Correct answer: 4

Bleeding gums require further evaluation in any event. Gingival hyperplasia, a side effect of phenytoin, can cause

Use the ABCs if you have no idea of a correct answer. Select option 4, which deals with circulation. You could also give a system to each

Rationales	Test-Taking Tips

overgrowth with softening and severe tenderness of the gums. Cavities are not a side effect of this medication. Hypotension, not hypertension, is a common side effect. Sedation, not agitation or confusion, is a common side effect.

option to help you select the correct answer. Option 1 is teeth, option 2 is cardiovascular, option 3 is mental status, and option 4 is circulation or bleeding. With these themes, it is evident that bleeding has precedence.

6. Correct answer: 3

An increase in the dopamine should decrease the symptoms of Parkinson's disease. Option 1 is the action of anticholinergic agents, which can be used but are not the drugs of choice. The dopaminergic system is already decreased in this disease. An increase in cholinergic activity will increase the symptoms of the disease.

A way to remember Parkinson's is to stutter "pddddddd." Parkinson's **d**isease is a **d**eficiency in **d**opamine with results of **d**ifferent mannerisms which make clients look **d**opey for which **d**rugs that increase **d**opamine are given to **d**iminish the findings.

7. Correct answer: 3

Because the brain normally blocks the entry of dopamine, conversion of levodopa within the brain into dopamine boosts the dopaminergic system. This is what happens with the use of levodopa and carbidopa (Sinemet). This combination increases the effectiveness but does not block all side effects of levodopa. With L-dopa (levodopa) by itself, the dopamine is mostly converted in the periphery. Then this dopamine does not cross the blood-brain barrier. Clients who use levodopa with carbidopa do not exhibit anticholinergic effects.

A common sense approach here helps you to make the correct option selection. Reread the question with each option. The one that makes most sense is option 3. If conversion of levadopa to dopamine occurs in the brain because of carbidopa, common sense and logical thinking tell you that the drug will have a better effect.

8. Correct answer: 2

The control of the symptoms fluctuates with the on-off phenomenon, despite repeat dosing. End-of-dose deterioration would manifest a return of symptoms *before each dose.* Extrapyramidal effects may be manifested with a return of symptoms but would not occur for only a short time period. The dawn phenomenon occurs with antidiabetic agents. Dawn phenomena in type 1 diabetics may require an increased insulin dose in the early morning hours because of an increase in serum glucose level, which is treated with extra insulin. In contrast, the Somogyi phenomenon is a rebound effect where too much insulin the evening before induces hypoglycemia around 2:00 AM to 3:00 AM, with results that the body breaks down glucose stores to increase serum glucose in response to the hypoglycemia. In doing so, it overshoots the actual need, so that by 6 AM the fasting glucose level is elevated.

The clue in the stem is the time. The important issue to contrast is the administration time of the medication in relation to the clinical findings. If the client had end-of-dose deterioration, the findings would occur mainly between the hours of 8 AM to 9 AM, 12 noon to 1:00 PM and 4:00 PM to 5:00 PM, not just from 12:30 PM to 4:30 PM.

9. Correct answer: 3

The action of these agents prolongs the effects of the acetylcholine, which diminishes the symptoms of the disease. The action of these agents involves the activation of the receptors at the neuromuscular junction and slows the destruction of acetylcholine. The action in option 2 describes antiparkinson drugs. Options 1 and 4 are false statements.

When you are tired and having difficulty in focusing and recalling information about the situation in the question, look at your options and do the cluster approach. Look for a theme of three of them as you reread them. In this situation "negative actions" is the theme for options 1, 2, and 4: deactivate, decrease, and destruction increased. Option 3 is more neutral. Select the odd option, which is 3. Common

Rationales	Test-Taking Tips

themes other than negative—positive, are internal—external, active—passive, nurse-focused–client-centered, assessment—intervention, and physical—psychosocial. Another recall tip is that the neuromuscular junction is also spoken of as the myoneural junction. Acetylcholine is needed for **a**ction of voluntary muscles at the **m**yoneural junction in **m**yasthenia gravis. Think **aa-mm.**

10. Correct answer: 4

The side effects could be from the dosage quantity. A visit to the physician is necessary for an adjustment in the amount of the medication. These are signs of major side effects of the medication, with a risk for cholinergic crisis. Cholinergic crisis occurs when the dosage is being initiated or increased to establish the correct dose for the patient: a larger dose is given than is needed. Cholinergic crisis is a pronounced muscle weakness and respiratory paralysis. In contrast, myasthenic crisis is the sudden return of the original clinical findings from an insufficient dose of the medication: a smaller dose is given than is needed. The medication should not be withheld without discussion with the physician. These symptoms do not warrant a diagnosis of cholinergic crisis but do need to be reported. Doses should not be changed unless recommended by the physician.

Eliminate options 1 and 3, since they break the basic rules of medication administration. Since the findings do not include any threat to the ABCs, no need exists for the client to go to the emergency department. The reasonable action is to advise as described in option 4. Recall that the tip for other initial findings of cholinergic crisis is to think of an overstimulation of the cholinergic or common functions of the body on a day-to-day basis. These common functions include salivation, modulation of the heart to keep the rate slow, and peristalsis. When these are overstimulated, you get increased salivation, secretions, peristalsis, intestinal cramps, bradycardia, nausea, and vomiting.

11. Correct answer: 2

These agents are given during surgery or to allow for total control of breathing while clients are on ventilators. The agents relax the skeletal muscles, yet do not interfere with the level of consciousness or affect perception of pain. Therefore, pain medication should be offered or routinely given along with these nondepolarizing blocking agents. A side effect is excess bronchial secretions, for which suctioning may be needed. Vital signs should be monitored more frequently, at least every 30 min. Bed rest is enforced, with the bed in low position and the side rails raised, while the client is under the influence of these agents. A calm environment with minimal visitors helps the client relax and may possibly lessen pain.

Recall that nondepolarizing blocking agents are neuromuscular paralyzers. Common ones are pancuronium bromide, gallamine triethiodide, pipecuronium bromide, and vecuronium. Thus these clients are unable to move voluntary and involuntary muscles. Therefore, in addition to airway maintenance and pain concerns, the eyes need protection, since blinking is absent. Given this information, the most reasonable answer is 2.

6

Drugs Affecting the Central Nervous System

FAST FACTS

1. Evaluation of the effectiveness of these drugs is completed by clinical assessment for changes in the following (listed in order of priority):
   - RR and pattern of respiration
   - LOC: excitement or dullness
   - HR, rhythm, and BP: increase or decrease, irregular or regular
   - MS: extremity strength, seizures, skin rash, extrapyramidal effects, which include tremors, tardive dyskinesia, dystonia, akathisia, rigidity
   - GI: swallowing, gag reflex, bowel sounds (increase or decrease)
   - Laboratory test results: serum creatinine level; CBC count; AST, ALT, sodium, and drug levels
2. Diazepam (Valium) cannot be mixed with any other drug or fluid. If given IV push, flush the line with NS before and after administration.
3. Hydroxyzine hydrochloride (Vistaril) requires Z-track administration, because it is an irritating drug.
4. The role of the nurse is not to administer anesthetic agents, but rather to know the nursing implications based on the effects of different anesthetic agents.
5. With mood stabilizers, side effects can occur at doses within the therapeutic serum level range.

CONTENT REVIEW

I. Preanesthetics
   #### A. Action: varies according to the classification

   B. Uses
1. Induce sedation and decrease anxiety
2. Decrease the risk of bradycardia
3. Allow for a smoother induction of anesthesia

   C. Nursing implications
1. Recognize that these are often given IM or IV
2. Know that usually a mix of two or more of these drugs produces the desired effect
3. Be aware that they may be ordered the night before or 30 to 60 minutes before the surgery
4. Use the Z-track method if medication is oil-based or is an irritating substance, and chart this technique, if applicable. Remember: Hydroxyzine hydrochloride (Vistaril) must be given Z-track.
5. Double-check the dosage, especially if given in a rushed situation
6. Know which drugs can be mixed together. Remember: Diazepam (Valium) cannot be mixed with other medications.
7. Check the client's drug allergies *before preparation* of medication
8. Verify the correct client by a check of the armband, and ask client to state his or her name
9. Know the correct time to administer the injection; secure the medicine and prepare the equipment ahead of time if possible. Many of these medications may be scheduled drugs and require signing out on a narcotic record.
10. Practice safety precautions, encourage client to void before medication administration. When medication is administered: place bed in low position, side rails up, and call light within reach. Give instructions to the client not to get up without assistance.

   D. Common drugs within each classification
1. Narcotics: morphine sulfate, meperidine (Demerol)
2. Anticholinergics: atropine sulfate
3. Neuromuscular blocking agents: succinylcholine chloride (Anectine), pancuronium bromide (Pavulon)
4. Antiemetics: promethazine (Phenergan), droperidol (Inapsine)
5. Antianxiety agents: diazepam (Valium)
6. Barbiturates: pentobarbital (Nembutal), secobarbital (Seconal)
7. Anticholinergics: glycopyrrolate (Robinol), atropine, scopolamine

II. Anesthetics

   A. Anesthesia is the loss of sensation as a result of reversible CNS depression

   B. Two basic categories
1. General anesthesia: loss of consciousness and loss of sensation
    a. Inhalation route
      (1) Gases
      (2) Volatile liquids
    b. Intravenous route

2. Local anesthesia: loss of sensation, particularly the inability to detect pain in a selected area
C. **Balanced anesthesia results from the selection of a combination of drugs to produce the desired effect for the type of surgery scheduled. This is required because there is no ideal anesthetic agent.**
D. **The role of the nurse is not to administer the agents but to know the nursing implications based on the effects of the agent used**

GENERAL ANESTHESIA

I. Three phases of anesthesia
A. Induction: a large amount of anesthetic agent is administered
B. Maintenance: the desired level is maintained
C. Recovery: the anesthetic agent is no longer administered, and its effects may be reversed

II. Anesthesia requires that critical concentration levels occur in the brain; the degree of effectiveness is dose-dependent

III. Anesthetic agents are administered until the client reaches the stage when loss of consciousness occurs and surgery may be performed
A. Clients are monitored by assessing respiration, pulse, blood pressure, pupil response, reflexes, and eye movement for maintenance levels during these stages
B. Diseases such as chronic airway limitation (chronic obstructive pulmonary disease [COPD], emphysema), and congestive heart failure (CHF) can increase or decrease the absorption of these agents

IV. Inhalation anesthetics
A. Actions: depression of the CNS, interference with nerve impulses, and relaxation of skeletal and smooth muscles. The exact mechanism of action is unknown.
B. Uses: rapid control and depth of anesthesia
C. Administered by semiclosed or closed method
D. Major side effects
   1. Cardiovascular depression: bradycardia, hypotension, dysrhythmias
   2. Respiratory depression: bradypnea, apnea, decreased oxygen saturation
   3. GI: nausea, vomiting
   4. Hypothermia
   5. CNS: confusion
   6. Shivering (from heat loss and the recovery of neurologic function)
   7. Toxicity: nephrotoxicity and hepatotoxicity

8. Malignant hyperthermia (a rare toxic reaction to inhaled anesthetics) manifests as tachycardia, hypertension, acidosis, hyperkalemia, muscle rigidity, and hyperthermia

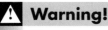 **Warning!**

These drugs are CNS depressants, except for nitrous oxide.

E. **Nursing implications**
   1. Encourage/evaluate turning, coughing, deep breathing, and the client's use of incentive spirometer to prevent hypostatic pneumonia after surgery
   2. Obtain a thorough nursing history before the surgery; note in particular any allergies or previous problems with anesthesia

⚠ Warning!

Diseases such as chronic airway limitation (COPD, emphysema), asthma, or CHF may increase or decrease the absorption

   3. Assess the client's neurologic status postoperatively and cautiously administer analgesics
   4. Practice and stress safety measures with the client, because psychomotor function is impaired. Set bed in low position; raise side rails; assist with ambulation; and place the call light within reach.
   5. Monitor VS; administer oxygen if indicated
   6. Assess for problems with elimination; client may have urinary retention as a result of preoperative or intraoperative medication
F. **Common anesthetic gases**
   1. Nitrous oxide (most common; weak gas and usually combined with other agents)
   2. Halothane (Fluothane): the prototype; often used for pediatric clients
   3. Enflurane (Enthrane): used for adults but not for children
   4. Methoxyflurane (Penthrane)
   5. Isoflurane (Forane): commonly used

V. Intravenous (IV) anesthetics
A. **Action: based on the individual agent group used**
B. **Uses**
   1. Before administration of inhalation agents
   2. Conscious sedation
      a. Diagnostic procedures
      b. Outpatient surgeries
   3. Reduce motor activity and anxiety and may cause an indifference to surroundings
C. **Major side effects**
   1. "Hangover" effect
   2. Apnea, laryngospasm, bronchospasm, coughing
   3. Depression of the cardiovascular system; however, this side effect occurs less with IV anesthetics than with inhalation agents

Warning!

Evaluate immediate effects on the pulmonary and CV systems.

D. Nursing implications

1. Have emergency equipment ready, IV fluids handy
2. Know each individual drug, since the classification varies
3. Practice and stress safety measures. Set bed in low position; raise side rails; assist with ambulation; and place the call light within reach.
4. Monitor vital signs, especially for respiratory depression
5. Monitor elimination status; in the first 24 hours, focus on urinary elimination; afterwards, monitor bowel movements
6. Administer cautiously any analgesics for pain in the recovery period while client is in the postanesthetic care unit

E. Common drugs within each classification

1. Neuroleptics: droperidol (Inapsine), fentanyl with droperidol (Innovar)
2. Opoid narcotics: fentanyl citrate (Sublimaze)
3. Barbiturates: thiopental sodium (Pentothal); methohexital (Brevital)
4. Benzodiazepines and related drugs, diazepam (Valium) or midazolam hydrochloride (Versed), are used more in outpatient surgery units
5. Sedative-hypnotic: propofol (Diprivan) (used for controlled mechanical ventilation), etomidate (Amidate)
6. Other: ketamine (Ketalar) is known as a dissociative anesthetic, an anesthesia characterized by analgesia and amnesia without loss of respiratory function or pharyngeal and laryngeal reflexes

LOCAL ANESTHESIA

I. General information

A. These drugs are given to affect either a small area of the body, such as a digit, or a larger area, such as an entire extremity. They may be applied topically, especially before peripheral IV insertion.

B. Methods of administration

1. Topical or surface: application of a topical anesthetic in the form of a solution, gel, spray, or ointment to the skin, mucous membrane, or cornea
2. Injection methods are as follows:
   a. Infiltration: the process whereby a local anesthetic is administered through the tissue. A field block produces anesthesia around the entire lesion or incision and is used in emergency rooms to repair lacerations.
   b. Regional: anesthesia of an area of the body by injection of a local anesthetic to block a group of sensory nerve fibers

    c. Spinal: injection of an analgesic or anesthetic drug into the subarachnoid space of the spinal column to achieve an insensitivity to pain in the lower part of the body

    d. Epidural: injection into the epidural space of the spinal cord

    e. Nerve block: injection of a local anesthetic along a nerve before it reaches the surgical site.

> ⚠️ **Warning!**
>
> These drugs may be combined with epinephrine hydrochloride (Adrenalin) to slow drug absorption, prolong the effect of the anesthetic, and reduce bleeding at site. Caution should be taken in clients with CV compromise.

II. Action: these agents block nerve impulses and decrease the ability of the cell to depolarize, which is necessary for impulse transmission

III. Uses

    A. Minor surgery

    B. Diagnostic procedures

    C. Minor treatments

    D. Toothaches

    E. Delivery

IV. Side effects

    A. Toxicity

    B. Interference with the organ involved

    C. Reversal of the block

    D. CV: bradycardia, hypotension, respiratory failure

    E. Frostbite with the topicals

    F. Skin irritation

> ⚠️ **Warning!**
>
> Many of these agents, if absorbed systemically, are cardiac depressants or CNS stimulants. Monitor closely. Protect the anesthetized area from trauma, since **motor function returns before sensory function.**

V. Nursing implications

    A. Monitor VS

    B. Use safety measures. Set bed in low position; raise side rails; assist with ambulation; and place the call light within reach.

    C. Properly position the extremity (regional) or body (spinal)

    D. Monitor the area anesthetized for return of motor function, sensation, and skin condition

    E. Caution clients to avoid eating if the throat is involved

VI. Common drugs
A. **Esters**
    1. Procaine (Novocain)
    2. Tetracaine (Pontocaine)
    3. Cocaine hydrochloride (Procaine)
B. **Amides**
    1. Lidocaine (Xylocaine)
    2. Prilocaine (Citanest)
    3. Mepivacaine (Polocaine)

CNS STIMULANTS

I. General information
A. **CNS stimulant: a substance that quickens the activity of the CNS by increasing the rate of neuronal discharge or by blocking an inhibitory neurotransmitter**
B. **Many drugs can stimulate, although few do so therapeutically. Therapeutic CNS stimulation involves the following:**
    1. Restoring mental alertness or consciousness
    2. Stimulating the respiratory center, or overcoming respiratory depression
    3. Treating hyperkinetic children by acting as a depressant in a child
C. **Classification of agents that stimulate therapeutically**
    1. **Amphetamines**
    2. **Anorexiants**
    3. **Analeptics**

 Warning!

Most of these agents are controlled (and highly abused) substances. Some agents are used to treat hyperkinetic children; these drugs have a reversed action as a depressant rather than a stimulant in children.

II. Amphetamines and amphetamine-like drugs
A. **Action: stimulate the release of norepinephrine, which causes increased alertness, less fatigue, and elevated mood**
B. **Uses**
    1. Narcolepsy: syndrome characterized by sudden sleep attacks. Stimulation of the CNS can alleviate these attacks and produce alertness.
    2. Endogenous obesity: obesity resulting from dysfunction of the endocrine or metabolic systems. Amphetamines suppress the appetite.
    3. Attention deficit hyperactivity disorder (ADHD): childhood condition involving inattention, impulsivity, and hyperactivity. Amphetamines increase attention span while decreasing the hyperactivity.

    4. Mental depression: amphetamines elevate mood, increase motor activity, and promote self-confidence

    5. Withdrawal syndromes: physical reactions after cessation or severe reduction in intake of a substance that has been used regularly to induce euphoria, intoxication, or relief from pain or distress. Amphetamines can enhance the effects of some narcotics and reduce the symptoms of withdrawal from abusive agents by their action to increase alertness, decrease fatigue, and elevate mood.

C. Major side effects

    1. Tolerance, dependence, abuse

    2. Tachyphylaxis: repeated administration of some drugs results in a marked decrease in effectiveness

    3. CNS: nervousness, irritability, increased motor activity

    4. Headaches, dizziness, insomnia

    5. CV: hypertension, palpitations, dysrhythmias

    6. Weight loss and fatigue from prolonged use

⚠ Warning!

Interactions may occur with antidepressants, which increase the effect of the amphetamine, and with urine alkalinizers, which increase the already lengthy half-life of these drugs. Contraindicated in epilepsy, many cardiac disorders, and thyroid diseases.

D. Nursing implications

    1. Support a weight-reduction diet and exercise program to accompany the use of these agents for obesity. Short-term use is recommended; usually less than a year.

    2. Teach the child and parents about the use of the drug for ADHD. Teach the following guidelines:

        a. Check with a pharmacist about all OTC medications

        b. Do not abruptly stop taking the drug

        c. Do not try to make up doses if one is skipped; call physician for instructions immediately if dose is skipped

        d. If the client is diabetic, check whether insulin or oral hypoglycemic requirements may be reduced or adjusted

    3. Avoid other stimulants while on these drugs

    4. Avoid taking the last dose after 6:00 PM to prevent insomnia

E. Common drugs

    1. Methylphenidate (Ritalin): most commonly used for ADHD

    2. Amphetamine complex (Biphetamine)

    3. Amphetamine sulfate

    4. Dextroamphetamine sulfate (Dexedrine)

    5. Pemoline (Cylert)

III. Anorexiants

A. Classification: sympathomimetics

B. Action: suppress appetite by acting on the hypothalamus

C. Use: weight reduction when accompanied by medical complications

D. **Side effects and nursing implications: similar to those of amphetamines. Tolerance and abuse are possible.**

 Warning!

These drugs are contraindicated in epilepsy and certain cardiac and thyroid disorders

E. **Common drugs**
   1. Benzphetamine (Didrex)
   2. Diethylpropion (Tenuate)
   3. Phenmetrazine (Preludin)
   4. Phentermine hydrochloride (Adipex-P)
   5. Phenylpropanolamine (Acutrim, Dexatrim)

IV. Analeptics and methylxanthines
A. **Action: stimulate the CNS by acting on the cerebral cortex and medulla**
B. **Uses**
   1. In OTC drugs, such as caffeine (Vivarin, NoDoz), to produce wakefulness and increase alertness. Also used in OTC cold medications and analgesics, such as acetylsalicylic acid (aspirin) with caffeine (Anacin), acetaminophen and caffeine (Excedrin), and phenylpropanolomine with chlorpheniramine (Triaminic).
   2. Overdose of **CNS depressants**
   3. Migraine headaches
   4. Respiratory depression
C. **Major side effects**
   1. Teratogenesis: fetal abnormalities
   2. CV: dysrhythmias, myocardial infarction, tachycardia, hypertension, tachypnea
   3. Caffeinism: restlessness, insomnia, nervousness, muscle twitching, headache
   4. Seizures
   5. Tolerance and abuse

⚠ **Warning!**

Sudden withdrawal of these agents could result in nausea, vomiting, and headaches

D. **Nursing implications**
   1. Monitor the dietary intake of caffeine
   2. Assess respiratory and cardiovascular systems
   3. Avoid other foods and drinks that contain stimulants
E. **Common drugs**
   1. Methylxanthines
      a. Caffeine
      b. Theophylline
      c. Theobromide
   2. Analeptic: doxapram hydrochloride (Dopram)

PSYCHOTROPICS

I. Classifications
A. **Antipsychotic agents (neuroleptics)**
B. **Antianxiety or anxiolytic agents**
C. **Antidepressants**
   1. Selective **serotonin** reuptake inhibitors: (SSRI)
   2. Tricyclic antidepressants
   3. **Monoamine oxidase (MAO)** inhibitors
   4. Heterocyclic (atypical) antidepressants
D. **Mood stabilizers**

II. Antipsychotic agents
A. **Action: block the dopamine receptors in the brain, which inhibits the dopamine response. This action results in lessened symptoms in the client with a psychiatric disorder. They also work as antiemetics by inhibiting the chemoreceptor trigger zones in the medulla.**
B. **Uses**
   1. Psychiatric disorders
      a. Schizophrenia: a psychiatric disorder characterized by gross distortion of reality, withdrawal, and disorganization of thought
      b. Bipolar disorder
      c. Delusional disorders
      d. Organic syndromes
   2. Antiemetic: prevention of emesis
C. **Major side effects**
   1. Serious movement disorders, extrapyramidal effects
      a. Tardive dyskinesia: involuntary repetitious movements of the muscles of the face, limbs, and trunk
      b. Dystonia: impairment of muscle tone
      c. Parkinsonism (see Chapter 5)
      d. Akathisia: restlessness, agitation, inability to sit still
      e. Neuroleptic malignant syndrome: a complication of psychotherapeutic drug regimens with neuroleptic drugs. Hypertonicity, pallor, dyskinesia, hyperthermia, incontinence, unstable BP, and pulmonary congestion characterize this syndrome.
      f. Tremors
   2. Addiction and tolerance
   3. Sedation
   4. Hypotension and tachycardia
   5. Anticholinergic effects: dry mouth, dilation of pupils, tachycardia, decrease in GI and GU motility
   6. **Photosensitivity.** Recall tip: remember the "S" in sensitivity for skin sensitivity to sun, compared with photophobia, which is sensitivity of the eyes to light.

> ⚠ **Warning!**
>
> Interactions include additive effect with other CNS depressants, especially alcohol, and delayed or blocked absorption when given with antacids.

D. **Nursing implications**
1. Obtain baseline psychological and physical assessments and reassess at intervals, as indicated, while client is taking the medicine
2. Monitor any controlled substances
3. Institute and teach safety measures due to the sedative effects
4. Document carefully the effects of the drug; monitor VS for a sustained HR of more than 100 beats/min and orthostatic hypotension
5. Teach the client about compliance and need for skin protection in the sun
6. Evaluate for effectiveness in treating nausea and vomiting
7. Teach the client about the side effects, especially how to monitor for extrapyramidal effects and anticholinergic effects

E. **Common drugs**
1. Phenothiazines
    a. Chlorpromazine (Thorazine)
    b. Acetophenazine maleate (Tindal)
    c. Prochlorperazine (Compazine)
    d. Mesoridazine besylate (Serentil)
    e. Triflupromazine hydrochloride (Vesprin)
2. Thioxanthines
    a. Chlorprothixene (Taractan)
    b. Thiothixene hydrochloride (Navane)
3. Butyrophenones: haloperidol (Haldol)
4. Dihydroindolones: molindone hydrochloride (Moban)
5. Atypical antispychotic agents
    a. Dibenzodiazepines: clozapine (Clozaril)
    b. Olanzapine (Zyprexa)
    c. Risperidone (Risperdal)

III. Antianxiety or anxiolytic agents

A. **Action: depression of the CNS, thereby increasing the effects of GABA, which produces relaxation and may depress the limbic system. The limbic system is activated by behavior and arousal and influences the endocrine system as well as the ANS. The limbic system is a major integrating system governing emotions.**
B. **Uses**
1. Anxiety states, muscle relaxant
2. Depression
3. Insomnia, as a hypnotic
4. Preanesthesia
5. Withdrawal syndromes

C. **Major side effects**
1. Abuse, dependence, tolerance
2. Sedation, which causes decreased motor skills
3. Hypotension
4. Respiratory depression

> ⚠ **Warning!**
>
> Interactions will occur with other CNS depressants, especially alcohol. *Flumazenil (Romazicon),* a benzodiazepine-receptor antagonist is indicated for treating benzodiazepine overdose or **to reverse the sedative but not the respiratory depressant effects.**

D. **Nursing implications**
1. Ensure the client is informed of the need for counseling and therapy to accompany treatment. These agents do not cure. They only treat the symptoms.
2. Monitor the amount of the medication taken
3. Use caution, because in higher doses, these drugs may be used as sedatives or hypnotics
4. Advise that most of these agents are not recommended during pregnancy (unless absolutely necessary) because of the risk to the fetus
5. Use cautiously with the older adult and debilitated clients, as well as those with pulmonary disorders, for whom complications may occur more frequently
6. Teach clients how to avoid effects of orthostatic hypotension
7. Ensure safety measures since an increased risk for injury exists from the sedative properties

E. **Common drug groups: many groups of drugs have the potential to lower anxiety**
1. Benzodiazepines
   a. Diazepam (Valium)
   b. Alprazolam (Xanax)
   c. Clorazeate dipotassium (Tranxene)
   d. Oxazepam (Serax)
2. Antihistamines: diphenhydramine hydrochloride (Benadryl)
3. Other agents
   a. Hydroxyzine hydrochloride (Atarax, Vistaril)
   b. Buspirone hydrochloride (BuSpar)

ANTIDEPRESSANTS

I. Selective serotonin reuptake inhibitors (SSRIs)

A. **Action: antidepressant response is from the inhibition of serotonin uptake into presynaptic terminals, thus increasing levels of serotonin at the nerve endings. Depression correlates with low levels of serotonin.**

B. **Uses**
1. Depression, **dysthymic disorder, dysthymia**
2. Obsessive-compulsive disorder
3. Appetite disorders
C. **Major side effects**
1. Nausea, diarrhea
2. CNS stimulation: insomnia, headache, nervousness, dizziness
3. Skin rash

⚠ Warning!

These agents are highly protein-bound and should be given cautiously with other protein-bound drugs, such as anticoagulants. Dosages may need to be reduced if the client has severe liver or kidney disease. Monitor the client for suicidal tendencies.

D. **Nursing implications**
1. Administer with meals to reduce the nausea
2. Teach the client to report the side effects. A rash, especially with fever, should be reported immediately. These together could signal serious complications.
3. Use cautiously in older adults
4. Monitor weight, since the agent can cause weight loss
5. Monitor the suicidal client, especially during improved mood and increased energy levels
6. Teach the client to take a single morning dose to avoid insomnia
7. Stress safety precautions if dizziness develops
8. Never abruptly withdraw without the physician's content
9. Stress the need for compliance
10. Know that these agents do not cure, they only treat the symptoms; other forms of therapy should be instituted
11. Inform clients that it may take 1 to 3 weeks before benefits occur
E. **Common drugs**
1. Fluoxetine hydrochloric (Prozac)
2. Sertraline hydrochloride (Zoloft)
3. Paroxetine (Paxil)
4. Venlafaxine (Effexor)
5. Fluvoxamine (Luvox)

II. Tricyclic antidepressants
A. **Action: increase neurotransmitter concentration levels of norepinephrine and serotonin**
B. **Uses**
1. Treat depression, **dysthymia**
2. Treat chronic headaches
3. Treat enuresis
4. Normalize sleep

　　5. Increase appetite
　　6. Elevate mood
C. **Major side effects**
　　1. Sedation or insomnia (agitation)
　　2. Orthostatic hypotension, dysrhythmias
　　3. Anticholinergic effects: dry mouth, dilated pupils (resulting in blurred vision), tachycardia, decreased GI and GU motility
　　4. Weight gain

⚠ Warning!

Interactions may occur with other CNS depressants, alcohol, and many medications. These drugs can mask suicidal tendencies.

D. **Nursing implications**
　　1. Know that these agents do not cure. They only treat the symptoms. Other forms of nondrug therapy should be instituted.
　　2. Instruct client that it may take 1 to 3 weeks before benefits occur
　　3. Teach client the need for compliance
　　4. Suggest that a single dose at bedtime may be beneficial, if daytime sedation is problematic
　　5. Institute safety measures: bed in low position, side rails up, safety around machinery or when driving
E. **Common drugs**
　　1. Amitriptyline hydrochloride (Elavil)
　　2. Doxepin hydrochloride (Sinequan)
　　3. Imipramine hydrochloride (Tofranil)
　　4. Perphenazine and amitriptyline (Triavil)
　　5. Chlordiazepoxide and amitriptyline (Limbitrol)
　　6. Nortriptyline hydrochloride (Pamelor)

III. Monoamine oxidase (MAO) inhibitors

A. **Action: inhibit monoamine oxidase (MAO) enzyme (present in the brain, blood platelets, liver, spleen, and kidneys), which metabolizes amines, norepinephrine, and serotonin. Thus, the concentration of these amines increases.**
B. **Uses**
　　1. As a last choice for depression
　　2. When depression is not responsive to SSRIs and tricyclic compounds
　　3. When the side effects of tricyclic compounds are intolerable
C. **Major side effects**
　　1. Hypertensive crisis, especially if food containing **tyramine** is eaten
　　2. Insomnia
　　3. CNS stimulation: anxiety, agitation, mania
　　4. Orthostatic hypotension

> ⚠ **Warning!**
>
> Interactions are numerous, with OTC drugs as well as prescription drugs. All medications should be approved by the physician while the client is on MAO inhibitors.

D. **Nursing implications**
  1. Teach client to avoid foods with tyramine, which may cause hypertensive crisis (Box 6-1)
  2. Instruct client to limit foods and beverages high in caffeine
  3. Teach about the need for compliance and the possible side effects if noncompliant with regimen
  4. Inform clients that it may take weeks before the benefits are experienced
  5. Instruct that if insomnia occurs, the drug should be taken early in the morning

E. **Common drugs**
  1. Phenelzine sulfate (Nardil)
  2. Tranylcypromine sulfate (Parnate)
  3. Isocarboxazid (Marplan)

IV. Heterocyclic (atypical) antidepressants

A. **Action: these agents are unrelated to the tricyclic antidepressants and are not classified as MAO inhibitors. The action is thought to be similar to that of SSRIs, in that serotonin reuptake is blocked.**

Box 6-1
Dietary Consideration: MAO Inhibitors and Tyramine

Clients taking MAO inhibitors may experience a hypertensive crisis if they ingest foods containing a large amount of tyramine. Foods high in tyramine include the following:

Avocadoes	Paté
Bananas	Pickled and kippered herring
Beer	Pepperoni
Bologna	Pods or broad beans (fava beans)
Canned figs	Raisins
Chocolate	Raw yeast or yeast extracts
Cheese (except cottage cheese)	Salami
Cheese-containing food (e.g., pizza or macaroni and cheese)	Sausage
	Sour cream
Liver	Soy sauce
Meat extracts (e.g., Marmite and Bovril)	Wine
Offal	Yogurt
Papaya products, including meat tenderizers	

Adapted from Clark JB, Queener SF, & Karb VB: *Pharmacologic basis of nursing practice,* ed 6, St Louis, 2000, Mosby.

They are thought to be weaker agents than SSRIs, and exhibit fewer side effects.

B. **Uses**
1. Depression
2. Anxiety
3. Trial use with schizophrenia disorders

C. **Side effects**
1. Drowsiness, headache, dizziness, or insomnia and agitation
2. Hypotension
3. Seizures

D. **Nursing implications**
1. Monitor vital signs at every clinic visit
2. Implement and caution clients about the sedative effects and the need for safety measures
3. Assess for a history of seizures or cardiovascular problems before administration

E. **Common drugs**
1. Bupropion (Wellbutrin, Zyban)
2. Nefazodone (Serzone)
3. Trazodone (Desyrel)

MOOD STABILIZERS

I. Action: normalize the catecholamine response in clients with bipolar, or manic-depressive, disorders

II. Use: bipolar illness

III. Major side effects

A. Minor toxicity: nausea, vomiting, diarrhea, fine hand tremors, GI upset, convulsions

B. Major toxicity: coarse tremors, severe thirst, tinnitus, diluted urine

C. Renal toxicity

D. Teratogenesis: physical defects in the embryo

E. Goiter: pronounced swelling in the neck, usually related to a hypertrophic thyroid gland

F. Metallic taste in mouth

⚠ Warning!

Interactions occurring include diuretics, sodium chloride, and nonsteroidal antiinflammatory drugs (NSAIDs). Toxicity is the major complication of lithium therapy, and serum levels should be checked every week initially until stable, then every 2 months. **Side effects can occur at doses within the therapeutic range.**

IV. Nursing implications

A. Teach the client the side effects and the need for close monitoring of serum lithium levels to prevent side effects and toxicity at serum levels above 2 mEq/L. Many of the side effects can occur at doses within the therapeutic range, which is 0.6 to 1.2 mEq/L.

B. Administer these agents in divided doses since the half-life is short. Doses should not be skipped. If skipped, advise client to contact physician.

C. Instruct client that benefits may not be seen for 1 to 2 weeks

D. Assess renal status and for elevations in serum creatinine level of more than 1.2 mg/dL.

E. Instruct client to avoid drugs that alter urinary elimination in any way

F. Know that these drugs are to be avoided in pregnant or lactating women

G. Prevent dehydration or low serum sodium levels, which may precipitate toxicity

H. Advise client that a high salt intake may diminish the therapeutic effects, since lithium is excreted with the sodium

V. Common drugs ~~Cousin Marc Manic-depression~~

A. Lithium carbonate (Lithane, Eskalith)

B. Lithium citrate syrup (Cibalith—S)

C. Other agents
   1. Carbamazepine (Tegretol)
   2. Divalproex (Depakote, Epival)

SKELETAL MUSCLE RELAXANTS

I. Classifications

A. Centrally acting

B. Peripherally acting

II. General information

A. Limited in usefulness because of the side effects

B. Relief may be obtained primarily because of the sedative properties

C. These agents do not cause loss of consciousness

D. Objective is to relieve musculoskeletal pain or spasm and severe musculoskeletal spasticity without causing loss of function

III. Centrally acting

A. Action: depression of the CNS, thereby altering the neurotransmitter function in the spinal cord and depressing selected areas of the brain that control skeletal muscle function

B. **Use: primary use of these agents is to relieve spasms associated with trauma, injury, inflammation, postsurgical procedures, anxiety, and pain. Some of the agents are used for spasticity of multiple sclerosis or spinal cord injuries.**

C. **Major side effects**
   1. Potential for dependency or addiction
   2. Drowsiness, dizziness
   3. Flaccid muscles
   4. Bradypnea, hypotension

D. **Interactions occur with all other CNS depressants and alcohol**

E. **Nursing implications**
   1. Check for allergies before administration
   2. Use safety precautions after administration: put bed in low position and side rails up, instruct client not to ambulate without assistance, and advise caution about driving or working around machinery
   3. Assess the amount (and effects) of medication being taken
   4. Instruct client about the use of heat, rest, and physical therapy as indicated to minimize or treat muscle spasms

F. **Common drugs**
   1. Cyclobenzaprine hydrochloride (Flexeril)
   2. Chlorzoxazone (Parafon Forte)
   3. Diazepam (Valium)
   4. Carisoprodol (Soma)
   5. Baclofen (Lioresal)
   6. Tizanidine (Zanaflex)
   7. Methocarbamol (Robaxin)

IV. Peripherally or direct-acting agents

A. **Action: work directly on the skeletal muscle, to decrease the availability of calcium in the muscle, and thereby decrease the contractility of the muscles**

B. **Uses**
   1. Decrease spasticity in chronic conditions such as multiple sclerosis, cerebral palsy, spinal cord injuries, and strokes
   2. Rehabilitation purposes when spasticity hinders muscle movement
   3. Malignant hyperthermia

C. **Major side effects**
   1. Muscle weakness in the nonspastic muscles, manifested by slurring of speech and drooling
   2. Drowsiness, dizziness, fatigue, malaise
   3. Severe hepatotoxicity

⚠ Warning!

Interactions with other CNS drugs and alcohol produce an additive effect. Cautious use of OTC cold products that contain alcohol. Dantrolene contains lactose and therefore may not be tolerated in lactose-intolerant clients.

   D. Nursing implications
      1. Know that it may be combined with diazepam to produce an additive effect. For this reason and because of the sedative potential, safety measures should be taken and taught to clients.
      2. Monitor liver function studies for elevations: ALT, AST
   E. Common drug
      1. Dantrolene sodium (Dantrium)

WEB Resources

http://health.yahoo.com/health/Diseases_and_Conditions/Disease_Feed_Data/
  Attention_deficit_disorder__ADD_/#Treatment
  Treatment for ADHD

http://www.bipolarhome.org/treatment/html
  Treatment for bipolar disorder

http://dir.yahoo.com/Health/Pharmacy/Drugs_and_Medications/Types/Antidepressants/
  Use of antidepressants

http://dir.yahoo.com/Health/Pharmacy/Drugs_and_Medications/Types/
  Selective_Serotonin_Reuptake_Inhibitors__SSRIs_/
  Use of SSRIs

REVIEW QUESTIONS

1. A client, age 40, enters the emergency department with a laceration to the left shoulder. The fitting from an oxygen tank had exploded and is embedded in the client's arm. The entry is at the elbow, and the fitting can be felt at the shoulder. The nurse anticipates a long procedure and the use of lidocaine hydrochloride (Xylocaine) with epinephrine based on which fact?
   1. Epinephrine stops the bleeding
   2. Epinephrine shortens the effect of the analgesia and can be repeated more often
   3. Epinephrine lengthens the effect of the analgesia
   4. Epinephrine is safe because the client is 40 years old

2. Which of these clients would benefit most from a preanesthetic?
   1. Sally, age 26, who is having her third knee operation
   2. Joe, age 39, who has never had surgery and is scheduled for open heart surgery
   3. John, age 79, who is having his shunt declotted
   4. Jimmy, age 2, who is having a tonsillectomy

3. Which of these groups of drugs is more likely to be questioned as a preanesthetic?
   1. Narcotics
   2. Anticholinergic agents
   3. Long-acting barbiturates
   4. Short-acting barbiturates

4. Which of these statements is true about amphetamines as a group?
   1. They have a low abuse potential
   2. They cause weight gain if used on long-term basis
   3. They are indicated in the treatment of narcolepsy
   4. They can promote a tired feeling

5. A nursing implication for clients on a MAO inhibitor would include which of these actions?
   1. Teach clients the side effects, especially of a hypertensive crisis
   2. Caution client's to stop eating foods high in sodium
   3. Administer the drug throughout the day if it causes sedation
   4. Advise clients to call for an appointment if no effect is noticed within a week

6. Which of these statements is true about lithium?
   1. The lithium concentration level must be monitored
   2. It is the drug of choice for depression
   3. Toxicity rarely occurs
   4. clients need to call for an appointment if no effect is noticed within a week

7. A client, age 45, takes an antipsychotic agent. The client asks the nurse if a glass of wine can be included with dinner each night. The nurse should tell the client to
1. Drink one or two glasses of wine daily
2. Consult the physician before the consumption of any alcohol
3. Drink in moderation because the wine will not interact with the medication
4. Drink wine because it will increase the drug's effectiveness

8. Amphetamines are potent stimulants with which of these actions?
1. Decrease the release of norepinephrine
2. Increase the release of norepinephrine
3. Depress the higher centers of the brain
4. Stimulate the CNS by acting directly on the cerebral cortex

ANSWERS, RATIONALES, AND TEST-TAKING TIPS

Rationales	Test-Taking Tips

1. Correct answer: 3

The epinephrine lengthens the effect of the lidocaine by slowing the absorption of it. Epinephrine slows the tendency to bleed but *does not stop* the bleeding. Epinephrine lengthens the effect of the analgesic. Age has no effect on the drug's action.

Use a common sense approach if you have no idea of the correct answer. Note the clue in the stem: "anticipates a long procedure." Then match the similar theme, option 3. Avoid reading too fast so that you do not misread the question as asking about bleeding and then make the selection of option 1 and not reading the other options. When you have the urge to make this error of not reading all the options, change the way you read the options. Immediately go to option 4 and read in a reverse order back to option 1. When you read in this reverse order your mind becomes more alert. Make a rule to always read all of the options. Then, read the options backwards as needed.

2. Correct answer: 2

A young man with no history of surgery who is now facing a major operation would probably most benefit from the calming effect of a preanesthetic. In option 1, there may be less anxiety after already having two operations. Declotting a shunt usually does not evoke serious anxiety. Children typically benefit from being awake with their parent(s) to accompany them to the surgery suite rather than being lethargic before surgery.

If you narrowed the options to either 2 or 4 because the surgery would be a new experience, reread the question and the two options. It will be evident that the 39-year-old instead of the 2-year-old would be more aware of the gravity of the procedure and need the preanesthetic.

3. Correct answer: 3

Short-acting agents are preferred so that there are no complications with the general anesthetic given. An agent such as

Use the clue in the option 3, "long-acting," to make your decision. Then go with what you know: preanesthetics are commonly

morphine sulfate is often used to decrease pain and relax the client before surgery. Anticholinergic agents are given to prevent the complications of bradycardia, atelectasis, or aspiration of gastric secretions. Barbiturates relieve anxiety, sedate, and decrease the complications of anesthetic agents.

short acting drugs. Thus, select option 3, which is the opposite. Avoid misreading the question. It is asking for a wrong classification: "more likely to be questioned."

4. Correct answer: 3

Amphetamines stimulate the CNS and produce wakefulness. Narcolepsy is the clinical condition where the client has sudden sleep attacks and amphetamines help maintain alertness. Amphetamines have a high potential for abuse, and tolerance develops quickly. Weight loss usually occurs if they are taken on a long-term basis. Amphetamines increase the energy level, unless abused. If abused and then stopped, clients will have feelings of tiredness.

If you narrowed the options to either 3 or 4, reread the question with each of the two options. Note that this is a "general question" about amphetamines. Therefore, the better answer is the disease that is a more general situation than the specific finding of tired feeling, which occurs in the specific situation of abuse and abrupt discontinuation of these drugs.

5. Correct answer: 1

Hypertension is a typical side effect and can be severe. Foods high in tyramine, which can cause hypertensive crisis, should be avoided. Insomnia is the typical side effect, not sedation. Usually a response to antidepressants is not evident for 1 to 3 weeks.

If you have no idea of the correct answer, go with what you know in general about teaching clients on drug therapies: teach the side effects. Select option 1.

6. Correct answer: 1

Lithium is one of the drugs that require the measurement of serum levels at regular intervals to check for toxicity. Other drugs in this category are

Toxic effects may occur when serum levels are in the therapeutic range of 0.6 to 1.2 mEq/L and definitely occur in the gray area between 1.2 to 2.0 mEq/L. With serum levels

Rationales	Test-Taking Tips
digoxin, theophylline, and phenytoin (Dilantin). Lithium, a mood stabilizer, is recommended for use in manic-depressive illness. Toxicity frequently occurs with this drug. A therapeutic effect is usually not seen until the medicine has been taken for 1 to 3 weeks.	greater than 2.0 mEq/L, clients exhibit definite clinical findings of toxicity. Minor toxicity findings are vomiting, diarrhea, poor coordination, fine motor tremors, weakness, and lassitude. Major toxicity findings are coarse tremors, severe thirst, tinnitus, and diluted urine. Fluid intake is essential during initial therapy, 2 to 3 L/day, and during maintenance, 1 to 2 L/day. Decreased sodium intake with decreased fluid intake may lead to lithium retention and toxicity, and visa versa. Recall tip: lithium requires levels.

7. Correct answer: 2

The combination of alcohol and other CNS depressants causes an additive effect. Alcohol, even in moderation, should not be mixed with antipsychotic agents. Wine will increase the drug's effectiveness; however, that is a reason *not* to drink it when taking these drugs.

If you have no idea of the correct answer, look at the options to find a common theme under which to cluster them. Three options suggest drinking alcohol. Therefore, the one option that doesn't is most likely the correct answer.

8. Correct answer: 2

This action of amphetamines increases norepinephrine, which increases HR, RR, and vasoconstriction. Option 1 is an incorrect action for amphetamines, which are CNS stimulants, not depressants. CNS stimulation is a result of the increase in norepinephrine, not of the direct action on the cerebral cortex.

Eliminate options 1 and 3, since these contradict the clue in the stem, "potent stimulants." Then make an educated guess: if these drugs are potent, they would act more generally to release a systemic substance rather than just acting locally on the cerebral cortex. Select option 2.

7

Drugs Affecting Sleep

FAST FACTS

1. Evaluation of the effectiveness of these drugs is completed by clinical assessment for changes in (listed in order of priority) the following:
   - rate, depth, and pattern of respiration
   - LOC: excitement or dullness; sleep or insomnia
   - HR, heart rhythm, & BP: an increase or decrease; irregular or regular
2. Patients should not be awakened to receive these drugs unless absolutely necessary. Uninterrupted sleep and rest should be provided as much as possible, preferably in blocks of 4 to 6 hours.
3. Patients who take **disulfiram** (Antabuse) may have severe complications within 30 minutes if the drug is taken along with alcohol
4. Fetal alchohol syndrome (FAS) can occur if pregnant women take as little as 3 drinks per day. The safe amount of alcohol to consume during pregnancy is unknown. Even small amounts consumed during critical periods may produce teratogenic effects.

CONTENT REVIEW

I. *Sedatives* and *hypnotics:* general considerations

  A. **Differences between classifications**
   1. **Sedative:** an agent that produces a state of calmness when given in divided doses. In high doses, a sedative becomes a hypnotic.
   2. **Hypnotic:** an agent given at bedtime (hs) to induce sleep, usually in a larger dose than a sedative
  B. **These agents alleviate symptoms but do not cure the cause**
  C. **All have the potential for producing *dependence***
  D. **Many of these agents induce rest by increasing the amount of sleep obtained, but do not necessarily produce restful *rapid eye movement (REM) sleep* (the type of sleep needed for physical and**

mental restoration). Some of these agents decrease REM sleep, while others do not affect REM at all.

E. **Additional agents affecting sleep patterns**
1. Antianxiety agents: see Chapter 6, p. 101
2. Amphetamines: see Chapter 6, p. 97
3. Antihistamines
4. Alcohol, p. 119

F. **Clients should not be awakened to receive these drugs unless absolutely necessary**

G. **Safety measures should be taken by the staff and taught to clients receiving these agents**
1. Place bed in a low position first, elevate side rails, and then document these actions
2. Encourage assistance in ambulation
3. Caution against driving or operating machinery within 4 to 6 hours of drug ingestion
4. Monitor for suicidal tendencies

⚠ Warning!

These agents should not be given late in the evening for elderly clients. In a hospital situation, late administration can lead to a reversal of day and night hours.

II. Barbiturates

A. **Action: produce various levels of CNS depression by decreasing the excitability of synaptic membranes in the cerebral cortex**

B. **Uses: particularly effective when sleep is interrupted early in the morning. Should be used only if nonbarbiturate does not work.**
1. Sedative (low dose) and hypnotic (high dose)
2. Preoperatively and as an anesthetic
3. Anticonvulsant agent

C. **Major side effects**
1. Excessive CNS depression: drowsiness, dizziness, hangover effect, confusion
2. CNS excitement: restlessness, delirium, disorientation
3. **Rebound insomnia:** the inability to sleep worsens after treatment
4. Anxiety
5. Hypersensitivity
6. Respiratory depression because of the effect on the CNS
7. Toxicity: pinpoint pupils, sluggish reflexes, irregular and slower pulse, slow respirations
8. Chronic poisoning: slow thought, incoherent speech, failing memory, weight loss

D. **Nursing implications**
1. Teach safety precautions to client (see general considerations)
2. Assess LOC, respiratory status, and effectiveness of the agent

3. Teach clients to monitor their use of the drug and not to abuse the medication
4. Know that chronic use is contraindicated because the agents lose their effectiveness in 2 to 3 weeks and suppress REM sleep
5. Hold if RR is less than 10/min and shallow or strained
6. Instruct client not to abruptly stop taking the medication. A weaning period of 2 to 3 weeks is needed.
7. Note that some are controlled substances

⚠ Warning!

Interactions include an additive effect with other CNS depressants (alcohol), increased metabolism of antidepressants and warfarin sodium; abrupt discontinuation of the drug is contraindicated

E. **Common drugs (Schedule II controlled substances)**
1. Phenobarbital (Luminal, Nembutal)
2. Secobarbital (Seconal)
3. Aprobarbital (Alurate)
4. Butabarbital sodium (Butisol Sodium)
5. Amobarbital (Amytal)

III. Nonbarbiturates

A. **Similar in all ways to barbiturates. except that the prescription drugs are a Schedule III or IV controlled substances. Some are available OTC.**
B. **Common drugs**
1. Prescription
   a. Chloral hydrate (Noctec)
   b. Ethchlorvynol (Placidyl)
   c. Methyprylon (Noludar)
   d. Paraldehyde (Paral)
   e. Buspirone (BuSpar)
2. Nonprescription
   a. Doxylamine succinate (Unisom)
   b. Diphenhydramine hydrochloride (Benadryl)

IV. Benzodiazepines

A. **Action: CNS depression by increasing the GABA neuronal inhibition**
B. **Uses**
1. Insomnia
2. Preoperative sedation
3. Anxiety
4. Sleep induction
5. Prolonged hypnotic therapy
6. Withdrawal syndromes

C. **Major side effects**
1. CNS changes: drowsiness, slurred speech, memory impairment, hangover effect, dizziness
2. Hypotension
3. Respiratory depression: bradypnea, shallow respirations
4. CNS excitement: nervousness, restlessness, euphoria, excitement, confusion (particularly in older adults)

D. **Nursing implications**
1. Follow safety measures and teach these to clients (see general considerations)
2. Monitor use, since these are controlled substances
3. Assess respiratory status; report RR of less than 10/min, oxygen saturation of less than 90%, shallow or labored respirations
4. Take measures to prevent clients from falling, because of the risk of injury when on these agents

⚠ **Warning!**

Contraindicated with other CNS depressants (alcohol). Interactions: additive effect with CNS depressants and decreased effectiveness with antacids; withdraw drugs slowly after prolonged use (over a 2- to 3-week period).

E. **Common drugs**
1. Flurazepam hydrochloride (Dalmane)
2. Temazepam (Restoril)
3. Haloperidol (Halcion)
4. Estazolam (ProSom)

V. Alcohol

A. **Action: CNS depressant that can produce sedation (low doses) and hypnotic effect or unconsciousness (high doses). Effects are as follows:**
1. Euphoria
2. Depressed learned inhibitions
3. Temporary increase in activity
4. Decreased fine motor skills
5. Decreased libido (in high doses)
6. Diuresis
7. Appetite stimulation (small doses) and inhibition of gastric secretions (larger concentrations)

B. **Used by older adult clients as a sedative and by younger clients as a muscle relaxant and antianxiety agent**

C. **Major side effects.**
1. CV: increased pulse and BP
2. Carcinogenic effects; toxicity to liver
3. CNS: hangover effect, disorientation, slurred speech, and decreased motor coordination, blackouts (lapse of memory of current events

or events within the past 24 hours). High blood alcohol levels can change a client's personality and enhance temperamental behavior. Toxicity is enhanced if large amounts are consumed on an empty stomach.

4. GI: nausea, vomiting (metabolism may take 24 hours)

> ⚠️ **Warning!**
>
> Fetal alcohol syndrome (FAS), a set of congenital psychological, behavioral, cognitive, and physical abnormalities that tends to appear in infants whose mothers consumed alcoholic beverages during pregnancy, may occur; as little as 8 ounces per day will be enough to cause fetal problems.

D. Nursing implications

1. Assess the amount and frequency of alcohol consumption as well as the type of alcohol used
2. Emphasize safety precautions if used by older adults
3. Monitor liver function tests: for increase in ALT, AST
4. Report any signs of alcohol abuse: change in client's appearance (unkempt), failure to report to school or work, excessive sleeping, staying in nightclothes during most or all of the day
5. Document blood alcohol and ammonia level
6. An elevated gamma-glutamyltranspeptidase (GGTP) level without elevation of other enzymes indicates long-term alcohol or drug consumption
7. Check VS and report sustained tachycardia of more than 120 beats/min and BP of higher than 140/90 mm Hg

> ⚠️ **Warning!**
>
> The drug, disulfiram **(Antabuse),** is used as a treatment for compliant clients who refrain from alcohol. Disulfram can cause severe complications within 30 minutes if taken along with alcohol; these include flushing, diaphoresis, hypoventilation, copious vomiting, confusion, chest pain, and difficulty in breathing. Its use in combination with alcohol can be fatal. Clients must be carefully screened and evaluated for compliance in alcohol withdrawal before disulfram is prescribed. Naltrexone (ReVia), an opoid antagonist, is prescribed to help prevent relapse and reduce the amount of cravings for alcohol.

WEB Resources

http://health.yahoo.com/health/Drugs_Tree/Medication_or_Drugs/0323/
  Information on various drugs, for example, Antabuse

http://health.yahoo.com
  For sleep medicines: assess the site and identify the drug under "Medicine" or "Drug"

REVIEW QUESTIONS

1. A barbiturate, pentobarbital (Nembutal), 100 mg PO at bedtime was prescribed for a client to aid in sleeping after an auto accident. The client comments that, after a month, sleep is a problem again. The nurse should recommend which of these actions?
   1. Stop taking the barbiturates because they have lost their effectiveness
   2. Take them only as needed and stop the routine dose every night
   3. See your physician, since the pills lose effectiveness after 2 weeks
   4. Take the agents with a small glass of wine

2. A client, age 63, is scheduled for open heart surgery in the morning. The physician has ordered secobarbital (Seconal), 100 mg PO at bedtime. After giving the tablet, the nurse knows that which of these actions are most important?
   1. Raise the side rails and instruct the client to try to rest
   2. Put the bed into low position, raise the side rails, and instruct the client not to get out of bed without assistance
   3. Instruct the client to use the bedside commode for safety and to have someone present during its use
   4. Inform the family member that they can assist the client to the bathroom if necessary

3. Which side effect would alert a nurse to hold a client's aprobarbital (Alura) at bedtime instead of giving the medicine as ordered?
   1. BP of 110/62 mm Hg
   2. Pulse of 92/min and regular
   3. RR of 8/min and shallow
   4. Pulse of 135/min and regular

4. While making rounds, the nurse finds a client confused, afraid of her daughter, and unable to remember her own name. The nurse should suspect which side effect of triazolam (Halcion)?
   1. CNS stimulation
   2. CNS depression
   3. Rebound CNS depression
   4. Respiratory excitement

5. Nursing implications while a client is taking a hypnotic or sedative would include which of these actions?
   1. Assess for signs of suicidal intention
   2. Assure the client that the hangover effect gets better over time
   3. Awaken the patient to take the medicine if he or she is asleep
   4. Assure the family that sluggish reflexes and slow respirations are normal responses to the agents

ANSWERS, RATIONALES, AND TEST-TAKING TIPS

Rationales	Test-Taking Tips

1. Correct answer: 3

Use of these agents longer than 2 to 3 weeks can cause suppression of REM sleep. Clients should never abruptly withdraw from a barbiturate. A daily routine is required to adjust to the level of sedation produced by the agents. Alcohol produces an additive effect and should not be combined with a barbiturate.

Think about what you know. The physician prescribed the medication. If problems occur afterward, refer the client back to the physician.

2. Correct answer: 2

The priority action is to put the bed into a low position. Therefore, even if the client should fall out of bed, the fall will not be very far. After sedation of clients, the second and third priorities are for the side rails to be up at all times and assistance given for any activity outside of the bed. Although option 1 is correct, the safety measures are a priority and should be strongly enforced. Assistance should be demanded and enforced, even for a bedside commode. A family member could assist the client to ambulate to the bathroom to prevent an accident. However, of the given options this is not the best choice.

This is a more difficult question, since all of the options are correct. Your clue in the stem is the format of the question, when it asks "which actions are most important." Thus, as you read the options, put them in order of priority rather than looking for three wrong options and one right option. Option 2 is more complete and contains more information, so it is most likely the best answer.

3. Correct answer: 3

Respiratory depression manifested by bradypnea is a concern with barbiturate agents. Options 1 and 2 list normal findings of BP and HR and should not prevent the client from taking the agent.

As you read the options for vital sign parameters, think about which options are normal or abnormal. This approach results in your elimination of options 1 and 2. Then look at what choices remain:

Rationales	Test-Taking Tips

An irregular pulse is a sign of toxicity. The tachycardia in option 4 is not a usual side effect and other causes, such as anxiety, fever, or fear, should be investigated.

option 3 is respiratory and option 4 is cardiac. Use the ABCs and select option 3—the one with the respiratory threat—as the priority.

4. Correct answer: 1

Excitement and confusion are signs of CNS stimulation, a side effect often seen in older clients taking triazolam (Halcion). The action of the drug is to depress the CNS. Rebound CNS depression is not a side effect of this agent. Respiratory depression, not excitement, is the typical side effect.

Look in the stem for clues. The important factors to identify in the stem are stimulation, confusion, and excitement of the client. Of the given options, only options 1 and 4 match with stimulation. It is obvious that the stimulation is not of the respiratory system but of the neurologic system.

5. Correct answer: 1

If sedatives or hypnotics are prescribed, the family and the staff should monitor the client for suicidal tendencies throughout therapy. Insomnia, for which these drugs are prescribed, is often a symptom of depression or other serious mental disorders. Suicidal tendencies could trigger the misuse of these agents. The hangover effect doesn't change over time. However, clients either adjust to it or have to try other interventions or medications. As much uninterrupted sleep as possible should be provided to facilitate REM sleep. In option 4, the two symptoms reported by family are abnormal effects of the agents and should be reported to the physician.

The approach to the selection of the correct answer is to eliminate options, since you know they are incorrect information. As you read the options you can use the "true or false" approach to each, and identify that options 2, 3, and 4 are false. Thus, you select option 1, even though it may be unknown or unfamiliar to you.

8

Drugs that Relieve Pain and Inflammation

FAST FACTS

1. Evaluation of the effectiveness of these drugs is completed by clinical assessment for changes in (listed in order of priority) the following:
   - CNS: relief of or decrease in pain
   - LOC: excitement or dullness
   - Rate, depth, and pattern of respiration
   - HR, rhythm, and BP: increase or decrease, irregular or regular
   - GI: increase or decrease in bowel sounds, constipation
   - Laboratory test results: serum creatinine level, CBC count, electrolyte levels, titers, uric acid level
2. Clients with narcotic toxicity have pinpoint pupils
3. Administer narcotics to client within the initial 24 to 48 hours after surgery before pain is too severe. Note that other actions, such as back rubs or positioning for comfort, are a supplement and not to be used as the primary source for pain relief.
4. Withdrawal from a dependence on narcotics includes these findings: nausea, vomiting, intestinal cramps, fever, faintness, and anorexia
5. If narcotic antagonist drugs are unknowingly given to clients who are addicted to opioid narcotic drugs, withdrawal symptoms begin within an hour of administration. Thus, in clients with a known addiction to opioid narcotics, narcotic antagonists should not be given.
6. If narcotic antagonists are given for respiration depression resulting from narcotic drugs, relapse of the respiratory depression occurs 15 to 20 minutes after administration of the antagonist, since the antagonist is shorter-acting than the narcotic agent.

CONTENT REVIEW

ANALGESICS

I. Narcotics

A. **Action: combine with opiate receptors to produce an analgesic effect by altering perception of pain**

B. **Uses**
1. Severe or chronic pain
2. Suppression of GI motility
3. Dyspnea
4. Antitussive effect

C. **Major side effects**
1. Toxicity: pinpoint pupils, coma
2. CNS: sedation, confusion, drowsiness, euphoria
3. Respiratory depression, hypotension
4. GI: nausea, vomiting, constipation after multiple doses
5. Tolerance and dependency

> ⚠️ **Warning!**
>
> Interactions include additive effects with other CNS depressants (alcohol) and a decreased effect with smoking. DO NOT administer to clients with head injuries or with increased intracranial pressure (ICP) since these agents may mask any deterioration. Use only with caution in clients with chronic airway limitations (CAL) or asthma to prevent respiratory depression.

D. **Nursing implications**
1. Assess respiratory status: depth, rate, and rhythm. Hold the medication if the RR is less than 10/min with shallow depth or labored effort.
2. Assess for hypotension and hold medication if systolic BP is less than 90 mm Hg
3. Monitor bowel elimination for constipation; offer stool softener if prescribed; offer fluids; increase dietary fiber; or increase assisted ambulation
4. Instruct clients to ask for the pain medication before the pain is too severe
5. Evaluate pain response to the analgesic with the use of a pain scale, usually a scale from 1 to 10
6. Implement and teach clients about safety: place bed in low position and then put side rails up; get assistance in ambulation; and refrain from the operation of machinery or driving within 3 to 5 hours of taking a dose of the medication
7. Advise clients not to abruptly withdraw or stop the medication
8. Administer antiemetics as needed
9. Monitor the use of the narcotics and maintain them in a locked area

10. Encourage other measures to relieve pain, if feasible with the client status: for example, rest, heat, decreased stress, back rubs, foot massage
11. Teach clients who use client-controlled analgesia (PCA) pumps how to administer the medicine; in particular, how to push the button when they are initially uncomfortable, without waiting until their pain is severe

E. Common drugs
1. Morphine sulfate (MS): immediate release tablet form (MSIR)
2. Meperidine hydrochloride (Demerol)
3. Codeine sulfate: added to cough medicine to suppress cough
4. Methadone hydrochloride (Dolophine)
5. Hydromorphone hydrochloride (Dilaudid): for severe pain or discomfort in terminal cancer
6. Oxymorphone hydrochloride (Numorphan)
7. Mixed agents: Brompton's cocktail (a mixture of morphine, cocaine, dextroamphetamine, and alcohol); used for severe pain in clients with terminal cancer
8. Oxycodone terephthalate (Percocet)
9. Propoxyphene hydrochloride (Darvon)

II. Mixed narcotic agonist-antagonist agents

A. Action: bind with specific receptors to prevent the opioid from remaining on opioid receptor sites. These agents have no antitussive effects and fewer GI effects than agonists do.

B. Uses
1. Mild to moderate pain
2. Respiratory depression
3. Reduction in the potential for narcotic abuse
4. Obstetric analgesia

C. Major side effects
1. Same as for narcotics
2. Withdrawal symptoms in clients who are dependent on narcotics: nausea, vomiting, cramps, fever, faintness, anorexia

D. Nursing implications
1. Same as for narcotics
2. Avoid administration to clients dependent on narcotics

⚠ Warning!

The same interactions with narcotics can occur with mixed agents. Abrupt withdrawal is contraindicated.

E. Common drugs
1. Butorphanol tartrate (Stadol)
2. Nalbuphine hydrochloride (Nubain)
3. Pentazocine hydrochloride (Talwin)
4. Buprenorphine hydrochloride (Buprenex)

III. **Narcotic antagonists**

A. **Action: compete with narcotics for receptor sites, thereby hindering the narcotic effect. These agents work only on opoid narcotic agonists.**

B. **Uses**
1. Respiratory depression (particularly drug-induced)
2. Opioid toxicity
3. Diagnosis of opioid overdose
4. Treatment of newborns from addicted mothers

C. **Major side effects**
1. Withdrawal symptoms in clients dependent on opiates or in infants of mothers addicted to opiates: nervousness, hypertension, palpitations, headache, shortness of breath
2. GI: nausea, vomiting
3. CV: tachycardia, hypertension
4. Return of pain or discomfort for which narcotic agonist was given

> ⚠ **Warning!**
>
> Relapse of respiratory depression occurs 15 to 20 minutes after administration of the antagonists, since antagonist is shorter-acting than the agonist. Never give these to a client addicted to opioid narcotics. If this drug is given IV and repeated once with no effect or change in clinical status, opioid narcotics are not the problem; do further assessment.

D. **Nursing implications**
1. Monitor clients closely for the return of respiratory depression
2. Assess and implement interventions to relieve pain and nausea
3. Assess vital signs every 5 minutes: RR and BP; report sustained HR of more than 120 beats/min and BP over 140/90 mm Hg
4. Know that you may repeat dose, which varies between drugs, within 30 minutes to 1 hour for acute respiratory depression; usually administered IV push
5. Assess for withdrawal findings and treat accordingly

E. **Common drugs and routes of administration**
1. Naloxone hydrochloride (Narcan), given IV, IM, or SC
2. Naltrexone (ReVia), given PO
3. Nalmefene (Revex), given IV, IM, or SC

IV. **Nonnarcotic analgesics**

A. **Actions: inhibit the enzyme necessary for the synthesis of prostaglandin, treat pain, and act on the hypothalamus to regulate body temperature**

B. **Uses**
1. Mild to moderate pain
2. Fever reduction
3. In combination with narcotics for an additive effect
4. Inflammation and inflammatory disorders: arthritis

     5. Transient ischemic attacks (TIA)

     6. Myocardial infarctions (MI)

     7. As additive effect with antiplatelet or anticoagulant drugs

C. Major side effects (rare with therapeutic use; if these side effects are found, suspect self-overmedication)

     1. Toxicity, which can cause liver and kidney damage: tinnitus, hearing loss, confusion, lethargy, hyperventilation

     2. Hypersensitivity

     3. GI distress: heartburn, dyspepsia

     4. GI bleeding

     5. Aspirin products given during or after viral infection can produce Reye's syndrome in children age 18 or under

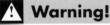 **Warning!**

Children can develop acetaminophen toxicity. Aspirin products are now combined with anticoagulants and antiplatelets to benefit from the additive effect. All aspirin products should be avoided in children under age 18, especially in those with chicken pox or during or after viral illnesses since Reye's syndrome may occur. These agents are highly protein-bound; competition is possible with other highly protein-bound agents (e.g., warfarin, digoxin, SSRIs). Contraindicated in clients with ulcers or those who consume alcohol. Cautious use with anticoagulant drugs.

D. Nursing implications

     1. Assess body temperature every 4 hours

     2. Administer acetylcysteine (Mucomyst), PO, as the antidote for acetaminophen toxicity, which should be treated immediately; usually given for 3 to 4 days

     3. Evaluate the degree of pain relief obtained, with a pain scale of 1 to 10

     4. Teach parents that "more is not better" with these agents, especially acetaminophen

     5. Assess for signs of bleeding: nasal; oral, with brushing teeth; pink-tinged urine; melena, or dark tarry stools; excessive or easy bruising; oozing from minor wounds or venipuncture sites

     6. Assess for allergies before administration

     7. Teach clients to avoid alcohol ingestion with these agents

     8. Teach clients to eat when taking these agents to prevent GI symptoms

     9. Same nursing implications as those listed under narcotics for those nonnarcotic analgesics that are combined with a narcotic*

E. Common drugs

     1. Acetaminophen (Tylenol, Datril, Panadol)

     2. Acetylsalicylic acid, or aspirin (Ecotrin); buffered aspirins (Alka-Seltzer, Bufferin)

     3. Oxycodone terephthalate (Percocet)*

*These drugs are a combination of narcotic and nonnarcotic analgesics.

4. Oxycodone hydrochloride and acetaminophen (Tylox)*
5. Hydrocodone bitartrate and acetaminophen (Vicodin)*
6. Others; diflunisal (Dolobid), salsalate (Amigesic)
7. "Super-aspirin": tirofiban hydrochloride (Aggrastat) (discussed in Chapter 11)

V. Nonsteroidal antiinflammatory drugs (NSAIDs) are nonnarcotic analgesics but are discussed at length under antiinflammatory agents, which follows

DRUGS USED TO TREAT INFLAMMATION

I. Antiinflammatory/antipyretic agents
A. **Actions: prevent the formation of prostaglandins, prevent platelet aggregation, and lower body temperature**
   1. Some have combination effects: acetylsalicylic acid (aspirin, or ASA) is a nonnarcotic analgesic (reduces pain), antiinflammatory (reduces inflammation), antiplatelet (increases coagulation time), and antipyretic agent (reduces temperature)
   2. Nonsteroidal antiinflammatory drugs (NSAIDs) inhibit the formation of prostaglandins; these include ibuprofen products
B. **Uses**
   1. Mild to moderate pain
   2. Arthritis
   3. Dysmenorrhea
   4. Fever reduction
   5. Minor postoperative procedures
   6. Decrease inflammation

> ⚠️ **Warning!**
>
> Interactions include an increased chance of bleeding when these drugs are used in clients with diseases in which bleeding can occur (ulcers), or in combination with alcohol consumption or other medications (anticoagulants). Contraindicated in clients with ulcers or those who have consumed alcohol, and cautious use in clients treated with anticoagulants. Reye's syndrome can occur with products containing acetylsalicylic acid (ASA) in clients under 18 years with high fevers or viral infections. These agents are highly protein-bound; competition is possible with other highly protein-bound agents (e.g., warfarin, digoxin, SSRIs).

C. **Major side effects**
   1. GI irritation: heartburn, GI bleeding, nausea, vomiting
   2. Hematologic: bone marrow depression, anemia, thrombocytopenia
   3. Toxicity: **tinnitus, ototoxicity,** respiratory alkalosis, tachypnea, nausea, vomiting, diarrhea, confusion, dizziness

---

*These drugs are a combination of narcotic and nonnarcotic analgesics.

4. Reye's syndrome
5. Hypersensitivity to NSAIDs: skin rashes, urticaria, hypotension, dyspnea, and angioedema (also called angioneurotic edema: acute painless swelling of short duration that involves swelling of the face, neck, lips, larynx, hands, feet, genitalia, or viscera)

D. Nursing implications
1. Give with food or antacids if GI upset occurs
2. Monitor CBC count and stress compliance with frequent visits for blood monitoring
3. Older adult clients should be monitored monthly
4. Carefully assess for serum changes, especially a decrease in hemoglobin level and hematocrit, as well as platelets
5. Assess the use of these products (early) if surgery is scheduled. These products may need to be discontinued 24 to 48 hours before major surgery. However, they are used before certain cardiovascular procedures.
6. Instruct mothers not to use ASA in children with high fevers or viral infections
7. Alternate NSAID products with acetaminophen (Tylenol) for extremely high or difficult-to-control fevers
8. Teach the client to report if a temperature does not decrease or subside after two doses, if bleeding occurs, or if the swelling and redness do not decrease
9. Administer with a full glass of water, food, or antacids, if GI upset occurs

E. Common drugs
1. Acetylsalicylic acid (aspirin) (ASA)
2. Ibuprofen (Advil, Motrin, Medipren, Nuprin)
3. Naproxen (Naprosyn, Aleve)
4. Fenoprofen calcium (Nalfon)
5. Flurbiprofen sodium (Ansaid)
6. Indomethacin (Indocin)
7. Tolmetin sodium (Tolectin)
8. Sulindac (Clinoril)
9. Nabumetone (Relafen)
10. Ketorolac (Toradol)
11. Diclofenac (Voltaren)
12. Piroxicam (Feldene)
13. Sulfasalazine (Azulfidine) acts as an NSAID

DRUGS USED TO TREAT ARTHRITIS

I. Antirheumatic agents
A. Major classifications
1. NSAIDs
2. Gold compounds
3. Antimalarial compounds

B. **Actions: suppress inflammation of synovial membrane in joints affected by arthritis during active stage of the disease; relieve pain, swelling, and stiffness, and can arrest the progression of the disease**
C. **Uses: arthritis and for arthritic clients who are not responsive to NSAID therapy alone**
D. **Major side effects**
1. Toxicity: nephrotoxicity, hepatotoxicity
2. GI: with gold compounds, a metallic taste in mouth, stomatitis, and mouth ulcers
3. Hematologic: thrombocytopenia, bone marrow depression
4. Skin changes: rash, dermatitis, changes in pigmentation
5. CNS: neuropathy, headache, dizziness

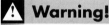 **Warning!**

> Toxicity and blood dyscrasias are important side effects to monitor in use of these agents. Teach clients the symptoms to assess and when to report them.

E. **Nursing implications**
1. Monitor CBC count for decreased platelets and elevated RBC levels, creatinine level, BUN level, and liver studies
2. Protect skin from overexposure to sun
3. Stress compliance with follow-up visits to the physician
4. Assess for mouth ulcers and refer for treatment accordingly
F. **Common drugs**
1. *NSAIDs* (see p. 128)
2. *Gold compounds*
     a. Gold sodium thiomalate (Myochrysine)
     b. Aurothioglycose (Solganal)
     c. Auranofin (Ridaura)
3. *Antimalarial medications*
     a. Chloroquine hydrochloride (Aralen)
     b. Hydroxychloroquine sulfate (Plaquenil)
4. Other agents
     a. Methotrexate (Rheumatrex), a folic acid antagonist (antiinflammatory properties)
     b. Penicillamine (Cuprimine, Depen), a chelating agent (immunosuppressive action)

II. Antigout agents
A. **Actions**
1. Control acute inflammation of the gout attack
2. Increase excretion of uric acid (uricosuric)
3. Decrease production of uric acid
B. **Uses**
1. Gouty arthritis, a disease associated with an increased production of, or interference with, the excretion of uric acid

2. Control uric acid production with antineoplastic drug therapy (allopurinol)

C. Major side effects
1. Renal: kidney stones
2. Hematologic: bone marrow depression, anemia
3. GI: nausea, vomiting, diarrhea

⚠ Warning!

To prevent recurrence of the disease, a low-purine diet should be maintained: limit beer, wine, shellfish, and legumes.

D. Nursing implications
1. Encourage fluid intake of at least 2 to 3 L/day to prevent kidney stone formation
2. Stress compliance with treatment and diet to prevent/control exacerbations
3. Monitor CBC count for decrease in all values to detect agranulocytosis, a decrease in neutrophil, eosinophils and basophils
4. Provide relief as needed for GI side effects

E. Common drugs
1. Colchicine
2. Probenecid (Benemid)
3. Sulfinpyrazone (Anturan)
4. Allopurinol (Zyloprim)

III. Antiinflammatory corticosteroids

A. Action: suppress the intensity of the inflammatory response

B. Uses
1. Myocarditis: inflammation of the myocardium
2. Pericarditis: inflammation of the pericardium
3. Arthritis: inflammation of joints manifested by pain and swelling
4. Tendinitis: inflammation of tendon
5. Bursitis: inflammation of bursa (tissue around joint)
6. Ulcerative colitis: chronic inflammation of the large intestine and rectum
7. Dermatitis: inflammation of skin, with erythema, pain, and pruritus
8. Collagen diseases: extensive disruption of connective tissue (systemic lupus erythematosus, rheumatoid arthritis)

C. Major side effects
1. Skin irritations: burning, allergic contact dermatitis, dryness, hypersensitivity
2. Other side effects are discussed in Chapter 13

⚠ Warning!

Hypersensitivity to these agents can occur: assess for allergies. Apply topical applications in a small portion before covering the entire area on the initial application.

D. **Nursing implications: discussed in Chapter 13**
   1. Assess for abnormalities of the area before application of the ointment
   2. Avoid the use of dressings since dressings may increase risk of systemic absorption; consult physician as needed
   3. Instruct client or parent(s) to follow the directions for application
   4. Instruct to avoid long-term use (more than 6 months) of the ointment, which can result in thin skin and spontaneous bruising
E. **Common drugs**
   1. Cortisone acetate (Cortistan)
   2. Hydrocortisone (Cortisol, Cortaid)
   3. Prednisone (Apo-Prednisone, Deltasone)
   4. Dexamethasone (Decadron)

DRUGS USED TO TREAT HEADACHES

I. Major groups used
A. **Analgesic combinations**
B. **Ergot-containing drugs**
C. **Triptans and serotonin antagonist**
D. **Beta blockers**

II. Analgesic combinations
A. **Action: specific to their group, which includes: narcotics, nonnarcotics, NSAIDs, acetaminophen, and aspirin (as discussed earlier). These agents all work to relieve headaches through their analgesic properties, and combining two or more agents within this group produces an additive effect.**
B. **Use: mild to moderate pain or migraine headaches**
C. **Side effects**
   1. GI: nausea and vomiting
   2. Specific to the group used
   3. CNS: sedation, drowsiness

> ### ⚠ Warning!
> Safety measures should be instituted and taught to clients on these medications: avoid driving or the use of machines, and caution should be taken with child care within 3 to 5 hours of taking a dose. Codeine may be combined with analgesics to enhance the effect of the analgesics.

D. **Nursing implications**
   1. Administer antiemetic before the agent, if necessary
E. **Common drugs**
   1. Butalbital, acetaminophen, and caffeine (Fioricet)
   2. Orphenadrine citrate, aspirin, and caffeine (Norgesic)
   3. Acetaminophen, dichloralphenazone, and isometheptene mucate (Midrin, Migrex)
   4. Hydrocodone bitartrate and acetaminophen (Vicodin)
   5. Oxycodone hydrochloride and acetaminophen (Percocet)

III. Ergot-containing drugs

A. **Action: discussed in Chapters 4 and 5. The caffeine added to many of these agents increases the rate and degree of absorption.**

B. **Use: migraine headaches**

C. **Side effects and nursing implications: discussed in Chapter 5**

⚠ Warning!

Ergotism can occur if drugs are not taken properly. Some of these agents contain caffeine.

D. **Common drugs**
   1. Ergotamine tartrate (Ergostat)
   2. Ergotamine tartrate with caffeine (Cafergot)
   3. Dihydroergotamine mesylate (DHE 45)

IV. Triptans and serotonin antagonist

A. **Action: stimulate the serotonin receptors, which results in the vasoconstriction of cerebral blood vessels and a block of the release of pain-producing inflammatory neuropeptides**

B. **Use: acute migraine headaches**

C. **Side effects**
   1. GI: nausea, malaise, dizziness, and weakness
   2. Tingling sensation
   3. Vasoconstriction: angina, hypertension, smoking, obesity

⚠ Warning!

The first dose of this medication should be administered with a physician's supervision. Avoid in clients with cardiovascular disease. Should never be used within 24 hours of ergotamine preparations.

D. **Nursing implications**
   1. Monitor for GI distress; administer an antiemetic as needed
   2. Identify if ergotamine preparations were used within the previous 24 hours
   3. Monitor the relief of the headache after these products are given
   4. Monitor HR and BP as needed, if indicated by significant changes from the client's baseline findings

E. **Common drugs**
   1. *Triptans*
      a. Sumatriptan (Imitrex)
      b. Zolmitriptan (Zomig)
   2. *Serotonin antagonist*
      a. Methysergide (Sansert)

V. *Beta blockers,* discussed in Chapters 4 and 9; used for prevention of migraine headaches; will not work in an acute attack

WEB Resources

http://www.arthritislink.com/
  Arthritis and related diseases.

http://www.bright.net/~reyessyn
  Reye's syndrome, about the disease.

http://www.bright.net/~reyessyn/aspirinlink.html
  Reye's syndrome, role of aspirin.

http://ink.yahoo.com/bin/query?p=List+of+NSAID%27s&hc=0&hs=0
http://www.dentaldigest.com/prescrip/nsaid.html
  Reye's syndrome, role of aspirin.

http://www.ncpanet.org/CONTEDU/cancer.html
http://home.ptd.net/~paulbarb/opioid.htm
http://health.yahoo.com/health/Diseases_and_Conditions/Disease_Feed_Data/Pain_medica-
  tions/index.html
http://www.headaches.org/
  Pain management.

REVIEW QUESTIONS

1. The day after a total abdominal hysterectomy, a client complains of pain. The nurse should withhold meperidine (Demerol) based on which of these observations?
   1. BP, 100/72 mm Hg; RR, 14/min; HR, 65 beats/min
   2. BP, 98/68 mm Hg; RR, 8/min; HR, 72 beats/min
   3. BP, 120/84 mm Hg; RR, 16/min; HR, 90 beats/min
   4. BP, 155/98 mm Hg; RR, 23/min; HR, 130 beats/min

2. A client, age 16, is brought into the emergency room unconscious without any explanation of cause. Narcotic overdose is suspected, and naloxone hydrochloride (Narcan) is administered based on which of these observations?
   1. Dilated pupils; BP, 200/98 mm Hg; RR, 8/min
   2. HR, 42 beats/min; RR, 18/min; BP, 118/62 mm Hg
   3. Pinpoint pupils; RR, 8/min
   4. HR, 88 beats/min; RR, 20/min; BP, 100/65 mm Hg

3. A migraine headache sufferer is seen frequently in the emergency department with the request for pain relief. Butorphanol tartrate (Stadol) might be administered instead of meperidine hydrochloride (Demerol) based on the fact that butorphanol tartrate is
   1. An effective analgesic for severe pain
   2. A narcotic antagonist
   3. Better and has few side effects
   4. A narcotic agonist-antagonist

4. Acetylcysteine (Mucomyst) is used as an antidote for which of these problems?
   1. Aspirin overdose
   2. Acetaminophen overdose
   3. Meperidine overdose
   4. NSAID toxicity

5. On discharge with a diagnosis of rheumatoid arthritis, a client should be taught which of these actions for the prevention of side effects with an NSAID?
   1. Take the NSAID every 4 hours and as needed
   2. Avoid antacids if the medication causes heartburn
   3. Cautiously operate machinery because of the sedative effect
   4. Report as requested for a CBC count and checkup

ANSWERS, RATIONALES, AND TEST-TAKING TIPS

Rationales	Test-Taking Tips

1. Correct answer: 2

Fewer than 10 respirations per minute should caution the nurse to avoid another dose. Respiratory depression will worsen with subsequent doses. The vital signs in options 1 and 3 are within normal limits. The vital signs in option 4 may indicate that the pain is still present or worsened and that the meperidine could help.

When you have a series format in the options, use the "vertical approach." Read down each first item of the series, the BPs. Eliminate options 1 and 3, since these BPs are within normal limits. Next reread the question to refresh in your mind that its focus is: what would cause the nurse to withhold a narcotic? Then read the second item, the RR, in the remaining options 2 and 4. At this point, it is obvious that a RR of 8/min versus a RR of 23/min is the reason to withhold the narcotic. Recall that the immediate side effect of narcotics is respiratory depression, and the side effect with repetitive doses over long periods of time is constipation and urinary retention.

2. Correct answer: 3

Both of these findings in option 3 are indicative of an opioid narcotic overdose. Narcotics cause pinpoint pupils and hypotension. The vital signs in options 2 and 4 are all within normal limits.

When you have a series format in the options use the "vertical approach." Read down each first item of the series. Eliminate the answers with indications of normal findings, options 2 and 4. Next, reread the question to refresh in your mind that its focus is that a narcotic overdose is suspected and which observations indicate this situation. Look at and compare option 1 and 3 to notice that both have the same RR, so your decision has to be based on the hypertension in option 1 and the size of the pupils. You can recall that when narcotics are given, the BP has the tendency to drop. Therefore, eliminate option 1 with the high BP reading. Avoid second-guessing yourself by going with what you know from your studies and experience.

3. Correct answer: 4

The agent relieves mild to moderate pain. It has similar major side effects as narcotics, and fewer GI effects than narcotics. However, these agents also have less of a potential for dependency and abuse. The general classification for butorphanol tartrate (Stadol) is narcotic analgesic and the specific classification is mixed narcotic agonist-antagonist. Butorphanol tartrate (Stadol) is not necessarily better with fewer side effects than meperidine. The narcotic, meperidine, is usually considered for severe pain.

If a client is dependent on narcotics and a mixed narcotic agonist-antagonist such as butorphanol tartrate (Stadol) is given, the client will most likely exhibit findings of narcotic withdrawal. These agents bind with specific receptors to prevent the opioid from remaining on the opioid receptor sites. Thus, acquisition of a history of specific medications that are taken for headaches is essential with these clients.

4. Correct answer: 2

Acetylcysteine (Mucomyst) works by decreasing the buildup of a metabolite that is hepatotoxic in acetaminophen poisoning. It is usually given orally for 3 to 4 days. When a client has overdosed on aspirin, modification of the pH in the urine with a urinary alkalinizer, acetazolamide (Diamox), a carbonic anhydrase inhibitor that decreases the reabsorption of sodium bicarbonate in the proximal tubule, can help eliminate acetylsalicylic acid. Naloxone hydrochloride (Narcan) is the recommended agent for a narcotic overdose, such as with meperidine (Demerol). Elimination of the NSAID will usually relieve symptoms of NSAID toxicity.

Associate **acet**ylcysteine with **acet**aminophen to recall the treatment for overdosage.

Rationales	Test-Taking Tips

5. Correct answer: 4

Anemias are common with the use of these agents. Regular monitoring of the CBC count is necessary to detect any major complications early on for the prevention of more severe side effects. Option 1 is the recommended dose and does not eliminate side effects. Heartburn is a common side effect and should be treated with antacids. NSAIDs typically do not cause excess sedation.

The clue in the stem is the key words "the prevention of side effects." Options 1, 2, and 3 focus on actions to minimize or to deal with side effects. So option 4 is the best answer.

9

Drugs Affecting the Cardiovascular System

FAST FACTS

1. Evaluation of the effectiveness of these drugs is completed by clinical assessment for changes in the following (listed in order of priority):
   - HR, heart rhythm: increase or decrease, regular or irregular
   - BP: check for orthostatic hypotension
   - GU: urine output volume equal to or greater than fluid intake volume; daily weight
   - LOC: drowsiness, confusion
   - RR, respiratory depth: wheezing, crackles
   - GI: nausea, vomiting, anorexia
   - Lab: PT, aPTT, ALT, AST, and drug levels; electrolyte (K, Mg, Na) levels; creatinine level; CBC count; creatine phosphokinase/lactate dehydrogenase (CPK/LDH) enzymes and isoenzymes; troponin level
2. Think BP and HR: most of these drugs vasodilate or vasoconstrict, which decrease and increase BP and HR, respectively.
3. The goal for most of the cardiovascular drugs is to decrease workload on the heart, to decrease **preload** and/or **afterload.**
4. An increase in preload is targeted for events of hypovolemia or generalized vasodilation, such as anaphylaxis.
5. NTG spray should be applied directly to the oral mucosa (avoid inhaling) on the same schedule as NTG tablets.
6. Safety: lie down or sit down when taking NTG for an acute attack to prevent falls from dizziness caused by the decreased preload, especially if 3 tablets are taken at 5-minute intervals.

7. Clients who take cardiac drugs, especially beta-adrenergic blockers, during exercise or other activity of cardiac rehabilitation, may not experience a rise in HR in response to the activity. Monitor the signs and symptoms rather than pulse rate in response to the exercise undertaken.
8. Antidysrhythmic agents require administration around the clock, since most require that a therapeutic level be maintained; the exception is any sustained release forms.
9. Some bile-sequestering agents taken to decrease hyperlipedemia bind with other acid drugs in the GI tract and thereby reduce the absorption of the fat-soluble vitamins A, D, E, and K.

CONTENT REVIEW

CARDIAC GLYCOSIDES AND SIMILAR DRUGS

I. **Actions: a positive inotropic, negative chronotropic, and negative dromotropic effect produced by the inhibition of the adenosine triphosphatase (ATPase) enzyme and the increase of calcium in the myocardial cytoplasm (Box 9-1)**

  A. Positive inotropic effect increases myocardial contraction, which may decrease heart size in clients with cardiomyopathy and CHF, and increases renal blood flow
  B. Negative chronotropic effect decreases heart rate
  C. Negative dromotropic effect slows conduction through the atrioventricular (AV) node
  D. Overall effects
    1. Increased cardiac output without increased oxygen demand in non–MI situations
    2. Decreased workload from the effect of a decreased heart rate
    3. Mild diuretic effect
    4. Decreased heart size in clients with cardiomyopathy
    5. The following actions are specific to amrinone lactate (Inocor), as a result of the vasodilation it causes:
      a. Decreased preload: decreased stretch of myocardial fiber at the end of diastole
      b. Decreased afterload and end-diastolic volume

Box 9-1
Effects of Drugs on the Heart

Inotropic: affects the force of contraction
Chronotropic: interferes with the rate of the heartbeat
Dromotropic: pertains to conduction

II. Uses
   A. CHF
   B. Atrial dysrhythmias, atrial flutter, supraventricular tachycardia

III. Side effects
   A. Digitalis toxicity
      1. GI disturbances: nausea, vomiting, anorexia, diarrhea (first signs of adult toxicity), upset stomach (first sign of toxicity in children), poor feeding (first sign of toxicity in infants)
      2. Neurologic symptoms: vertigo, headache, drowsiness, irritability, weakness, and convulsions
      3. Ophthalmologic disorders: photophobia, disturbances in color vision (yellow vision), yellow-green halos around objects, flickering lights
      4. CV: ECG changes, extra beats, bradycardia (first sign of toxicity in older children), heart block, tachycardia (first sign of toxicity in young children)
   B. **GI disturbances similar to those listed above may occur without toxicity. If toxicity is not present by verified serum levels, these side effects disappear with continued therapy.**

IV. Nursing implications
   A. **Monitor blood levels of drug and for initial signs of toxicity. Digitalis has a low therapeutic index which is 0.5 to 2 ng/ml, and toxicity occurs quickly.**
   B. **Because of the long half-life, monitor for associated factors of toxicity**
      1. Hypokalemia (< 3.5 mEq/L), hypercalcemia (> 10.5 mg/dl), hypomagnesemia (< 1.8 mg/dl)
      2. Hypothyroidism or hyperthyroidism
      3. Recent MI, ventricular tachycardia, or heart block
      4. Impaired renal function with creatinine level of more than 1.2 mg/dl, dehydration, low serum albumin level
      5. Rapid administration IV: if given too fast, the therapeutic level rises too fast with bolus
   C. **Monitor older adults carefully for possible interactions with other drugs, diseases, and slower absorption, which may lead to toxicity**
   D. **Assess HR by taking an apical pulse for 1 full minute. *Hold* the drug for heart rates of less than 60 beats/min (adult) and less than 110 beats/min (children) and less than 90 beats/min (infant); and *report* to the physician if HR exceeds 120 beats/min (adults) and 140 beats/min (children) and 160 beats/min (infants), unless other parameters have been set by the physician.**
   E. **Assess use of concurrent medications**
      1. Give separately from antacids (at least 1 to 2 hours apart)
      2. Use cautiously with other calcium channel blockers or beta blockers to prevent severe bradycardia or heart block

    F. Assess renal status, monitor I&O

    G. Assess for findings of increasing CHF: for right-sided CHF–NVD, weight gain, edema of feet and ankles; for left-sided CHF–lung congestion, S_3 or S_4 heart sounds, SOB

    H. Know that these drugs usually require digitalizing doses before beginning a maintenance dose. The preferred routes are IV and PO. These drugs are extremely painful if given IM. Digitalization requires loading doses that range from 0.50-1.25 mg/day. The digitalizing doses are usually given 8 to 12 hours apart on the initial day.

    I. Monitor hospitalized clients for electrolyte imbalances, ECG changes, creatinine and BUN level elevations

    J. Anticipate the use of digoxin immune FAB (Digibind) to treat toxicity if dysrhythmias are life-threatening. FAB, fragments of antidigitoxin antibodies, are used instead of whole antibodies to permit faster and more extensive distribution in the body.

    K. Teach the client the following:

        1. Proper dose, time of day to take the medication, and other medications to avoid

        2. How and when to count a pulse rate and when to notify the physician of changes. Take the pulse daily before getting out of bed from sleep. This is the time of the day when the pulse would be at its lowest point: the greatest time of relaxation.

        3. When to report to the physician: extra beats, fast heart rates, signs of toxicity, excess coughing, weight gain (report gain of more than 2 lb/week or 2 lb/day)

        4. Information about toxicity and the importance of knowing what dose to take if the physician changes the prescription

V. Interactions can occur with prescription and OTC medications. Nurses should review the current medication record, and clients should be sure to tell any physician they visit that they are taking a digitalis preparation. A pharmacist should be consulted before clients take OTC preparations. Interactions have occurred with quinidine, beta blockers, calcium channel blockers, loop diuretics, and thyroid preparations.

⚠ Warning!

Digitalis preparations are contraindicated in idiopathic hypertrophic subaortic stenosis (hypertrophic cardiomyopathy), Wolf-Parkinson-White syndrome, and heart block. **Hypokalemic clients have a greater incidence of toxicity.** There is a narrow window between a toxic level and therapeutic level for some clients.

VI. Common drugs
    A. Digitalis preparations
        1. Digoxin (Lanoxin, Lanoxicaps)
        2. Deslanoxide (Cedilanid-D), given IV only
        3. Digitoxin (Digitaline)
    B. Amrinone lactate (Inocor) is similar to cardiac glycosides but differs in the following ways
        1. Does not cause dysrhythmias in large doses
        2. Side effects also include thrombocytopenia and hypotension
        3. Used in CHF when cardiac glycosides fail
        4. Should not be diluted in dextrose products
        5. Should not be given with furosemide (Lasix)

ANTIANGINALS

I. Classifications of drugs used to treat angina
    A. Nitrates
    B. Beta-adrenergic blockers
    C. Calcium channel blockers

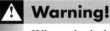

⚠ Warning!
When alcohol consumption is combined with taking beta blockers or calcium channel blockers, hypotension can be severe.

II. Nitrates
    A. Actions
        1. Decrease oxygen demand
        2. Decrease preload by dilating veins
        3. Higher doses dilate all major systemic arteries, which decreases afterload: the resistance against which the left ventricle must eject its volume of blood during contraction
    B. Uses: first line treatment for immediate and long-term prevention of angina: chest pain from lack of oxygenated blood supply to the heart
    C. Major side effects
        1. CNS: Headache (most common), syncope, flushed feeling, dizziness, weakness
        2. CV: Hypotension or postural hypotension
    D. Nursing implications
        1. Know how to administer nitrates in all available forms: PO (tablet or chewable); IV; sublingual (SL) tablet; topical (ointment or patch); inhalation (spray)
        2. Assess the frequency and nature of the angina before drug therapy and what degree of relief is obtained
        3. Monitor BP *before any dose.* BP should be taken *before, during,*

and after therapy. Parameters for administration should be ordered by the physician and documented thoroughly by the nurse.

4. Provide instructions for patches and ointment application
    a. Use a nonhairy area
    b. Rotate sites
    c. Remove the old patch and clean off old ointment immediately before applying a new dose
    d. Use gloves to avoid getting ointment on hands
    e. Squeeze the prescribed amount of ointment onto the paper and apply to the skin without rubbing. Tape the paper in place or apply a plastic wrap over the paper to increase absorption.
    f. Date the patch on the outside
    g. Avoid using the lower legs as an application site, especially in clients with a history of arteriosclerosis. Poor circulation to the legs will inhibit the absorption and distribution of the nitrate and result in a subtherapeutic response. Be aware that clients like to use this site because it causes less intense headaches. Tell them why the site is not ideal and suggest different sites.

5. Provide instructions for SL and spray preparations of nitroglycerin
    a. May take up to 3 SL tablets, 3 to 5 minutes apart to obtain pain relief. Tell client "if relief is not obtained, seek medical attention; either call an ambulance or have someone take you to the nearest emergency room."
    b. Tablets should be protected from light, heat, and moisture
    c. Tablets or spray should always be available. Teach clients to carry them at all times on their person.
    d. Tablets should be replaced 3 to 6 months after bottle is opened. A burning sensation should occur when taken SL.
    e. Spray should be applied directly to the oral mucosa (client to avoid inhaling) on the same schedule as tablets are taken
    f. Cotton should be removed from all new bottles, and expiration dates on bottles should be checked

6. IV nitroglycerin (Tridil) should be mixed with 5% dextrose, in water (D5W) or normal saline in a glass bottle with *the manufacturer-supplied tubing.* A pump should be used and the dose titrated every 3 to 5 minutes according to pain assessment and blood pressure and pulse measurements. Do not mix any other drug with IV nitroglycerin (Tridil). IV nitroglycerin (Tridil) interferes with the effects of IV heparin, so IV heparin rates usually need to be increased to obtain a therapeutic effect.

7. Client teaching
    a. Take nitroglycerin (Nitrostat) tablets at the first sign of an anginal attack

    b. Nitrates are not habit-forming, but tolerance can develop

    c. Safety: lie or sit down while taking NTG for an acute attack to prevent falls from potential dizziness from the decreased preload, especially if three tablets are taken at 5-minute intervals

    d. To prevent angina, take one dose of agent 5 to 10 minutes before stressful physical activity known to cause angina, such as exercise or sexual activity

    e. Teach the specifics about the form of NTG prescribed

    f. Monitor BP if equipment available at home; rise slowly if orthostatic hypotension occurs

    g. Client should be compliant with use of NTG even if headache occurs

> ⚠️ **Warning!**
>
> Avoid use in clients who have sustained head trauma and cases of increased ICP or cerebral hemorrhage. Interactions can occur with alcohol and other vasodilators.

  E. Common drugs

    1. NTG (Nitro-bid, Nitrostat, Tridil, Transderm-Nitro, Nitrodisc, Nitro-dur, Nitrogard, Deponit, Minitran)

    2. Erythrityl tertanitrate (Cardilate)

    3. Isosorbide dinitrate (Isordil); isosorbide mononitrate (Monoket, ISMO)

    4. Pentaerythritol tetranitrate (Peritrate)

III. Beta-adrenergic blockers *low / slow / gurgly*

  A. Actions: block beta receptor sites in the heart, which decreases the force of the contraction and lowers oxygen demand. These actions result in the following

    1. Lowered heart rate

    2. Decreased cardiac output

    3. Decreased contractility

    4. Prevention of exercise-induced tachycardia

    5. Decreased dysrhythmias

  B. Uses: for long-term prevention of angina. These agents assist chronic angina clients to increase their exercise potential. These agents are not used for acute attacks. Beta blockers are also used after an MI to prevent further infarcts, for hypertension, and as antidysrhythmics (Table 9-1).

  C. Side effects

    1. CV: hypotension, bradycardia, worsening of CHF, heart block

    2. Mood: beta blocker "blues," which includes decreased libido, depression, fatigue

    3. Respiratory: bronchospasm

    4. GI: constipation

TABLE 9-1 **Clinical Uses for Beta Blockers and Calcium Channel Blockers**

Classification	Antianginal	Antihypertensive	Antidysrhythmic
Beta blockers	Relieve pain by • decreasing HR • decreasing contractility • decreasing oxygen demand • producing negative inotropic effect • producing negative chronotropic effect	Lower BP by • blocking sympathetic stimulation • decreasing cardiac output	Stop dysrhythmias by • decreasing ischemia by lowering oxygen demand due to decreasing HR (negative chronotropic effect)
Calcium channel blockers	Relieve pain by • decreasing intracellular calcium, which decreases myocardial contractility, which then lowers oxygen demand	Lower BP by • decreasing peripheral vascular resistance • decreasing calcium transport across cells	Stop dysrhythmias by • decreasing conduction rate (negative dromotropic effect) • blocking calcium influx, which decreases irritability

HR, heart rate; BP, blood pressure

D. Nursing implications
1. Monitor BP and pulse *before, during, and after therapy.* If BP is less than 100 mm Hg systolic or the apical pulse is below 60 beats/min for a full minute, consult the physician, unless other parameters have been given.
2. Assess other medications the client is taking. Avoid administering at the same time as antacids (wait 1 to 2 hours), calcium channel blockers, or cardiac glycosides.
3. Monitor the ECG status of the client
4. Client teaching
   a. Do not abruptly withdraw the medication without consulting the physician first; abrupt withdrawal may result in angina with the risk of MI
   b. Take the medication at the same time each day
   c. If a dose is forgotten, do not double the dose; contact the physician for specific instructions
   d. Report any side effects to the physician
   e. Do not take hot baths, sit in hot tubs, or be exposed to the hot sun for long periods of time, usually for no longer than 10 to 20 minutes
   f. Monitor the pulse at the same time daily; count for 1 full minute; suggest the best time is before getting out of bed after sleep
   g. Eat a high-fiber diet, with plenty of fluid to lessen constipation; a stool softener may be needed
5. Monitor triglyceride and cholesterol level (LDL) for elevations
6. Clients exercising or attending cardiac rehabilitation may not experience a rise in HR in response to the activity. Monitor the *signs and symptoms of the client rather than pulse rate* in response to the exercise undertaken.

⚠ **Warning!**

Use cautiously in clients with CHF, heart block, and peripheral vascular insufficiency. Because of the risk of bronchospasm, use cautiously in clients with Chronic Airflow Limitation (CAL) and asthma. Interactions: increased potential for bradycardia with concurrent use of cardiac glycosides and calcium channel blockers, and an increased hypotensive effect with diuretics.

E. Common drugs: these drugs end in "lol"
1. Propranolol hydrochloride (Inderal)
2. Nadolol (Corgard)
3. Metoprolol tartrate (Lopressor)
4. Atenolol (Tenormin)
5. Pindolol (Viskin)
6. Timolol maleate (Blocadren)

    7. Sotalol (Betapace)

    8. Labetalol (Trandate)

IV. Calcium channel blockers

  A. **Actions**

    1. Decrease myocardial contractility by preventing the influx of calcium ions into the cells

    2. Decrease oxygen demand

    3. Dilate coronary and peripheral arteries

  B. **Uses (see Table 9-1)**

    1. Prevention of complications after MI

    2. Acute and long-term prevention of angina attacks

    3. Angina caused by vasospasm

    4. Conversion of supraventricular tachycardia (SVT) rates of more than 150 beats/min to normal sinus rhythm (NSR)

    5. As an antihypertensive.

  C. **Major side effects**

    1. CV: hypotension, bradycardia, heart block

    2. Respiratory: dyspnea, wheezing, worsening CHF

    3. GI: distress

⚠ Warning!

Interactions: increased effects if taken with a beta blocker and increased digoxin level if taken with digoxin products. When giving IV push or piggyback, have a bedside monitor available or telemetry access; record monitor strip and vital signs every 5 to 10 minutes during administration. Use cautiously in clients with a compromised respiratory status.

  D. **Nursing implications**

    1. Monitor BP and pulse *before, during, and after* administration. Limits (high and low) should be set for acceptable BP and HR by the physician.

    2. Monitor ECG pattern and avoid giving the medication when heart block is present

    3. Administer these oral medications with meals or milk

    4. Monitor renal status: for increased serum creatinine and decreased urine output

    5. Assess lung sounds as indicated by client status

    6. Know that the nifedipine (Procardia) capsule might be given for an event of acute severe hypertension. This use is considered investigational. The end of the gel capsule is punctured with a 16- or 18-gauge needle three to four times. The liquid is then squeezed under the tongue of the client. Another method is for the client to put the gel capsule between the back teeth and bite down so the liquid flows onto the mucous membranes of the mouth. The BP should be checked within 5 minutes of administration and every 5 to 10 minutes after the BP starts to

drop. Once a stabilized BP is obtained, the nurse can resume
regular frequency of measuring VS.

E. **Common drugs**
1. Diltiazem hydrochloride (Cardizem), IV and PO
2. Nicardipine hydrochloride (Cardene), PO
3. Nifedipine (Procardia, Adalat), PO and SL
4. Verapamil hydrochloride (Calan, Isoptin), PO and IV
5. Felodipine (Plendil), PO
6. Amiodipine (Norvasc), PO

ANTIDYSRHYTHMIC AGENTS

I. Actions: separated into classes I through IV based on the action and type of dysrhythmia the drug treats. A dysrhythmia is a deviation from the normal pattern of the heartbeat. These drugs work by one or more of the following ways:

A. Decrease *automaticity:* decreases the ability of any cell in the myocardium to self-activate through spontaneous development of an action potential. The ability of cells to fire an impulse accounts for many of the dysrhythmias and extra (premature) beats.

B. Decrease reentry phenomena: decreases the reactivation of myocardial tissue for the second or subsequent time by the same impulse

C. Decrease conduction: slows HR

II. Specific actions, uses, side effects, and nursing implications for each class are identified in Table 9-2

III. Nursing implications

A. Monitor vital signs *before, during, and after* treatment

B. Make sure IV forms of antidysrhythmic drugs are always on an IV controller or pump

C. Monitor ECG patterns during therapy and withhold if heart block occurs

D. Administer around-the-clock, since most require that a therapeutic level be maintained, *unless a sustained release form is available*

E. Monitor electrolytes, especially potassium and magnesium values

F. Dilute these agents in IV fluids to produce the following concentrations if possible:
1. 1:1 drip (1 mg/ml); 1 g/L
2. 2:1 drip (2 mg/ml); 2 g/L or 1 g/500 ml
3. 4:1 drip (4 mg/ml); 2 g/500 ml, or 1 g/250 ml

TABLE 9-2 Antidysrhythmics: Class, Action, Side Effects, and Nursing Implications

Class/Name	Action/Use	Side Effects	Nursing Implications
Class I Moricizine hydrochloride (Ethmozine)	• Classes I, IA, IB, and IC decrease conduction by blocking sodium channels in cardiac cells • Used for life-threatening ventricular dysrhythmias	Exacerbation of existing dysrhythmias or additional dysrhythmias, dizziness, nausea, fatigue, palpitations, dyspnea, angina, CHF	• Monitor for findings of CHF • Observe for additional dysrhythmias
Class IA Quinidine sulfate* (Quinidine) Quinidine gluconate (Quinaglute) Polygalacturonate (Cardioquin) Procainimide* hydrochloride (Pronestyl Procain ET 1000) Disopyramide phosphate* (Norpace)	• Depress contractility • Depress myocardial excitability • Depress the refractory period • Used for atrial dysrhythmias (atrial fibrillation) and ventricular dysrhythmias	Cinchonism (tinnitus, headache, vertigo, fever, visual disturbances) Hypotension GI upset (anorexia, diarrhea, cramping) Cardiotoxicity: widening of the QRS complex and QT interval Can cause *torsades de pointes*	• Monitor for QRS > 0.12 and widening of QT interval • If GI upset occurs, especially diarrhea, immediate attention is needed • Extended release tabs may help with compliance
Class IB Xylocaine hydrochloride (Lidocaine) (IV) Mexiletine hydrochloride (Mexitil) (PO) Tocainide hydrochloride (Tonocard) (PO)	• Accelerate repolarization, cell membrane stabilizers • Used to suppress or prevent ventricular dysrhythmias, to suppress ventricular ectopic beats • First-line drug of choice	CNS disturbances: *drowsiness* (lst sign of toxicity),* confusion, light-headedness, slurred-speech GI distress Hypotension, bradycardia *Seizures* (sign of severe toxicity) *Drowsiness* (lst sign of toxicity) *Seizures* (sign of severe toxicity) Lidocaine toxicity, especially if administered with cimetidine (Tagamet) or propranolol (Inderal)	• Check allergies to local anesthetics • Give Mexitil and Tonocard with food • Administer Lidocaine IV • Read labels carefully to be sure of administering correct IV form of drug • Monitor LOC • Implement safety measures • Monitor VS carefully

Class IC

Flecainide acetate (Tambocor)
Encainide hydrochloride (Enkaid)
Propafenone hydrochloride (Rythmol)

- Interrupts reentry, stabilizes cell membrane, decreases depolarization
- Used for ventricular dysrhythmias and to prevent sustained ventricular tachycardia
- Used when unresponsive to class IB

- CNS disturbances: dizziness, headache, visual disturbances
- Dyspnea
- Abdominal and leg pain
- Worsen CHF
- Exacerbate existing dysrhythmias and create new ones

- Monitor therapeutic serum levels
- Maximum dose of Lidocaine is 300 mg IVP
- Monitor K levels
- Assess BP
- Assess for signs of CHF
- Give with food if GI upset occurs
- Assess lung sounds
- Monitor ECG pattern

Class II (beta blockers)**

Propranolol hydrochloride (Inderal)
Acebutolol hydrochloride (Sectral)
Esmolol hydrochloride (Brivibloc)
Nadolol (Corgard)

- Decreases ischemia by decreasing oxygen demand and decreasing HR (negative chronotropic effect)
- These actions cause less irritability and fewer dysrhythmias
- Used for controlling atrial and ventricular ectopy and sudden atrial or ventricular tachycardia. Any arrhythmia caused by sympathetic activity or catecholamine release.

- Bradycardia, hypotension, syncope, precipitate CHF, decreased libido, fatigue, lassitude
- (see beta blockers, under antianginals)

- Use cautiously in clients with heart block, CHF, COPD
- Withhold if HR < 60 beats/min
- Monitor for signs of CHF
- Do not abruptly withdraw: angina may result
- May not see an increase in HR with exercise, need to assess signs and symptoms of fatigue

Continued

GI, gastrointestinal; CHF, congestive heart failure; LOC, level of consciousness; VS, vital signs; K, potassium; BP, blood pressure; HR, heart rate; IV, intravenous; ECG, electrocardiogram; CNS, central nervous system; AV, atrioventricular; MI, myocardial infarction; HS, at bedtime; CXR, chest X-ray; PFS, pulmonary function studies.

*Can cause *torsades de pointes*

**Drugs ending in "lol" are typically beta blockers

TABLE 9-2 Antidysrhythmics: Class, Action, Side Effects, and Nursing Implications—cont'd

Class/Name	Action/Use	Side Effects	Nursing Implications
Class III Amiodarone hydrochloride (Cordarone) (fast-acting) Bretylium tosylate (Bretylol) (slow-acting) Sotalol (Betapace)* Ibutilide fumarate (Corvert)*	• Decreases automaticity, stops reentry, delays repolarization of fast potentials • All three can affect the heart in different ways; therefore they are not interchangeable • Used for life-threatening ventricular dysrhythmias unresponsive to IB and IC	Orthostatic hypotension, dizziness, can aggravate existing dysrhythmias, fatigue, malaise Can cause torsades de pointes* Toxicity and dysrhythmias are increased by hypokalemia: widens QRS, prolongs PR and QT intervals Photosensitivity	• Monitor BP and pulse • Monitor ECG for changes • Teach client to use sunscreens • Implement safety measures • These agents can affect the heart in different ways; therefore they are not interchangeable
Class IV (calcium channel blockers) Verapamil hydrochloride (Calan, Isoptin, Covera HS) Nifedipine (Procardia XL) Diltiazem (Cardizem CD)	• Blocks calcium influx across myocardial cell and decreases conduction rate (negative dromotropic effect) • Used for controlling ventricular rate in clients with supraventricular dysrhythmias • Will not convert atrial fibrillation but slows down ventricular HR	Severe orthostatic hypotension, especially when administered IV Sinus and AV blocks Worsen CHF Flushing, headache, leg and muscle cramps Can precipitate MI Hepatotoxicity and pulmonary toxicity	• Use cautiously in clients with bradycardia, CHF clients, and sick sinus syndrome • Give IV slowly, over 2 to 3 minutes • Assess BP • Assess signs of CHF • Monitor ECG during IV administration • Monitor CXR, PFS, and liver studies every 3 mo • New forms are longer-acting and help with compliance • Covera HS is beneficial in peaking during morning hours, but must watch BP and HR for one full hour when begin dose • Teach client to rise slowly

ANTIHYPERTENSIVES

I. **The stepped-care approach (Table 9-3) for the treatment of high BP has been recommended for many years. Newer research recommends the same initial step, but with a choice of the classifications of drugs used for hypertension according to the BP readings, race, and risk factors identified for HTN (Table 9-4). Monotherapy (use of low doses of two or more of the antihypertensive agents) is highly recommended in the literature. Diuretics and beta blockers are still the most commonly recommended initial drug therapy. Race has been an initiating factor for monotherapy. For example, African-Americans respond best to diuretics or calcium channel blockers as monotherapy. Caucasians seem to respond better to ACE inhibitors and beta blockers. Regardless of which plan is used, initial steps should begin with life-style modification (Step 1), consisting of the following:**
   A. Exercise
   B. Reduction of stress

TABLE 9-3   Stepped-Care Approach (1993)

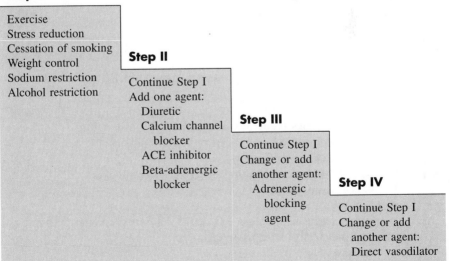

Step I
Exercise
Stress reduction
Cessation of smoking
Weight control
Sodium restriction
Alcohol restriction

Step II
Continue Step I
Add one agent:
   Diuretic
   Calcium channel
      blocker
   ACE inhibitor
   Beta-adrenergic
      blocker

Step III
Continue Step I
Change or add
   another agent:
   Adrenergic
      blocking
      agent

Step IV
Continue Step I
Change or add
   another agent:
   Direct vasodilator

Adapted from National Heart, Lung, and Blood Institute (NHLBI): *The fifth report of the Joint National Committee on detection, evaluation and treatment of high blood pressure.* Bethesda, MD, 1993, National Institutes of Health, US Department of Health and Human Services.
ACE, angiotensin-converting enzyme.

TABLE 9-4	Stepped-Care Approach (1997)

Step I

Exercise
Stress reduction
Cessation of smoking
Weight control
Sodium restriction
Alcohol restriction

Step II

Continue Step I
Add one agent from the list
  below or combine two of
  the drug classes in low
  doses:
  Diuretic
  Calcium channel blocker
  ACE inhibitor
  Beta-adrenergic blocker
  Adrenergic blocking agent

Step III

Continue Step I
Change or add another
  agent:
  Adrenergic blocking
  agent

Adapted from National Heart, Lung, and Blood Institute (NHLBI): *The sixth report of the Joint National Committee on detection, evaluation and treatment of high blood pressure.* Bethesda, MD, 1997, National Institutes of Health, US Department of Health and Human Services.

    C. Cessation of smoking
    D. Loss of excess weight
    E. Restriction of sodium
    F. Decrease in alcohol intake

II. Classifications of drugs used beyond Step 1
    A. Diuretics
    B. Beta-adrenergic blockers
    C. Sympatholytics (centrally acting, peripherally acting, alpha-adrenergic blockers, ganglionic blockers)
    D. Calcium channel blockers
    E. ACE inhibitors or angiotensin II receptor blockers
    F. Direct vasodilators

III. Diuretics (see Chapter 10, p. 171) are often tried first, especially in older adults
    A. Actions
       1. Increase sodium and water excretion
       2. Decrease cardiac output
       3. Directly vasodilate arterioles

4. Decrease peripheral vascular resistance (PVR): a resistance to the flow of blood determined by the tone of the systemic vascular musculature and the diameter of the blood vessels

B. Uses

1. Essential hypertension (HTN): thiazides and loop diuretics
2. Potassium-sparing diuretics: often combined with other agents to lower BP

C. Side effects, nursing implications, and common drugs (see Chapter 10, pp. 171-182)

1. Remember to measure BP and electrolyte levels before administering the drug. Postural hypotension may occur, and BP readings when lying, sitting, and standing may be necessary.
2. Remember the mnemonic: DIURETIC

D = daily weight

I = I&O

U = urine output

R = response of BP

E = electrolytes

T = take pulse

I = ischemic episodes (TIA)

C = complications: CAD, chronic renal failure (CRF), CHF, CVA

> ⚠ **Warning!**
>
> Avoid use of these drugs in anuric clients. Assess for allergies to sulfonamides. Schedule the last daily dose early enough to prevent nocturia.

IV. Beta-adrenergic blockers

A. Actions: inhibit sympathetic stimulation, which lowers HR and decreases cardiac output to lower BP (see Table 9-1)

B. Often used in combination with a diuretic to lower BP

C. Side effects and nursing implications (see antianginals, p. 145)

1. Monitor the BP before administering the agent
2. Monitor the pulse daily for 1 full minute; hold if HR is less than 60/min

> ⚠ **Warning!**
>
> Avoid administering at the same time as antacids; wait 1 to 2 hours between these medications. Increased potential for bradycardia exists with concurrent use of cardiac glycosides and calcium channel blockers, as well as an increased hypotensive effect with diuretics. Never abruptly withdraw the medication. Avoid hot tubs or exposure to the sun for long periods (no longer than 10 to 20 minutes at one time).

D. Common drugs—those drugs end in "lol"

1. Atenolol (Tenormin)

   2. Labetalol (Normodyne)
   3. Metoprolol tartrate (Lopressor)
   4. Nadolol (Corgard)
   5. Pindolol (Viskin)
   6. Propranolol hydrochloride (Inderal)
   7. Carvedilol (CoReg)
   8. Bisoprolol (Zebeta)
   9. Sotalol hydrochloride (Betapace)
   10. Timolol maleate (Blocadren)

V. Calcium channel blockers

   A. **Actions: inhibit release of intracellular calcium, which decreases the force of contraction and prevents entry of calcium ions into smooth muscle; this lowers arteriolar constriction, thereby lowering PVR and decreasing BP (see Table 9-1)**
   B. **Uses: mild to moderate HTN alone or in combination with diuretics**
   C. **Side effects and nursing implications (see antianginals, p. 148)**
   1. Monitor VS before, during, and after administration of medication
   2. Know that SL use of nifedipine (Procardia) is investigational for acute HTN events
   3. Monitor for worsening CHF, hypotension, and bradycardia

> ### ⚠ Warning!
>
> Increased effects can occur if taken with a beta blocker and increased digoxin level may occur if taken with digoxin products. When giving IV push or piggyback, have a bedside monitor available or telemetry access; record monitor strip and VS every 5 to 10 minutes during administration.

   D. **Common drugs**
   1. Diltiazem hydrochloride (Cardizem)
   2. Amlodipine besylate (Norvasc)
   3. Nicardipine hydrochloride (Cardene)
   4. Verapamil hydrochloride (Isoptin)
   5. Nifedipine (Procardia)
   6. Felodipine (Plendil)
   7. Nisoldipine (Sular)

VI. Angiotensin antagonists (angiotension-converting enzyme [ACE] inhibitors)

   A. **Actions: interrupt the renin-angiotensin-aldosterone system in one of three ways (Box 9-2)**
   1. Inhibit conversion of angiotensin I to angiotensin II
   2. Decrease aldosterone secretion
   3. Compete with angiotensin II to block its effect

Box 9-2
Three Mechanisms of Action from ACE Inhibitors in Relation to Normal Physiology

Long-Term Regulation of Blood Pressure

With a decrease in BP, stimulation of the kidneys occurs to excrete renin, an enzyme

((1) inhibits)

involved in the formation of angiotensin I. Angiotensin I is converted to

((3) competes with)

angiotensin II (potent vasoconstrictor). Angiotensin II produces two effects: elevation

((2) decreases)

of BP by potency, or a release in aldosterone, which decreases the excretion of sodium

and water and thereby elevates BP.

Key: (Mechanism of drug action)

_____
BP, blood pressure.

B. **Uses: mild to moderate HTN**
C. **Side effects**
    1. CV: chest pain, palpitations, hypotension, tachycardia
    2. Proteinuria: large quantities of protein in the urine, associated with renal disease, hypertension, heart failure
    3. Rash
    4. Hematologic
       a. Neutropenia: an abnormal decrease in the number of neutrophils in the blood, associated with leukemia, infection, rheumatoid arthritis
       b. Agranulocytosis: reduction in the number of basophils, esosinophils, and neutrophils
    5. Hyperkalemia: potassium level of greater than 5.0 mEq/L
    6. Elevated magnesium level

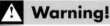 Warning!

Instruct client not to abruptly stop taking the medication; rebound HTN may result. Clients should check with their physician before taking OTC medications, which can interfere with the drugs. A benign, dry cough may occur; if clients find this irritating, encourage them to consult physician for a medication change.

D. Nursing implications
1. Monitor CBC count and electrolytes, especially elevated potassium and magnesium levels
2. Assess for signs of infection, low WBC count, fever, malaise
3. Instruct client to check BP and HR daily and keep a monthly log as needed; note sustained elevations in BP of more than 140/90 mm Hg and HR of more than 100 beats/min
4. Instruct client to do the following:
   a. Inform any new physician about the medication taken
   b. Avoid excess intake of foods rich in potassium and potassium supplements (see Box 10-1 in Ch. 10, p. 175)
   c. Avoid OTC medications without approval of the physician
   d. Take NTG for chest pains if client has this drug available; otherwise go immediately to the emergency department

E. Common drugs
1. ACE inhibitors: these drugs end in "ril"
   a. Captopril (Capoten)
   b. Enalapril maleate (Vasotec)
   c. Losartan potassium (Cozaar)
   d. Benazepril hydrochloride (Lotensin)
   e. Trandolapril (Mavik)
   f. Fosinopril sodium (Monopril)
   g. Lisinopril (Zestril)
   h. Moexipril (Univasc)
   i. Quinapril hydrochloride (Accupril)
   j. Ramipril (Altace)
2. Angiotensin II receptor blockers
   a. Valsartan (Diovan)
   b. Losartan potassium (Cozaar)

VII. Sympatholytics and adrenergic blocking agents
A. Groups of drugs within this class
1. Centrally acting adrenergic blocking agents
2. Peripherally acting antiadrenergic agents
3. Ganglionic blockers
4. Alpha-adrenergic blocking agents

B. Actions: vary depending on the group
1. Centrally acting adrenergic inhibitors: stimulate the alpha$_2$ receptors in the CNS, which decreases sympathetic outflow of norepinephrine; this lowers blood pressure by decreasing cardiac output (CO)
2. Peripherally acting antiadrenergic agents: decrease vascular tone to decrease the BP and decrease the PVR
3. Ganglionic blockers: block both parasympathetic and sympathetic ganglia and decrease PVR

    4. Alpha-adrenergic blockers: lower BP by preventing norepinephrine from activating $alpha_1$ receptors on vascular smooth muscle to produce vasoconstriction

C. Uses

    1. Mild to moderate essential hypertension: peripherally acting antiadrenergic agents; alpha-adrenergic blockers

    2. Mild to severe essential hypertension: ganglionic blockers and centrally acting adrenergic blockers

D. Side effects

    1. Centrally acting: bradycardia, sodium retention, edema, anticholinergic effects

    2. Peripherally acting: orthostatic hypotension, weakness, edema, GI distress, diarrhea

    3. Ganglionic blockers: severe hypotension, respiratory arrest, anticholinergic effects, pseudotolerance to IV form

    4. Alpha-adrenergic blockers: sudden hypotension, tachycardia, fluid retention, dizziness

⚠ Warning!

Use cautiously in clients who have coronary insufficiency, recent MI, cerebrovascular disease, CRF, or a history of mental depression. Monitor closely in clients with impaired renal function: check serum creatinine for elevations above 1.2 mg/dl.

E. Nursing implications

    1. Monitor BP and HR; monitor BP in lying, sitting, and standing positions as needed; obtain baseline VS before beginning therapy

    2. Monitor I&O, weight, assess for edema

    3. Offer ice chips and hard candy if anticholinergic effects occur

    4. Monitor elimination patterns, offer stool softener or antidiarrheal as needed

    5. Teach client the following:

        a. Eat low-sodium foods

        b. Rise slowly if orthostatic hypotension occurs

        c. Be compliant with therapy; some drugs may take weeks to reach a peak effect

        d. Avoid OTC medications without first checking with your physician

    6. Use an infusion pump to give these drugs IV and convert to PO form as quickly as possible

F. Common drugs

    1. **Centrally acting adrenergic agents**

        a. Methyldopa (Aldomet)

        b. Quanfacine (Tenex)

        c. Guanadrel (Hylorel)

        d. Guanabenz acetate (Wytensin)

        e. Clonidine hydrochloride (Catapres)

2. **Peripherally acting antiadrenergic agents**
   a. Reserpine (Serpalan)
   b. Guanethidine sulfate (Ismelin)
3. **Ganglionic blockers**
   a. Trimethaphan camsylate (Arfonad)
4. **Alpha-arenergic blocking agents**
   a. Prazosin hydrochloride (Minipress)
   b. Phentolamine mesylate (Regitine)
   c. Terazosin (Hytrin)
   d. Doxazosin mesylate (Cardura)

VIII. Direct vasodilating agents

A. **Actions: relax arteriolar smooth muscle, dilate arteries, and decrease PVR**
B. **Uses: moderate to severe HTN and *hypertensive crisis***
C. **Side effects**
   1. Neurologic: headache
   2. Renal: sodium retention
   3. CV: rebound HTN, increased workload of heart, tachycardia, palpitations
   4. GI: nausea, vomiting, abdominal pain

> ## ⚠ Warning!
>
> Sodium nitroprusside (Nipride) must be protected from light; wrap IV bag and tubing with foil. Use of an IV controller or pump is essential. Do not mix with other drugs. Know that if the IV drip is stopped, within 1 to 2 minutes the BP rises, since the drug has a short half-life.

D. **Nursing implications**
   1. Monitor VS every 5 to 15 minutes, titrate dose to BP, and do not leave client unmonitored
   2. Monitor I&O, preferably with a urethral urinary catheter in the critical care setting
   3. Give hydralazine hydrochloride (Apresoline) slowly IV push; have a continuous BP monitor if available
E. **Common drugs**
   1. Sodium nitroprusside (Nipride)
   2. Hydralazine hydrochloride (Apresoline)
   3. Diazoxide (Hyperstat)

IX. General nursing implications for all antihypertensives

A. **Monitor baseline BP and pulse *before, during, and after* therapy**
B. **Monitor I&O and renal function by following creatinine clearance or serum creatinine levels**

C. Encourage lifestyle changes (see Step 1 of Stepped-Care Approach, Table 9-3)
D. Teach the client how to check the BP at home; offer parameters from which to report abnormal values. Explain orthostatic BP and, if present, emphasize the need to rise slowly from a lying or sitting position.
E. Teach the client to report edema, cough (both productive and nonproductive), and weight gain of more than 2 pounds per week
F. Stress need to comply with taking and documenting the BP readings and medication
G. Stress need to avoid all OTC products unless physician has been consulted

ANTIHYPERLIPIDEMIA AGENTS

I. **Therapy for high cholesterol levels (> 200 mg/dl in adults) and triglyceride levels (> 140 to 160 mg/dl, depending on the client's age). Remember: low-density lipoprotein (LDL) → want low levels; high-density lipoprotein (HDL) → want high levels. Treatment is recommended based on the LDL level rather than on the total cholesterol level.**
   A. First line of therapy: nondrug treatment
      1. Diet management
      2. Exercise program
      3. Reduction of other risk factors
   B. Second line of therapy is to treat with medications that lower cholesterol, lower triglycerides, or lower both
      1. Hepatic hydroxymethylglutaryl coenzyme A (HMG-CoA) reductase inhibitors
      2. Bile acid sequestrants
      3. Fibric acid derivatives

II. **HMG-CoA reductase inhibitors (called "statins")**
   A. Action: Decrease the rate of cholesterol production by inhibiting HMG-CoA reductase. The liver requires HMG-CoA reductase to produce cholesterol. Agents are very potent and effective to decrease LDL levels.
   B. Used to reduce LDL, total cholesterol, and very low-density lipoprotein (VLDL) levels and to increase HDL level
   C. Side effects
      1. GI: dyspepsia, flatulence, constipation, and abdominal cramps
      2. Myopathy: soreness, weakness, increase in CPK level
      3. Unexplained altered liver function tests, especially with atorvastatin (Lipitor)

> ⚠️ **Warning!**
>
> Avoid use in pregnancy because these agents block the synthesis of cholesterol, which is needed for growth and maintenance. This could cause harm to the fetus. Administration with digoxin may cause slight elevation of digoxin levels, which may need to be checked more frequently.

D. **Nursing implications**
   1. Teach clients that these agents should be used as an adjunct to diet therapy
   2. Monitor renal function: I&O, creatinine level/clearance, and BUN levels
   3. Stress compliance and follow-up visits for further cholesterol evaluation
   4. Teach clients to have liver function tests (ALT, AST) checked within 3 months after initial therapy and then every 6 to 12 months while on therapy or with a dosage change

E. **Common drugs (all of the generic names end in "statin")**
   1. Atorvastatin (Lipitor)
   2. Fluvastatin (Lescol)
   3. Lovastatin (Mevacor)
   4. Simvastatin (Zocor)

III. Bile-sequestering agents

A. **Action: form insoluble complexes with the bile acids in the GI tract, which causes cholesterol to replace the lost bile acids, thereby lowering the cholesterol level**

B. **Uses: when dietary management does not lower cholesterol and the LDL cholesterol is high. These are often used together with the statins to reduce severe hypercholesterolemia.**

C. **Side effects**
   1. Gl: constipation, abdominal pain, nausea, and diarrhea
   2. Headache
   3. Hepatotoxicity
   4. Alteration of PT

> ⚠️ **Warning!**
>
> These agents bind with other acid drugs in the GI tract and thereby reduce the absorption of the fat-soluble vitamins A, D, E, and K. These agents can increase the triglyceride level as a result of increased hepatic very low-density lipoprotein (VLDL) production. Therefore these drugs should not be used in clients with a triglyceride level of more than 200 mg/dl.

D. **Nursing implications**
   1. Instruct the client how to mix the powder or granules in a liquid or food

    2. Monitor PT monthly

    3. Assess cholesterol levels frequently (at least monthly), triglyceride levels, liver function tests

    4. Monitor for GI distress, especially bowel elimination patterns

E. Common drugs

    1. Cholestyramine (Questran)

    2. Colestipol hydrochloride (Colestid)

IV. Fibric acid derivatives

A. Actions: Activate lipoprotein lipase, an enzyme responsible for the breakdown of cholesterol, suppress the release of free fatty acid from adipose tissue, inhibit the synthesis of triglycerides in the liver, and increase the secretion of cholesterol into bile. These agents also increase HDL level.

B. Uses: decrease high levels of triglycerides and lower cholesterol levels

C. Side effects

    1. GI: nausea, vomiting, and diarrhea

    2. Cholelithiasis

    3. Benign and malignant liver tumors

    4. Bleeding tendencies

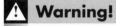 **⚠ Warning!**

These agents are for short-term use only.

D. Nursing implications

    1. Monitor use since they are best used for short term only

    2. Monitor PT

    3. Assess for a history of gallstones and liver disease

    4. Teach the client about dietary compliance with a low-fat, low-cholesterol diet

E. Common drugs

    1. Gemfibrozil (Lopid)

    2. Fenofibrate (Lipidil)

WEB Resources

Internet access to cardiac drugs is available by searching for drugs by disease or by name.
http://www.medscape.com/FirstDataBank/cfdocs/fdb_bydism.cfm?qt=dis&disease=cardiac
   Medscape does require a "free" registration; open site and choose "drugs by disease" or "drugs by name" in the green box to the left.

http://www.cyber-nurse.com/veetac/cham3.htm

http://www.vh.org/Providers/Publications/RXUpdate/1995/09.September.95.html

http://www.vh.org/Providers/Lectures/EmergencyMed/Hypertension/Management.html
   Access "cardiac drugs" through a *Yahoo* search; an abundance of websites exist.

REVIEW QUESTIONS

1. Which finding would be of concern to the nurse if a client was taking calcium channel blocker nicardipine hydrochloride (Cardene)?
   1. "My mouth is so dry"
   2. "I haven't had a BM in 4 days"
   3. BP 200/100 mm Hg
   4. BP 80/50 mm Hg

2. What is the initial treatment for a client with essential hypertension?
   1. A diuretic agent
   2. A diuretic agent, low-fat diet, and exercise
   3. Low-sodium diet, weight reduction, and an exercise program
   4. Adrenergic blocking agent and weight reduction

3. How should the nurse respond when a client asks how a beta blocker lowers the BP?
   1. "The drug decreases the amount of oxygen demanded by the heart"
   2. "The drug dilates veins, which increases the workload of the heart"
   3. "You'll have to discuss this with your doctor"
   4. "The drug slows the HR and decreases cardiac output and thereby lowers the BP"

4. Which of these are the drugs of choice for the reduction of triglycerides in clients who do not respond to dietary management?
   1. Bile-sequestering agents
   2. Fibric acid derivatives
   3. HMG-CoA Reductace Inhibitors
   4. Bile-sequestering agents and HMG-CoA Reductace Inhibitors

5. A loading dose of digoxin (Lanoxin), 0.5 mg PO, is administered and followed by 0.25 mg PO daily. The positive inotropic and negative chronotropic effect is reflected in which of these sets of data?
   1. BP 150/70 mm Hg, HR 92 beats/min, RR 24/min, decrease in urine output
   2. BP 130/80 mm Hg, HR 60 beats/min, RR 22/min, increase in urine output
   3. BP 80/50 mm Hg, HR 60 beats/min, RR 22/min, no effect on urine output
   4. BP 80/50 mm Hg, HR 92 beats/min, RR 24/min, decrease in urine output

6. The nurse should suspect digoxin (Lanoxin) toxicity if a client makes which of these statements?
   1. "I can't have a BM"
   2. "The lights seem very bright"

3. "I have no appetite"
4. "My BP has been elevated lately"

7. Which of these levels should alert the nurse to consider digoxin (Lanoxin) toxicity?
1. Potassium level 5.5 mEq/L
2. Sodium level 146 mEq/L
3. Magnesium level 1.5 mEq/L
4. Potassium level 2.3 mEq/L

8. After the administration of the first SL NTG (Nitrostat) to a client, the nurse checks the blood pressure and gets 80/50 mm Hg. The client still complains of chest pain. The nurse should do which of these actions next?
1. Give the SL NTG (Nitrostat) tablet anyway and notify the physician
2. Hold the SL NTG (Nitrostat) tablet and notify the physician
3. Apply a NTG (Transderm-Nitro) transdermal patch instead
4. Wait 5 minutes, recheck the BP, and if elevated give the NTG (Nitrostat)

9. After application of a NTG (Nitrodur) patch, which of these statements would be considered to fall into the category of a common side effect?
1. "My skin itches all over"
2. "I see halos around everything"
3. "My head is pounding"
4. "I feel tired"

10. A client is admitted with ventricular tachycardia in an emergency situation. The physician orders a bolus of lidocaine hydrochloride (Xylocaine) followed by an IV infusion of the same drug, a Class I-B antidysrhythmic. Which of these statements is true about this medication?
1. Lidocaine is the drug of choice for ventricular dysrhythmias
2. Lidocaine seldom causes drowsiness or confusion
3. Lidocaine is indicated in the above dysrhythmia and heart block
4. Lidocaine can be mixed with epinephrine (Adrenalin) to slow the absorption

11. After several bolus doses of lidocaine hydrochloride (Xylocaine), a Class I-B drug, the ventricular tachycardia does not stop. The nurse anticipates the use of which of these drugs?
1. Class I-C, encainide hydrochloride (Enkaid)
2. Class I-A, quinidine sulfate
3. Class II, esmolol hydrochloride (Brevibloc)
4. Class IV, verapamil hydrochloride (Isoptin)

ANSWERS, RATIONALES, AND TEST-TAKING TIPS

Rationales	Test-Taking Tips

1. Correct answer: 4

The dilation of coronary and peripheral arteries causes the hypotensive effect. Options 1 and 3 are not known side effects of these agents. Option 1 is a side effect of anticholinergics. Option 2, which suggests constipation, is a common side effect of multiple doses of narcotics. This drug is given to control hypertension. Option 3, even though it is a high reading, might be considered a controlled reading for selected clients.

Calcium channel blockers act on the vascular system to relax smooth muscle or the walls of the vessels. Thus, narrow the options to either 3 or 4. Then reread the question to refocus that the question is about a concern of the drug and not the use of the drug. With this drug group, hypotension is more of a problem than hypertension. If the question asked about indications for a subtherapeutic response, then option 3 would have been the correct answer.

2. Correct answer: 3

In Step I, diet, weight reduction, and exercise are indicated before drug therapy is begun, unless the BP is elevated to a level so high that there is a risk of complications, such as stroke. Then medication is given first. The drug in option 1 is a step II drug, which should be added to step I. Option 2 is the step II phase. Adrenergic blocking agents are step III agents that are used in combination with step II drugs or else alone when actions in steps I and II are not effective for BP control.

The clue in the stem is the key words "initial treatment." As with most other therapies, a noninvasive or more natural approach is used first. Be cautious not to read too quickly and read over the diuretic in option 2, since the other two items are correct initial actions.

3. Correct answer: 4

The decrease in cardiac output lowers the BP. In option 1, the described action is true but does not answer the question. Option 1 explains the agent's

If you have narrowed the options to 1 or 4, reread the question. The clue is usually in the question when you have narrowed the options to two. Note that the client is taking the antianginal and antiarrhythmic effect but not the antihypertensive effect. In option 2, the description is for the function of nitrates in lower levels. The workload of the heart is increased since the preload would be decreased and the heart will have to increase HR and contractility to maintain the BP. Option 3 is an inappropriate and nontherapeutic response by the nurse.

drug to decrease the BP. Thus, option 4 is the best. If you had no idea of a correct answer, you can use the match technique. The question is about BP so select the option with the BP, which is option 4.

4. Correct answer: 2

These agents lower cholesterol and triglycerides. In options 1, 3, and 4, the listed agents only lower cholesterol.

Focus on what you know after your initial reading of the given drug classifications. Look for clues in the options. In options 3 and 4, the word "cholesterol" is the clue that these are incorrect answers, since the question is about the reduction of triglycerides. Eliminate these two options. Next, think about what you know about bile; it is formed in the liver, stored in the gall bladder, and has some component of cholesterol as well as bilirubin. Therefore, with an educated guess, eliminate option 1 and select the only option left, option 2.

5. Correct answer: 2

The decrease in pulse indicates the negative chronotropic effect: a decrease in HR, and the increase in urine indicates the positive inotropic effect of an increase in contractility. Information in option 1 indicates a negative inotropic and positive chronotropic effect. The positive inotropic effect influences the urine output. Option 4 represents an effect directly opposite of these agents.

Recall the association of chronotropic with chronologic or with numbers which would be the heart rate. Then think the other is the opposite; inotropic is contraction.

Rationales | Test-Taking Tips

6. Correct answer: 3

Anorexia is a first indicator of toxicity in digoxin and in many other drugs. Diarrhea rather than constipation can indicate toxicity. Halos around objects, disturbances in color vision, a yellow or a yellow-green tint to vision, and the perception of flickering lights are symptoms of toxicity, not bright lights. BP is usually not affected in digoxin toxicity.

If you have no idea of the correct answer, think about most drugs and their side effects on the body, which are commonly problems with the GI tract. Thus, narrow options to 1 and 3. Reread each option and think about time. Anorexia would be an earlier finding than constipation, since it may take up to a week or longer to determine if clients are constipated. Select the option that seems most logical, which is option 3.

7. Correct answer: 4

Hypokalemia, or low potassium levels of less than 3.0 mEq/L, usually indicates a risk for toxicity. Normal potassium level is 3.5 to 5.0 mEq/L. Sodium levels are usually not altered with events of digitalis toxicity. Hypomagnesemia may be evident with hypokalemia. Normal magnesium is 1.5 to 2.5 mEq/L. However, hypokalemia increases the risk of digoxin toxicity.

If you have no idea of a correct answer, look at the serum levels for what is normal and abnormal. Options 2 and 3 are within normal parameters. Eliminate them. Of the remaining options, note that option 4 (2.3 mEq/L) is farther from the normal value of 3.5 mEq/L than option 1, which is 5.5 mEq/L as contrasted to a normal potassium of 5.0 mEq/L. Select the most abnormal value, option 4. Recall tip: the minimum magnesium level is about one-half of the minimum potassium level of 3.5 mEq/L, when divided by 2 equals 1.7 mEq/L, a minimum level for magnesium.

8. Correct answer: 2

A medication such as morphine, other than NTG, can be administered to relieve the pain. The significant drop in the BP and the continued pain are ominous signs that the client may have multiple problems. If repeated, the NTG will continue to lower the BP. The NTG patch would have the

The clue in the stem is that it was the "first" dose, a drastic or significant physiologic effect occurred and the client still has pain. Any client is in danger when the systolic blood pressure falls below 100 mm Hg because of the risk of insufficient blood flow to the vital organs—the brain, the heart, and the kidneys. If the client had other findings from

same side effects as the SL tablet. Waiting 5 minutes for a cardiac client with chest pain is contraindicated.

the effects of this cardiac decompensation, such as dizziness, nausea, or vomiting, the nurse could elevate the client's legs in an attempt to raise the BP to at least 100 mm Hg systolic.

9. Correct answer: 3

A headache is common because of the vasodilation properties of the drug. The patch could cause irritation to the skin directly under the patch. However, that is not a common finding. A yellow-green tint in vision or halos in the vision is a sign of digitalis toxicity. Fatigue is not a common side effect of the drug. Fatigue is a first indication of possible heart failure.

The clue in the stem is "common side effect." Another technique to use is to give each option a theme about the effect: option 1, skin; option 2, vision; option 3, circulation; option 4, comfort. Think about what you know: NTG alters circulation. Think logically to select option 3. Warning: only use this technique in situations when you have no idea of a correct answer.

10. Correct answer: 1

Lidocaine suppresses ventricular irritability and thereby stops ventricular tachycardia. Drowsiness or confusion in option 2 are initial signs of lidociane toxicity, particularly in older clients. Lidocaine is contraindicated in heart block because of the suppressive nature of the drug. Heart block may be a side effect of this drug. IV lidocaine is not mixed with epinephrine (Adrenalin). The topical subcutaneous lidocaine injection may have epinephrine in it to cause local vasoconstriction and minimize bleeding during the suturing of lacerations.

Use caution! Did you read all of the options? A common error is to select option 1 without reading all of the options, since you know option 1 is the correct answer. When you get the impulse to do this, immediately jump down to option 4. Read it, then option 3, then option 2, then reread option 1. Reread the question and the option selected, which is most likely option 1. After this verification of your selected option, chose it and go on to the next question. Beware! Avoid knee-jerk actions, for they can result in your failing tests.

11. Correct answer: 1

Class I-C drugs include flecainide and encainide, which interrupt reentry and stabilize irritable

This type of question may increase your anxiety. Rather than focus on the classes, look at the specific

Rationales	Test-Taking Tips

tissue. Class I-A drugs, such as quinidine sulfate, are administered PO except for pronestyl, which can also be given by IV drip. Class II drugs are beta blockers, which are indicated for ventricular dysrhythmias once they are stabilized. Class IV drugs, such as verapamil, are calcium channel blockers, which are used for controlling ventricular "rates."

drugs, which might give you a clue to the correct answer. Recall that drugs that end in "lol" are beta blockers, which are not usually indicated in acute ventricular events. Eliminate option 3. Recall that the drug **v**erapamil is given when normally conducted cardiac impulses are going **v**ery fast, such as in a situation of atrial tachycardia. Recall the tip that the drug **q**uinidine is given when normally conducted cardiac impulses are going **q**uickly, such as in a situation of atrial flutter or fibrillation. Otherwise, if you could only eliminate one or two options, the best approach is make a guess and go on to the next question. Expect that you will not be familiar with all the questions on the examination. After difficult questions like this one, do your favorite relaxation exercise to clear you mind and reduce the tension in your muscles. Go on to the next question with a refreshed mind and body.

10

Drugs Affecting the Renal System

FAST FACTS

1. Evaluation of the effectiveness of these drugs is accomplished by clinical assessment for changes in (listed in order of priority) the following:
   - BP: check for orthostatic hypotension
   - Urine: output > or = intake; daily weight
   - HR, heart rhythm: increase or decrease; irregular or regular
   - LOC: drowsiness, confusion
   - RR and respiratory depth: wheezing, crackles
   - GI: nausea, vomiting, anorexia, stools (diarrhea)
   - Laboratory test results: PT, aPTT; ALT, AST; serum drug levels; CBC count; electrolytes (potassium [K], magnesium [Mg], sodium [Na]); creatinine and glucose levels; blood urea nitrogen (BUN)
   - General: chest pain, palpitations, malaise, headache, faintness, bleeding: gums, bruises
2. Toxicity of digoxin and lithium can occur with some diuretics
3. Loop diuretics are the most powerful or potent and carbonic anhydrase inhibitors, such as acetazolamide (Diamox), are the weakest
4. Carbonic anhydrase inhibitors are also used as an anticonvulsant or, in some drug overdoses, to alkalinize the urine to enhance the excretion of an overdosed drug
5. Many older adults are generally dehydrated so that when diuretics are given a minimal response occurs. Check the hydration status of these clients by bedside clinical assessments: look for the degree of moistness of the mucous membranes in the mouth; check for the presence of orthostatic hypotension, also called "a positive tilt." Although it may indicate hypovolemia, the nurse should check the client's cardiac medications, because some have orthostatic hypotension as a side effect. Dry mucous membranes and a positive tilt point to dehydration in the vascular compartment.

CONTENT REVIEW

DIURETICS

I. Major classifications
  A. Thiazide and thiazide-like agents
  B. Loop diuretics
  C. Potassium-sparing diuretics
  D. Carbonic anhydrase inhibitors
  E. Osmotic agents

II. Thiazide and thiazide-like agents
  A. Actions: inhibit sodium and chloride reabsorption in the distal tubule and lower peripheral vascular resistance (PVR)
  B. Used to treat the following:
    1. Hypertension
    2. **Edema** associated with: CHF, pregnancy, kidney failure, and liver disease
    3. Decreased urine output in diabetics
  C. Side effects
    1. CV: orthostatic hypotension
    2. Electrolyte imbalance: **hypokalemia, hypomagnesemia**
    3. GI: anorexia, nausea, vomiting, dry mouth, thirst
    4. Glucose intolerance: high glucose levels

> ⚠️ **Warning!**
>
> Interactions include decreased excretion of lithium, which could cause lithium toxicity; increased dysrhythmias with digitalis in the presence of hypokalemia; increased potassium loss with corticosteroids and some penicillins; orthostatic hypotension if taken with alcohol or other antihypertensives; hyponatremia and hyperglycemia, which may be caused by oral hypoglycemic agents and insulin. Check for allergies to sulfonamides.

  D. Nursing implications
    1. See general nursing implications at the end of this chapter
    2. Monitor potassium levels for changes
    3. Monitor closely in the presence of renal or liver dysfunction
    4. Monitor serum glucose for levels higher than 120 mg/dl
    5. Teach clients to take these drugs with or immediately after meals
    6. Instruct clients that the GI symptoms, if persistent over more than 72 hours, can indicate hypokalemia or digitalis toxicity and they should promptly notify their physician
  E. Common drugs (not all thiazides, of which there are many, are listed)
    1. Chlorothiazide (Diuril). Clue: remember, Diuril acts in the distal tubule.
    2. Hydrochlorothiazide (Esidrix, HydroDiuril)

TABLE 10-1	**Thiazide Diuretics Combined with Other Antihypertensive or Diuretic Agents***

Components	Trade Names
Thiazide with ACE Inhibitors	
Hydrochlorothiazide + captopril	Vaseretic
Hydrochlorothiazide + lisinopril	Prinzide, zestoretic
Thiazide with Alpha Blocker	
Polythiazide + prazosin	Minizide
Thiazide with Beta Blocker	
Bendroflumethiazide + nadolol	Corzide
Chlorthalidone + atenolol	Tenoretic
Hydrochlorothiazide + metoprolol	Loperssor HCT
Hydrochlorothiazide + timolol	Timolide
Thiazide with Centrally Acting Antihypertensives	
Chlorthalidone + clonidine	Combipress
Thiazide with Potassium-sparing Diuretics	
Hydrochlorothiazide + amiloride	Modiuretic
Hydrochlorothiazide + spironolactone	Maxzide
Thiazide with Rauwolfia	
Hydrochlorothiazide + reserpine	Hydropres
Trichlormethiazide + reserpine	Metatensin
Thiazide with Vasodilator	
Hydrochlorothiazide + hydralazine	Apresazide, hydrazide
Thiazide with Rauwolfia and Vasodilator	
Hydrochlorothiazide + reserpine + hydralazine	Ser-Ap-Es

*Condensed list of combination drugs including thiazides; there are more drugs than listed in this table.
Adapted from Clark, JB, Queener, SF, & Karb, VB: *Pharmacologic basis of nursing practice,* ed 6, St. Louis, 2000, Mosby.

    3. Methyclothiazide (Aquatensen)
    4. Combinations of thiazides and other agents are used frequently (see Table 10-1)

III. Loop diuretics (potent diuretics)

    A. Actions: block the reabsorption of Na in the loop of Henle, the ascending loop where the greatest Na reabsorption normally occurs; also reduce preload and afterload in the heart
    B. Uses
        1. Edema: CHF, renal or hepatic dysfunction
        2. Hypertension (HTN)
        3. Whenever a potent diuretic is needed

C. **Side effects**
1. Increased electrolyte depletion because of potency: hypokalemia, **hypochloremic alkalosis**
2. Excessive diuresis (urination), which could lead to circulatory collapse
3. High doses: transient hearing loss, abdominal pain
4. Hematologic:
   a. Leukopenia: abnormal decrease in white blood cells to less than 5000/cm^3
   b. Thrombocytopenia: reduction in platelets to less than 150,000/mm^3
5. CV: postural hypotension and tachycardia

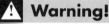
⚠ Warning!

Interactions include hypotension with alcohol; lithium toxicity with lithium; GI bleeding with anticoagulants; digitalis toxicity with digitalis; hyponatremia with oral hypoglycemics; hypotension with NSAIDs. Assess for allergies to sulfonamides. Give IM by Z-track method because of the pain at the injection site.

D. **Nursing implications**
1. See general nursing implications at the end of this chapter
2. Schedule the last dose early enough to prevent nocturia
3. Avoid this class if client becomes anuric
4. Teach the client to do the following:
   a. Consume potassium-rich foods (Box 10-1)
   b. Report muscle cramps, which are usually in the calves of the legs (especially at night) that indicate low serum potassium levels
   c. Take tablets that have changed color, since they are still effective
5. Assess for signs of dehydration, especially in older adults
6. Caution client about switching brands without physician consent; this may change bioavailability and the clinical effects
7. Monitor CBC count for decreased WBCs and platelets
8. If given IV push or piggyback, maintain a rate no faster than 10 mg/min; if given faster and in large doses, transient hearing loss may occur

E. **Common drugs**
1. Furosemide (Lasix). Clue: Remember loop diuretic and the way it acts in the ascending loop of Henle.
2. Ethacrynate sodium (Edecrin), an old drug being used more often
3. Bumetanide (Bumex)
4. Torsemide (Demadex)

IV. Potassium-sparing agents

A. **Actions: inhibit the pump mechanism that normally exchanges potassium for sodium in the distal convoluted tubule. Spironolactone (Aldactone) antagonizes aldosterone, which mediates Na^+ and K^+ exchange. This mechanism reduces Na**

Box 10-1
Dietary Consideration: Potassium Sources

Some drugs, especially the loop and thiazide diuretics, corticosteroids, and amphotericin B, cause excessive loss of potassium, resulting in hypokalemia, which may go unnoticed, but in severe cases, may contribute to toxicity from other drugs, as well as cardiac toxicity. Good dietary sources of potassium include:
Citrus fruits and juices
Bananas, watermelon
Grape, cranberry, apple, pear, and apricot juices
Cereals
Leafy vegetables, dried beans, baked potatoes
Meat, fish, and fowl
Salt substitutes (read label)
Coffee, tea, and cola beverages
Nuts and peanut butter
  Some sources of potassium may be contraindicated in persons who must also limit sodium intake. Licorice can cause potassium excretion and should be avoided by clients experiencing hypokalemia.

Clark J, Queener S, & Karb V: *Pharmacologic basis of nursing practice,* ed 6, St Louis, 2000, Mosby.

reabsorption while retaining K^+. The other drugs within this class produce the same effects as spironolactone (Aldactone) but do not depend on aldosterone.

B. Uses
1. Edema
2. Diuretic-induced hypokalemia
3. Hyperaldosteronism: hypersecretion of aldosterone
4. Corticosteroid-induced edema
5. In combination with other potassium-losing diuretics
6. Ascites in liver failure

C. Side effects
1. **Hyperkalemia** if used alone and with a high-potassium diet or potassium supplements
2. CV: hypotension
3. GI upset: nausea, vomiting, diarrhea, abdominal cramps
4. CNS: weakness, fatigue, paresthesia of hands and feet; numbness or tingling
5. Megaloblastic anemia

⚠ Warning!

Interactions include hyperkalemia with K^+ supplements; lithium toxicity with lithium; nephrotoxicity with indomethacin (Indocin). Assess potassium levels closely if client is receiving blood; blood can contain more than 30 mEq/L of K^+ when stored.

D. Nursing implications
1. See general nursing implications at the end of this chapter
2. Teach that a high-potassium diet is contraindicated; a regular diet is appropriate
3. Monitor other medications for potassium sources
4. Frequently monitor CBC count
5. Teach the client the symptoms of hyperkalemia and to report these as soon as noticed
6. Advise client to keep tablets stored in a dark container

E. Common drugs
1. Spironolactone (Aldactone)
2. Amiloride hydrochloride (Midamor)
3. Triamterene (Dyrenium)

V. Carbonic anhydrase inhibitors (CAI) (weak diuretics)

A. Actions: inhibit the enzyme carbonic anhydrase, which prevents the secretion of hydrogen ions and causes an alkaline urine. The Na^+ is excreted along with the bicarbonate.

B. Uses
1. Glaucoma: lower intraocular pressure (internal pressure of the eye)
2. Edema
3. Control of premenstrual syndrome (PMS)
4. Alkalinize the urine in an overdosed drug
5. Anticonvulsant

C. Side effects
1. Electrolyte imbalance; hyperglycemia
2. Hemolytic anemia
3. Frequent moderate headaches
4. CNS: nervousness, depression, malaise
5. GI: nausea, vomiting, anorexia

⚠ Warning!

Interactions are limited but include increased effect of amphetamines and toxicity of salicylates. Assess for allergy to sulfonamides.

D. Nursing implications
1. See general nursing implications at the end of this chapter
2. Monitor glucose and electrolyte levels and CBC count
3. Do not mix with fruit juices; use honey or syrup to disguise the bitter taste
4. Avoid IM injection, which is painful
5. Administer with antacids to lower GI distress

E. Common drug: acetazolamide (Diamox)

VI. Osmotics

A. Action: increase osmotic pressure, which decreases water reabsorption

B. Uses
1. Prevent oliguria in early stages of acute **renal failure**
2. Lower ICP in cerebral edema
3. Lower intraocular pressure (IOP)
4. Lower pressure in CSF
5. Treat certain drug intoxications or overdoses
6. Emergency management of any of the above

C. Side effects
1. CV: transient expansion of plasma volume, which can lead to circulatory overload; increased blood volume, which can lead to heart failure or pulmonary edema
2. Rebound ICP 8 to 12 hours after initial diuresis
3. Irritation at IV site, including sloughing of tissue with infiltration
4. Headache from cerebral dehydration
5. Thrombophlebitis: inflammation of a vein
6. Electrolyte imbalance
7. Neurologic: headache, cerebral dehydration

⚠ Warning!

Contraindicated in clients with acute renal failure, CHF, intracranial hemorrhage, pregnancy, or severe dehydration. Do not mix with blood products or other drugs.

D. Nursing implications
1. Monitor urinary output closely: should be more than 50 ml/hr with effective therapy
2. Monitor electrolyte and BUN levels
3. Assess IV site frequently during administration; avoid extravasation
4. Warm mannitol (Osmitrol) vial or bottle under hot water and shake vigorously if crystallized; obtain a new vial or bottle if unsuccessful in dissolving of crystals
5. Monitor with ECG for ectopy and vital signs: HR more than 20 beats/min over baseline rate, increase in BP and RR

E. Common drugs
1. Mannitol (Osmitrol)
2. Isosorbide (Ismotic)

VII. General nursing implications (all diuretics)

A. Assess weight (gain or loss) at the same time each day and in the same clothes

B. Monitor I&O carefully as needed, based on the client's condition

C. Monitor food consumption and offer instructions according to potassium-rich or low potassium foods (Box 10-1)

D. Advise clients to avoid all alcohol products because of their diuretic effect and potential for a drop in the BP

E. Assess for findings of hypokalemia and hyperkalemia. Monitor electrolyte levels.

F. Administer early in the day to avoid nocturia (9 AM and 5 PM if ordered bid)

G. Instruct client to limit Na$^+$ if diuretic is used for hypertension

H. Monitor pulse and BP; caution client about rising too abruptly, to avoid or minimize orthostatic hypotension

I. Instruct the client in the signs of decreased effectiveness: weight gain, edema, coughing, return of original symptoms

J. Instruct client to take with or after meals if GI distress occurs. Caution the client that nausea and vomiting may be indicative of an electrolyte disturbance.

K. Monitor for abuse of diuretics, especially by overweight clients

L. Know that older adults may need lower doses and dietary counseling, as well as more frequent accurate assessment of BP and electrolyte levels

Web Resources

http://www.gradstudies.musc.edu/dentistry/top40/lecture_pages/alphablockers.htm

http://ink.yahoo.com/bin/query?p=Lasix&z=2&hc=0&hs=0

http://mayohealth.org/mayo/9708/htm/hype_1sb.htm

http://search.yahoo.com/bin/search?p=hypertension
Internet resources for diuretic therapy with additional choices at the bottom of each website.

REVIEW QUESTIONS

1. Administering furosemide (Lasix), a loop diuretic, too fast IV push or piggyback could result in which of these problems?
    1. Hypertension
    2. Permanent hearing loss
    3. Transient hearing loss
    4. Hyperkalemia

2. While on a potassium-sparing diuretic, spironolactone (Aldactone), a client should be instructed to avoid which foods?
    1. Bananas, meat, peanut butter
    2. Fish, red beans, bread
    3. Carrots, green beans, apple juice
    4. Tomato juice, potatoes, beets

3. When a client received daily spironolactone (Aldactone) and 3 units of packed red blood cells (RBCs), the nurse would be most concerned with which laboratory test result?
    1. Potassium level of 2.3 mEq/L
    2. Magnesium level of 1.5 mEq/L
    3. Sodium level of 145 mEq/L
    4. Potassium level of 5.8 mEq/L

4. A client, age 39, is diagnosed with glaucoma and can no longer drive an eighteen-wheeler truck. The nurse anticipates the use of which of these medications?
    1. Thiazide: hydrochlorothiazide (Hydrodiuril)
    2. Loop diuretic: bumetanide (Bumex)
    3. Carbonic anhydrase inhibitor: acetazolamide (Diamox)
    4. Potassium-sparing diuretic: spironolactone (Aldactone)

5. During the preparation of mannitol (Osmitrol), the nurse notices crystals in the ampule. The nurse should take which action?
    1. Return the ampule to the pharmacy
    2. Hold the ampule under cold tap water
    3. Hold the ampule under warm tap water
    4. Shake vigorously

ANSWERS, RATIONALES, AND TEST-TAKING TIPS

Rationales	Test-Taking Tips

1. Correct answer: 3

Temporary hearing loss may occur from an excessive dosage of the drug or an overly rapid administration. Postural hypotension is a side effect, not hypertension. In clients taking loop diuretics, hypokalemia is a common side effect.

If you had no idea of the correct answer, use this technique. Cluster options 1 and 4 under the umbrella of "hyper" and eliminate them. Then decide between options 2 and 3. Select option 3 based on your knowledge that effects of drugs, especially when given IV, are more likely to be transient than permanent.

2. Correct answer: 1

In option 1, all three foods are high in potassium. In option 2, fish and beans are high in potassium. In option 3, only apple juice is high in potassium. Tomato juice is high in sodium and potassium.

Go with what you know. If you only identified that bananas and peanut butter are high in potassium, select option 1. It is not advisable to select an option about which you know little.

3. Correct answer: 4

Potassium is not lost while a client is on spironolactone, a potassium-sparing diuretic. Stored blood can be high in potassium. Both the drug and the blood would raise the potassium level. The magnesium and sodium level should not be affected by blood administration.

First read the options to see which ones you would be concerned about in general. Options 2 and 3 are normal values for magnesium and sodium, so eliminate them. Of the two remaining options, 1 and 4, both potassium levels are of a concern with one being elevated and the other being low. The clue is in the medication, it is a potassium-sparing diuretic. Therefore, option 4 is the correct answer. Recall tip for **A**ldactone is to associate the **A** with its action to **a**dd potassium to the blood.

4. Correct answer: 3

Carbonic anhydrase inhibitors are used primarily to lower intraocular pressure (IOP) in

Think about what you know about the given diuretics. Cluster three of the options, 1, 2, and 4, under glaucoma. Thiazides are not recommended for glaucoma. Loop diuretics are extremely potent and not recommended for glaucoma. Spironolactone is not recommended for glaucoma.

"common diuretics for heart failure or fluid overload." The one left, option 3, must be used for the eyes.

5. Correct answer: 3

Warm tap water will dissolve the crystals so the drug can be used. Crystals form in the bottle or ampule while the drug is stored. The bottle or ampule would be returned to the pharmacy for a replacement if the nurse was unsuccessful in dissolving the crystals. Cold water will not dissolve the crystals. Shaking the bottle or ampule will not dissolve the crystals.

Use common sense as to what dissolves substances. Use the warm water. Eliminate option 4 because of the word "vigorously." Most medications in containers can be shaken, but not vigorously shaken. In the event of an emergency, the nurse should get another ampule without crystals from the pharmacy. Returning the bottle or ampule to pharmacy is an incomplete answer. Avoid reading into the given statement that option 1 means to obtain a new bottle or ampule.

11

Drugs Affecting the Hematologic System

FAST FACTS

1. Evaluation of the effectiveness of these drugs is accomplished by clinical assessment for changes in the following (listed in order of priority):
   - Laboratory test results: PT, PTT, and aPTT levels and international normalized ratio (INR)
   - General: bleeding in gums, urine, stool, venipuncture sites, nose, or ecchymosis
2. A greater incidence of bleeding occurs with oral anticoagulants than with parenteral anticoagulants.
3. Oral anticoagulants take 48 to 72 hours to reach therapeutic levels. During this time the client's parenteral anticoagulant is usually continued.
4. Doses of low-molecular-weight heparin (LMWH) are not interchangeable, and some are ordered in units per hour and others in milligrams.
5. Protamine sulfate is the antidote for heparin and some of the LMWH's.
6. No antidote is available at this time for the LMWH danaparoid (Orgaran).
7. NTG IV can decrease the effects of IV heparin and can compromise the effects of thrombolytics.
8. Oral forms of iron have increased absorption when taken with ascorbic acid or Vitamin C.

CONTENT REVIEW

DOSAGE MONITORING WITH ANTICOAGULANTS

I. Use of laboratory test results: PT, PTT, aPTT, INR

    A. *Prothrombin time (PT):* **used with oral anticoagulants, such as warfarin sodium (Coumadin)**

B. *Partial thromboplastin time (PTT):* used with parenteral anticoagulants, such as heparin

C. *Activated partial thromboplastin time (aPTT):* more accurate than PTT

D. *International normalized ratio (INR):* used with either oral or parenteral anticoagulants, primarily warfarin sodium (Coumadin)

II. Ways to monitor dosing

A. Results of laboratory test results compared to control

1. The client's results for PT, PTT, or aPTT are compared with the control value set by the laboratory. The client's value should be 1.5 to 2.5 times the control for a therapeutic effect.

2. The client's results for the INR value are analyzed with the PT, PTT, or aPTT. A value for therapeutic anticoagulant therapy ranges between 2 and 3. Some physicians may exceed this and want a slower clotting time, with an INR range of 2.5 to 3.5. The INR adjusts for the reagent used in the preparation of the PT, PTT, or aPTT.

B. Sliding scale: a sliding scale can be established by a physician or agency to use in analyzing the results of the PT, PTT, or aPTT. The scale will usually set a low and high parameter for the lab tests and the amount (dosage) to adjust the anticoagulant according to the scale. For example: the sliding scale may state: "If PT is less than 50, increase the heparin by 200 u/hr and if more than 80, decrease the heparin by 200 u/hr." Usually a daily PT or PTT value is obtained and may be obtained more often during initial therapy.

C. Weight-based dosing: client is weighed on a daily basis and the dose is adjusted according to the weight and the laboratory results of the PT or PTT tests. This method is thought to be more accurate but involves obtaining a daily weight, which may be more hazardous, depending on the position or severity of the clot in the client.

ANTICOAGULANTS

I. Oral anticoagulants

A. Action: inhibits blood clotting by depressing synthesis of clotting factors VII, IX, and X, thereby preventing the use of vitamin K by the liver

B. Uses

1. Slow down or prevent the extension of a blood clot
   a. Deep vein thrombosis (DVT)
   b. Pulmonary embolism
   c. Coronary artery disease (CAD), cardiovascular thrombosis
   d. Atrial fibrillation

    2. Rheumatic heart disease

    3. Prophylactically: major surgery, periods of prolonged immobilization when coagulation complications are possible, and prosthetic heart valves

C. Side effects

    1. Greater incidence of bleeding than with parenteral anticoagulants

        a. **Hematuria:** blood in the urine

        b. Epistaxis: nosebleed

        c. Ecchymosis: bruising

        d. Tarry stools: black, sticky

        e. Bleeding gums

    2. Leukopenia: a decreased white blood cell (WBC) count; agranulocytosis: decreased counts of neutrophils, basophils, and eosinophils

    3. Hypersensitivity

    4. GI upset: diarrhea, nausea, vomiting

> ⚠️ **WARNING!**
>
> Interactions include increased effect with glucocorticoids, acetylsalicylic acid (aspirin), alcohol, and antibiotics; decreased effect with barbiturates, estrogens, and oral contraceptives. Clients should avoid foods high in vitamin K, such as green leafy vegetables, tomatoes, fish, liver, cheese, egg yolks, and red meats. A food-to-drug interaction could occur and increase the coagulation process from a decrease in the drug's effectiveness. Have vitamin K (AquaMephyton) injectable available as an antidote. Vitamin K activates the precursors in the liver needed for clotting. Contraindicated in pregnancy or conditions in which hemorrhage is possible, such as ulcers or situations threatening hemorrhage, liver, and renal diseases.

D. Nursing implications

    1. Assess for bleeding

    2. Monitor the PT, at 1.5 to 2.5 times the control, and INR range of 2 to 3. Careful monitoring for bleeding is necessary when the PT values are more than 2.0 times the control and the INR is > 3.

    3. Give by mouth only; may be started while parenteral form is infusing. Use extreme caution to monitor for bleeding. Takes 2 to 3 days to reach therapeutic levels.

    4. Monitor for bleeding: hematuria, hematoma, epistaxis, eccyhmosis

    5. Instruct clients to do the following:

        a. Protect themselves from excessive bruising or cuts. Use an electric razor and a soft toothbrush.

        b. Wear a medical alert bracelet

        c. Consult a physician before taking any OTC drugs

        d. Avoid acetylsalicylic acid (aspirin and aspirin products) in excess unless prescribed by the physician. These cause an additive effect.

        e. Report any excess bruising, pink urine, tarry stools

      f. Take bleeding precautions for 9 to 10 days after the last dose of the drug

  6. Monitor the client's medication record sheet for the following items:

      a. Acetylsalicylic acid (aspirin) and aspirin products. Pay particular attention to the frequency and type of pain relievers.

      b. Avoid IM injections if possible. If used, hold pressure for several (3 to 5) minutes after the injection.

  7. Closely observe the other medications prescribed and the client's protein level, since anticoagulants are highly protein-bound, if a therapeutic effect is not seen. Suspect a competition for the protein-binding sites.

  8. Label the head of the bed if hospitalized or recommend a bracelet that indicates that client is on an anticoagulant to alert staff in other departments

  9. Monitor the CBC count

  10. Investigate the use of OTC herbal products, as many of these have Coumadin-like properties and produce anticoagulant effects

E. Common drugs

  1. Warfarin sodium (Coumadin)

  2. Dicumarol (Bishydroxycoumarin)

II. Parenteral anticoagulants

A. Action

  1. Heparin: combines with antithrombin III to retard thrombin activity

  2. LMWH: a fragment of standardized heparin that binds to antithrombin III complex to prevent the ultimate conversion of fibrinogen to fibrin in the clotting cycle and prevents conversion of clotting factor X to thrombin. Advantage is that it is as effective as heparin in preventing thrombosis with fewer bleeding complications, particularly thrombocytopenia. LMWH causes less bleeding because it does not significantly change fibrinogen levels and does not significantly inhibit platelet aggregation at the site of a vascular injury.

  3. Parenteral warfarin sodium, anisindione (Miradon): same as oral warfarin sodium

B. Uses

  1. Heparin

      a. Short-term or emergency treatment

      b. All of the situations listed for oral anticoagulants

      c. Myocardial infarction (MI)

      d. After coronary artery bypass graft (CABG) surgery

      e. Hemodialysis

  2. LMWH

      a. Prophylactically, in DVT, especially after hip surgery or abdominal surgery

    b. Extended prevention of DVT for 3 weeks after hip, abdominal, or CABG surgeries

    c. Prophylaxis of ischemic complications in unstable angina and non-Q-wave MI with aspirin therapy

    d. No FDA approval for these indications: heparin-induced thrombocytopenia, ischemic stroke, catheter-induced thrombosis, and pulmonary embolism

  3. Anisindione (Miradon), the form of warfarin sodium given IV: same uses as oral anticoagulants

C. Side effects

  1. Hemorrhage (same as with oral products)

  2. Heparin-induced thrombosis: white clot syndrome

  3. Thrombocytopenia: platelets decreased to less than $150,000/mm^3$

  4. **Angioedema** (life-threatening)

⚠ WARNING!

Interactions include increased effect with acetylsalicylic acid (aspirin), alcohol, antibiotics, some OTC herbal products; decreased effect with NTG products, digoxin (Lanoxin), antihistamines, and other anticoagulants. Contraindicated in ulcers or situations threatening hemorrhage, liver, and renal diseases. Have protamine sulfate available as an antidote for heparin and some of the LMWH. No antidote at this time for LMWH: (danaparoid) Orgaran. Most of these agents are incompatible with other drugs given IV. Avoid foods containing vitamin K with anisindione (Miradon), the IV form of warfarin sodium.

D. Nursing implications

  1. Assess for bleeding in urine, stool, venipuncture sites, nose, gums, incisions (wounds)

  2. Know proper application for SC or IV route; rotate the sites for SC and do not rub the injection site

  3. Always keep continuous IV administration on a controller or pump

  4. Monitor the PT or aPTT, which should be maintained at 1.5 to 2.5 times the control for a therapeutic effect

  5. Monitor the INR: should be maintained between 2 and 3 for a therapeutic effect

  6. Let workers in other disciplines know that client is receiving a parenteral anticoagulant

  7. Instruct clients to avoid falls or abrasions to the skin, and to use caution with sharp utensils while eating. The physician should be consulted about the use of razors. Usually electric or battery-operated razors are preferred.

  8. Monitor the medication record (same as with oral products)

  9. Monitor the CBC count

 10. Instruct clients to report any signs of bleeding

E. **Common drugs**
1. Heparin sodium (Liquaemin Sodium)
2. LMWH
    a. Dalteparin (Fragmin)
    b. Danaparoid (Orgaran)
    c. Enoxaprin (Lovenox)
    d. Ardeparin (Normiflo)
3. Warfarin sodium (Coumadin), parenteral form: anisindione (Miradon)

THROMBOLYTIC AGENTS

I. Thrombolytic agents

A. **Actions: dissolve the clot by converting plasminogen to plasmin, which lyses the thrombi, and fibrinogen. Activity of the newer agents is dependent on the presence of fibrin. Minimal amounts of plasminogen are converted to plasmin in the absence of fibrin.**
B. **Uses**
1. Acute thromboembolic disorders
2. Pulmonary embolus
3. DVT
4. MI
5. Arterial or coronary thrombosis
6. Thrombi in parenteral cannulas
C. **Side effects**
1. **Hemorrhage**
2. Allergic reaction: usually with streptokinase only
3. Febrile reaction
4. CV: dysrhythmias and chest pain
5. Reocclusion: occlusion of a vessel that had been occluded and opened

> ⚠ **WARNING!**
>
> Interactions: increased tendency to bleed with any drug that alters coagulation or platelets. Contraindicated in clients with **hemophilia,** intracranial disorders, recent GI bleeds, uncontrolled HTN, high-risk situations for hemorrhage, organ biopsy, or trauma within past 10 days and in clients who bruise easily. Have the antifibrinolytic agent, aminocaproic acid (Amicar), available as an antidote. Fresh frozen plasma or cryoprecipitate can slow the bleeding by providing more clotting factors. IV NTG can compromise the effects. Can be administered with aspirin or anticoagulants; watch for hemorrhage.

D. **Nursing implications**
1. Monitor bleeding closely, especially during the loading dose period. Hidden bleeding can occur in the brain (watch for

neurologic changes) and in the retroperitoneal area (watch for findings of back pain, leg weakness, and weak peripheral pulses).
2. Know how to mix properly for IV administration. Many of these agents are expensive. IV bags that are mixed should be used within 24 hours. Carefully calculate the dosage.
3. Administer with a controller or pump, minidrip, and filter
4. Alert workers in all other disciplines that these agents were infused; post sign on client's door, on chart, or over bed if possible
5. Check with physician about all acetylsalicylic acid (aspirin) and aspirin products: additive effect will occur
6. Monitor the PT, PTT, aPTT, fibrin level, and CBC count
7. Assess the client for reperfusion dysrhythmias within the initial 1 to 2 hours of the loading dose; reoccurrence of angina may indicate reocclusion
8. Hold excess pressure for 5 to 10 minutes on all discontinued IV sites
9. Follow same safety measures for clients as with anticoagulants
10. Monitor the client carefully for hemorrhage during the 24 to 48 hours of the infusion. These agents have a short half-life, but bleeding risk may persist for 24 to 48 hours *after* infusion.
11. Know that diphenhydramine (Benadryl) or hydrocortisone sodium succinate (Solu-Cortef) may be given before streptokinase to prevent allergic reactions
12. Monitor VS every 5 to 15 minutes during infusion and notify physician if fever occurs
13. Investigate the use of OTC herbal products, since many of these have Coumadin-like properties and produce anticoagulant effects

E. Common drugs
1. Streptokinase (Streptase)
2. Alteplase (Activase), also known as t-PA
3. Urokinase (Abbokinase)
4. Anistreplase (Eminase, Retavase or r-PA)

OTHER AGENTS

I. Antiplatelet agents

A. Actions: interfere or inhibit the adherence of platelets to exposed collagen at sites of vascular injury; hinders platelet aggregation

B. Uses
1. Cerebral vascular accidents (CVA)
2. MI
3. Before or after angioplasty or coronary artery stent placements
4. Prophylactically: TIAs, prosthetic heart valves, CABG, stable or unstable angina

C. Side effects differ and are specific to the drug
1. Bleeding tendencies: bruises easily, inability to stop bleeding after minor cut

  2. Hematologic: agranulocytosis, leukopenia, thrombocytopenia
  3. GI: nausea, vomiting, cramps, and diarrhea

> ⚠ **WARNING!**
>
> Use cautiously in clients with ulcers, liver impairment, and the elderly; these agents should not be used with any condition that places the client at risk for bleeding. Many of these agents are highly protein-bound; assessment of the client's medication regimen should be made with evaluations of each medication for their therapeutic effects.

D. Nursing implications
  1. Advise clients to take these drugs with or immediately after food if GI upset occurs
  2. Monitor CBC count and PT and PTT values for increases
  3. Monitor for bleeding gums during oral care
  4. Initiate safety measures to prevent bleeding or cuts
  5. Instruct clients that they may be at risk for infection
  6. Investigate the use of OTC herbal products, since many of these have Coumadin-like properties and produce anticoagulant effects

E. Common drugs
  1. Acetylsalicylic acid (aspirin)
  2. Dipyridamole (Persantine)
  3. Ticlopidine (Ticlid)
  4. Sulfinpyrazone (Anturane)
  5. Tirofiban (Aggrastat)
  6. Clopidogrel (Plavix)
  7. Abciximab (ReoPro)

II. Hemostatic agents

A. Actions: hasten clotting of blood by inhibiting the substances that activate plasminogen and inhibit plasmin

B. Uses
  1. Stop bleeding during surgery or after a procedure
  2. Stop bleeding in emergencies
  3. Control bleeding in wound care

C. Side effects are minimal and depend on whether the agent is used topically or systemically
  1. CV: thrombophlebitis, dizziness, hypotension, bradycardia, dysrhythmias
  2. GI: nausea, vomiting, diarrhea

> ⚠ **WARNING!**
>
> Some agents may be left in the wound (Gelfoam) and are self-absorbing; others will not absorb (oxidized cellulose).

D. Nursing implications depend on the agent
  1. Know how to administer or mix the drug
  2. Assess for cessation of bleeding, which should occur within minutes

3. Monitor for signs of thrombosis, positive Homan's sign, leg or chest pain, color and temperature of skin and assess circulation to the extremities
4. Monitor vital signs: BP, HR
5. Monitor ECG for ectopy

E. Common drugs
1. Systemic agents
   a. Vitamin K (AquaMephyton)
   b. Aminocaproic acid (Amicar)
   c. Aprotinin (Traysylol)
   d. Tranexamic acid (Cyklokapron)
2. Local agents
   a. Gelfoam, Gelfilm: absorbable gelatin sponge or film
   b. Thrombin (Thrombostat)
   c. Oxidized cellulose (Surgicel)
   d. Oxidized cellulose (Oxycel)
   e. Microfibrillar collagen hemostat (Avitene)

HEMATINIC AGENTS

I. Iron products

A. Actions: replace the depleted iron stores and raise the iron level in hemoglobin

B. Uses
1. Iron deficiency anemia
2. Premature infants
3. Pregnant women
4. Lactating women
5. Bleeding disorders
6. Menses with heavy blood loss

C. Side effects
1. GI upset (most common): anorexia, nausea, vomiting, diarrhea, constipation
2. Dark stools: black or dark-green
3. Potential for staining of the teeth and the skin
4. Pain and soreness if given IM

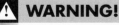 **WARNING!**

Interactions include increased absorption with ascorbic acid (vitamin C); decreased absorption with antacids, tetracyclines, and milk. Iron poisoning in children: symptoms are lethargy, vomiting, bloody diarrhea, cyanosis, and gastric and intestinal pain. Antidote for iron toxicity is deferoxamine mesylate (Desferal), given IM or IV.

D. Nursing implications
1. If given IM, use Z-track method; IM injections can stain the skin and be extremely painful

    2. Advise clients to take oral form of the drug before or after eating

    3. Instruct clients about which foods are high in iron. Refer to nursing implications under vitamin B_{12}.

    4. Have clients sip iron-containing liquids through a straw to prevent staining teeth

    5. Instruct clients about bloody, tarry stools, which are abnormal. Darker stools are normal with the intake of iron supplements.

    6. Monitor a CBC count

    7. Teach clients the symptoms of accidental poisoning: lethargy, nausea, vomiting, abdominal pain, diarrhea, pallor, cyanosis, or convulsions

E. Common drugs

    1. Ferrous sulfate (Feosol, Fer-Iron)

    2. Ferrous gluconate (Fergon, InFed)

    3. Iron dextran (Imferon, DexIron)

    4. Ferrous fumarate (Feostat)

II. Hydroxocobalamin (vitamin B_{12}-alpha)

A. Actions: replaces B_{12}-alpha not found in diet. Essential for cell growth and the nervous system.

B. Uses: treats megaloblastic anemia, a hemolytic disorder characterized by the production and peripheral proliferation of immature, large, dysfunctional erythrocytes; these megaloblasts are usually associated with severe pernicious anemia or folic-acid deficiency anemia

C. Side effects

    1. Hypersensitivity

    2. Hematologic reactions

> ⚠ **WARNING!**
>
> Monitor folate levels; large doses mask folate deficiency. Use cautiously in pregnant and lactating women. Cimetidine (Tagamet) impairs absorption.

D. Nursing implications

    1. Know that, in some conditions, the injectable form is only used because GI absorption depends on an intrinsic factor in the gastric mucosa

    2. Stress compliance: monthly injections are usually required for life

    3. Include dietary teaching about the following items:

        a. Consume foods high in iron if intrinsic factor is available from parietal cells in stomach: egg yolks, wheat germ, fish, fowl, cereal grains, dried beans, and green leafy vegetables

        b. Avoid foods low in iron: milk, vegetables that are not green and leafy

    4. Monitor CBC count for changes in hemoglobin level and hematocrit

III. Folic acid (vitamin B$_9$)

A. **Action: required for normal erythrocyte production and growth**

B. **Uses**
   1. Folic acid anemia (megaloblastic anemia)
   2. Prophylactically: pregnancy, alcoholism, renal disease, liver disease

C. **Side effect: allergic responses**

⚠ WARNING!

Interactions include decreased metabolism with anticonvulsants or contraceptives.

D. **Nursing implications**
   1. Dietary teaching to include foods rich in folic acid: bran, yeast, dried beans, nuts, fruits, fresh vegetables, asparagus
   2. Monitoring for B$_{12}$ deficiency, which may be masked

E. **Common drugs**
   1. Folic acid (Folvite)
   2. Leucovorin calcium (Wellcovorin)

IV. Human hormone for anemia

A. **Action: Stimulates the production of RBCs. It is a protein, administered IV or SC, and is the human hormone erythropoietin.**

B. **Uses: anemia with chronic renal failure. It is in the evaluation stage for use as treatment with anemias of various sources: HIV therapy and cancer therapy.**

C. **Side effects**
   1. Headaches
   2. Joint pain
   3. HTN

⚠ WARNING!

Should not be administered in individuals with uncontrolled hypertension. Abuse among athletes has been reported from the increased ability to perform because of the increased ability of RBCs to carry oxygen. Death from heart block has been reported with abuse.

D. **Nursing implications**
   1. Administer analgesic as needed for headache and joint pain
   2. Monitor BP

E. **Common drug: epoetin alfa (Epogen, Eprex, Procrit)**

WEB Resources

http://www.stjames.ie/nmic/warfarin/warfuoo.html

http://www.gradstudies.musc.edu/dentistry/top40/lecture_pages/anticoagulants.htm
   Anticoagulants

REVIEW QUESTIONS

1. A client is on warfarin sodium (Coumadin) every day at 9 AM. The laboratory result comes back with the PT four times the control. The nurse notices that the client's laboratory results were within normal limits for a therapeutic effect the day before. The nurse's first action would be to
   1. Call the physician
   2. Call the physician and prepare vitamin K
   3. Check when the laboratory sample was drawn
   4. Call the laboratory to draw another sample

2. A client has an infusion of heparin sodium (Liquaemin) for a DVT. The physician orders the dose to be lowered and starts the client on warfarin sodium (Coumadin), 5 mg PO every day. Why should the nurse be concerned about bleeding?
   1. Heparin sodium (Liquaemin) is a potent anticoagulant, and bleeding potential is high
   2. Warfarin sodium (Coumadin) has a greater risk of bleeding than heparin sodium (Liquaemin) does
   3. The warfarin sodium (Coumadin) dose is too high
   4. Heparin sodium (Liquaemin) has a short half-life, but the bleeding tendencies last beyond the half-life

3. At 4 AM, a client, who is on a heparin IV drip and has had the initial dose of warfarin sodium (Coumadin) given at 5 PM the previous day, notices oozing of blood from the IV site and at the site where the laboratory drew blood at 7 AM the previous day. The nurse would expect the physician to order which of these medications?
   1. Aminocaproic acid (Amicar)
   2. Protamine sulfate
   3. Vitamin K (AquaMephyton)
   4. Hydroxocobalamin (vitamin B_{12}-alpha)

4. A client is diagnosed with a coronary thrombosis after a heart catheterization. The physician plans to infuse alteplase (t-PA) to prevent a myocardial infarction. This medicine exerts its fibrinolytic action by which of these actions?
   1. Preventing the use of vitamin K
   2. Retarding the extension of the clot
   3. Using hemostatic action
   4. Retarding thrombin formation and lysing the clot

5. Discharge instructions for a client going home on warfarin sodium (Coumadin), 10 mg/day PO, would be which of these items?
   1. Eat plenty of foods rich in vitamin K
   2. If easier bruising is noted, stop taking the medicine and call the physician
   3. Wear a medical alert bracelet and use caution with sharp instruments
   4. Report to the physician as ordered for blood studies

ANSWERS, RATIONALES, AND TEST-TAKING TIPS

Rationales	Test-Taking Tips

1. Correct answer: 3

The laboratory sample could have been drawn after the 9 AM dose, especially since the value for the previous day was normal. A registered nurse would be expected to investigate the time the laboratory sample was drawn. The physician would need to be notified of this value if the blood sample was drawn at the proper time. Vitamin K would be needed if bleeding were to occur. The nurse would first need to check with the physician before any medication preparation or laboratory sample is drawn.

Pay attention to any information given in the stem. The clues to guide you to select option 3 are the fact that the laboratory results were within normal limits for therapy the day before and the fact that the client has been getting a daily maintenance dose of the medication. Recall that it takes warfarin 48 to 72 hours to reach a therapeutic level. Once this level is reached, the physician establishes a maintenance dose. Thus no changes were likely in the dosage. Another way to select the correct answer is to use the nursing process to do further assessment of the situation before doing an intervention.

2. Correct answer: 2

Warfarin, an oral anticoagulant, has a greater potential for bleeding than heparin. Also, the warfarin dose will be increased while the heparin dose is decreased. Option 1 is correct. However, note that the heparin dose is being lowered. Option 3 is incorrect, since the dose is within normal. Option 4 is a correct statement about thrombolytic agents, not anticoagulants.

A clue in the stem is that the heparin dose has been lowered. Eliminate option 1. Option 4 is a false statement for heparin. In deciding between options 2 and 3, if you are not certain about the dose of a medication, don't select it as an answer. Go with option 2, which is a reasonable answer. Think about the situation in a different way. Recall the length of each of the drugs' effects: heparin has an effect for 4 to 6 hours and warfarin has effects for 7 to 10 days after it is stopped. Now it is obvious which of the drugs might have more problems with bleeding, the warfarin.

3. Correct answer: 2

This is the antidote for heparin therapy, which the client has been on for a longer period of time. Both agents would

Make an educated guess. The heparin has been given the longest, so select the antidote for it, option 2.

Rationales	Test-Taking Tips

probably be stopped for a period of time. Option 1 is the antidote for thrombolytic agents. Only one dose has been given of the warfarin, which has peak action from 1 to 3 days. It's too early for warfarin to have peaked. In option 4, vitamin B_{12}-alpha does not correct bleeding tendencies.

4. Correct answer: 4

Thrombolytics dissolve or lyse clots. Option 1 is the action of oral anticoagulants. Option 2 is the action of parenteral anticoagulants. Hemostatic agents hasten the clotting of blood.

Think about what you know. The physician wants to prevent an MI, which is commonly caused by clots. Therefore it is logical to choose the option that refers to the lysing of the clot. Select option 4. Avoid making the question harder than it is because of information in the options that you may not recall or be familiar with.

5. Correct answer: 3

A medical alert bracelet is needed in case of an emergency. Cuts could result in bleeding problems and safety is needed. In option 1, a food-to-drug interaction could occur. With a high intake of vitamin K, the action of the warfarin would be hindered. The client should notify the physician before stopping an anticoagulant. A reduced dose may be all that is necessary if the client has easy bruising. A visit to the physician would probably be for a PT or aPTT level.

Eliminate option 4 since it is too general with the clue of "blood studies." Eliminate option 1 with your knowledge that vitamin K is an antidote for excessive warfarin. Eliminate option 2 since you noticed the clue "stop taking the medicine." General protocol for medication administration is to check with the physician first before discontinuation of any drug.

12

Drugs Affecting the Immune System

FAST FACTS

1. Immunity is either natural or acquired from natural or artificial sources.
2. The goals of immunization are to prevent contagious illnesses from becoming epidemic and causing serious life-changing consequences.

CONTENT REVIEW

IMMUNOLOGIC AGENTS

I. General considerations

    A. *Immunity* can be innate or acquired; natural or artificial (Table 12-1)

    B. Scheduling (Box 12-1). A current schedule of the recommended immunizations for children and adults can be retrieved from the CDC website. The updated schedule is revised after the first of each year and can be obtained from the address in the resources list at the end of the content review.

        1. Children must have a current schedule to enter and attend school in the United States

        2. Schedules should be followed as closely as possible. Schedules should be altered or exemptions granted for the following situations:

            a. An ill, febrile child

            b. An **immunosuppressed** child

            c. Use of certain medications or other recent immunizations

        3. Instruct parents to keep the immunization schedule in a safe place

    C. Public emphasis: provide pamphlets; use local health units as resources. Critical ages are between 2 and 5 years of age.

TABLE 12-1 Sources of Immunity

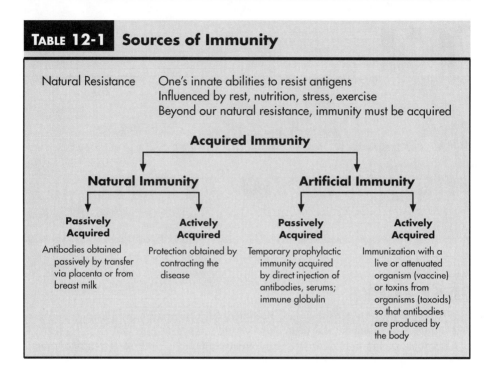

Natural Resistance	One's innate abilities to resist antigens Influenced by rest, nutrition, stress, exercise Beyond our natural resistance, immunity must be acquired

Acquired Immunity

Natural Immunity | **Artificial Immunity**

Passively Acquired	**Actively Acquired**	**Passively Acquired**	**Actively Acquired**
Antibodies obtained passively by transfer via placenta or from breast milk	Protection obtained by contracting the disease	Temporary prophylactic immunity acquired by direct injection of antibodies, serums; immune globulin	Immunization with a live or attenuated organism (vaccine) or toxins from organisms (toxoids) so that antibodies are produced by the body

D. High-risk groups
1. Unimmunized parents and children
2. Refugees and immigrants
3. Healthcare providers

E. Side effects
1. Common—teach to care provider of child and/or recipient
   a. Low-grade fever
   b. Soreness at site
   c. Joint pain
   d. Minor rash
   e. Malaise: fatigue
   f. Raised red area at site
   g. Symptoms of the disease
2. Uncommon, but more severe; report immediately
   a. Convulsions
   b. Anaphylaxis: an exaggerated, life-threatening hypersensitivity reaction
   c. Encephalitis: an inflammatory condition of the brain
   d. Serum sickness: an immunologic disorder that may occur 2 to 3 weeks after the administration of an antiserum
   e. Allergic response
   f. Guillain-Barré syndrome: an idiopathic, peripheral polyneuritis occurring between 1 and 3 weeks after a mild episode of fever

Box 12-1
2000 Immunization Schedule for Children from Birth to 16 Years

	Hep B	DTaP	IPV	Hib	MMR	Other
Birth	#1					
2 mo		#1	#1	#1		
4 mo	#2	#2	#2	#2		
6 mo		#3		#3		
12 mo	#3		#3	#4	#1	Var #1
15 mo		#4				
18 mo						
4-6 yr		#5			#2	
11-12 yr	*	Td	#4		**	***
14-16 yr						

*Hep B recommended if previously recommended doses were missed or given earlier than the recommended minimum age.
**MMR may be required by state law before admittance into kindergarten. This can be different state-to-state. CDC guidelines recommend it at 11-12 years if not taken at 4-5 years.
***Varicella should be taken at 11-12 years if not taken at the scheduled time.
Key: Hep B, hepatitis B vaccine; DTaP, diphtheria and tetanus toxoids, and acellular pertussis vaccine; IPV, inactivated poliovirus vaccine; Hib, *Haemophilus influenzae;* MMR, measles, mumps, rubella vaccines; Var, varicella vaccine; Td, tetanus and diphtheria toxoids.
Source: http://www.cdc.gov/nip/recs/child-schedule.pdf

associated with a viral infection or with immunization; characterized by an ascending paralysis from the feet up in a bilateral ascension

F. Role of the nurse
1. Know proper administration: dose, route, and site
2. Conduct a history interview to assess for these items:
   a. Allergies to eggs or egg products; if allergic to eggs, ask what type of reaction occurred; know that the live form of the immunizations cannot be used; know that giving antihistamines may be necessary before the killed form of the virus is given
   b. Current acute or febrile illness
   c. Immunosuppressive therapy in progress
   d. Recent injection of an **immune globulin** or a blood transfusion
   e. History of malignancies, antineoplastic therapy
   f. Possibility of pregnancy
3. Check the expiration date on all vials
4. Properly store immunization vials in the refrigerator or freezer, but not in the doors of the appliances
5. Change needles after drawing up the injection and always aspirate

      6. Observe the child for 30 minutes after immunization is given

      7. Properly restrain the child during the injection and be truthful about pain

      8. Report abnormal or severe reactions with the lot number and the symptoms experienced to the CDC

  G. Teach parents the following

      1. Expected and unexpected side effects, and when to call the physician

      2. How to use antipyretics for side effects

      3. Closely observe the child for the first 24 hours after the injection

      4. Encourage the child to rest for the first 24 hours after the injection

      5. Ask the nurse any questions about the injections and express any fears about harmful side effects

II. Passive immunity agents

  A. Source: serums obtained from humans or animals in which antibodies have been formed against a pathogenic organism

  B. Action: provide temporary immunity

  C. Uses: prevent infectious disease from occuring or relieve symptoms of the disease after suspected or actual exposure

  D. Side effects

      1. Hypersensitivity, allergic reaction, and anaphylaxis

      2. Local pain and erythema at the injection site

      3. Serum sickness

      4. CV: hypotension (immune globulins)

⚠ WARNING!

Many of these agents should be administered within a certain time period from exposure or a bite: consult the literature. IV administration of some of these agents should be slow (over 5 minutes). Assess for pregnancy; many of these agents should not be given if the client is expecting. Large doses may be required for some of the venoms: consult the literature.

  E. Nursing implications

      1. Perform a skin or conjunctiva hypersensitivity test (usually to horse serum)

      2. Advise parents to use acetaminophen as needed for pain

      3. Document the lot number and report serum sickness to the CDC

      4. Monitor BP in the initial 24 hours

  F. Common agents

      1. Immune globulin: exposure to hepatitis A, immunodeficiency syndromes

      2. Agents with known antibodies

          a. Hepatitis B immune globulin (HBIG): exposure to hepatitis B

          b. Tetanus immune globulin (Hyper-Tet): treatment of tetanus or prophylaxis after exposure; may be given in emergency departments for severe massive trauma or to clients with burns

     c. Varicella-zoster immune globulin (VZIG): prevention of varicella, chickenpox

     d. RhoD immune globulin (RhoGAM): for Rh-negative pregnant women or women who deliver an Rh-positive baby

     e. Vaccine immune globulin: for prevention of vaccine infection

3. **Antitoxins** and **antivenins**

     a. Antitoxin: an agent prepared from the serum of horses immunized against a particular toxin-producing organism

       (1) Diphtheria antitoxin: treatment of diphtheria

       (2) Tetanus antitoxin: treatment of tetanus when immune globulin is not available

     b. Antivenin: a suspension of venom-neutralizing antibodies prepared from the serum of immunized horses

       (1) Rabies immune globulin: exposure to rabies

       (2) Antivenin for snake and spider bites

III. Active immunity agents

    A. *Vaccines:* **biologic agents that stimulate antibodies to be produced in the body. Clue: remember the "a" in vaccine refers to active immunity; the body acts to produce antibodies and it takes about 2 to 3 weeks.**

1. Live vaccine: live microorganisms that are altered but will still multiply in the body over time and cause a reaction

     a. Measles, mumps, rubella (MMR)

     b. Poliovirus (Sabin, OPV), used only in special circumstances to eliminate the risk of vaccine-associated paralytic polio (VAPP). Refer to CDC web site.

     c. Yellow fever

2. **Attenuated vaccines**: microorganisms that are killed, inactivated, or altered in such a way that their virulence is reduced

     a. *Hemophilus influenzae* **vaccine (Hib)**

     b. **Hepatitis B vaccine (Heptavax, HBV)**

     c. Inactivated poliovirus vaccine (IPV)

     d. Influenza vaccine

     e. Rabies vaccine

     f. Cholera vaccine

     g. Typhoid vaccine

     h. Rubella vaccine: instruct women to wait at least 3 months before attempting to get pregnant

     i. Havarix vaccine: for hepatitis A

     j. Varivax vaccine: for chicken pox

     k. BCG vaccine (TICE BCG): for tuberculosis (TB)

     l. DTaP vaccine: diphtheria, tetanus toxoid, and acellular pertussis vaccine, or DTP (whole-cell diphtheria, tetanus, and pertussis vaccine)

     m. Pneumococci polyvalent vaccine: for pneumonia

B. **Toxoids: toxins that have been treated to eliminate the toxic properties but retain the ability to stimulate antibodies**
   1. Tetanus toxoid: administer every 10 years
   2. Diphtheria toxoid
   3. Diphtheria, tetanus, pertussis (DTP)
   4. Diphtheria and tetanus (Td): recommended for 7-year-olds, teens, and adults
C. **Uses: prevent the occurrence of specific communicable diseases and infectious processes**
D. **Side effects**
   1. Low-grade fever, joint pain, minor rash and malaise
   2. Soreness and raised red area at the site
   3. Uncommon: convulsions, anaphylaxis, encephalitis, serum sickness, allergic response, Guillain-Barré syndrome

> ⚠️ **WARNING!**
>
> Check the expiration date on all vials. Teach the parents to observe the child for the first 24 hours for any changes. Avoid immunizing ill or immunosuppressed children.

E. **Nursing implications**
   1. Teach the parents about the recommended schedule. Use pamphlets to educate.
   2. Teach about the common side effects, to encourage rest and to use acetaminophen for minor discomforts
   3. Report any uncommon reactions to the CDC
   4. Observe the child for 30 minutes after the injection is given
   5. Check for allergies to eggs before the injection is given. If allergic to eggs, the agent in the live form cannot be given. If the killed form is given, antihistamine agents may be given before the injection to minimize or prevent allergic reactions.
   6. Recall tip: *va*ccine has an *a*ctive immunity

IMMUNOSUPPRESSIVE AND IMMUNOMODULATING AGENTS

I. Immunosuppressive agents
A. **Action: lessen or prevent an immune response. Specific drug groups also act as immunosuppressive agents and are discussed in other chapters: corticosteroids, antimetabolites, and certain antibiotics.**
B. **Uses: organ transplantation and autoimmune diseases**
C. **Side effects**
   1. Infections
   2. Cancerous lymphomas
   3. GI: nausea, vomiting
   4. Hematologic: anemias, leukopenia, thrombocytopenia
   5. Irritation at IV site

> ⚠️ **WARNING!**
>
> Contraindications: live vaccines, combination immunosuppressive therapy. Serum sickness can occur 2 to 3 weeks after therapy: fever, skin rash, joint pain, swollen lymph nodes.

D. Nursing implications

1. Monitor CBC count and liver enzymes: AST, ALT, GGT
2. Assess for transplant rejection and signs of infection, report fever of 99° F or higher
3. Advise to give oral forms with food or milk to reduce GI upset
4. Monitor IV site carefully; avoid extravasation
5. Frequently assess major body systems, including oral cavity
6. Monitor CBC count for drops in hemoglobin level and hematocrit, WBC count, and platelets

E. Common drugs

1. Azathioprine (Imuran)
2. Tacrolimus (FK506, Prograf)
3. Muromonab-CD3 (Orthoclone OKT3)
4. Cyclosporine (Sandimmune)
5. Mycophenolate mofetil (CellCept)

II. Immunomodulating agents

A. Interferons

1. Action: possess antiviral and antineoplastic effects, directly inhibit effects on DNA and protein synthesis, and increase cancer cell antigens on the cell surface, thus enabling the immune system to recognize the cancer cells more easily. These actions stop virus replication and prevent penetration into healthy cells. They enhance the action of other cells of the immune system and stop the division of cancer cells.

2. Uses
   a. Treatment of viral infections: rhinovirus, papillovirus, retrovirus, hepatitis, condyloma—a wart-like growth in the perineal area; transmitted sexually
   b. Treatment of various cancers: Kaposi's sarcoma, multiple myeloma, renal cell carcinoma, melanoma, bladder cancer, T-cell lymphoma
   c. Treatment of some autoimmune diseases: multiple sclerosis

3. Side effects
   a. Flu-like effects: fever, chills, headache, malaise, myalgia, and fatigue
   b. GI: nausea, vomiting, diarrhea, anorexia
   c. CNS: dizziness, confusion, paranoia
   d. CV: tachycardia, cyanosis, tachypnea
   e. Hematologic: neutropenia, thrombocytopenia
   f. Renal: increased BUN and creatinine levels, proteinuria, altered results on liver function tests

> **⚠ WARNING!**
>
> Interactions can occur with aminophylline therapy, and there are additive effects with other antiviral agents

4. Nursing implications
   a. Assess allergies to egg proteins or neomycin. If allergic, then these substances are not given. However, if the allergic reaction to eggs or neomycin was mild, such as a rash, and these substances are required for therapy, they may be given along with antihistamines to prevent severe reactions.
   b. Monitor CBC count, renal studies
   c. Monitor VS at each visit
   d. Caution the client about the potential for bleeding and infections
   e. Implement safety precautions if CNS effects occur
   f. Use nonopoid analgesics as needed for flulike symptoms
5. Common drugs
   a. Interferon-alfa (Roferon-A, Alferon N)
   b. Interferon-beta (Betaseron)
   c. Interferon-gamma (Actimunne)

B. Interleukins (or lymphokines)
1. Action: enhances multiplication of the activated killer T-cell, which recognizes cancer cells as nonself and ignores normal cells, thus destroying cancer cells; also increases production of B-cells
2. Uses
   a. Renal cell carcinoma
   b. Malignant melanoma
   c. Colorectal adenocarcinoma
   d. Limited use in Hodgkin's disease, cancer of the female reproductive organs, and lung cancer
3. Side effects
   a. Severe toxicity caused by capillary leak syndrome: capillaries lose their ability to retain important proteins and other essential components of blood vessels. The leaking of these substances into the surrounding tissue causes fluid retention (weight gain of 20 to 30 pounds) with edema.
   b. Fluid retention can lead to: CHF, arrhythmias, MI
   c. Flu-like symptoms: fever, chills, rash, fatigue, headache, myalgias

> **⚠ WARNING!**
>
> Interaction can occur with antihypertensives, corticosteroids, several of the chemotherapeutic agents and antibiotics.

4. Nursing implications
   a. Monitor fluid balance: I&O, weight gain, edema
   b. Treat flulike symptoms as necessary with nonopioid analgesics
5. Common drug: aldesleukin (Proleukin)

C. Colony-stimulating factors (CSFs)

1. Action: bind to receptors on the cell surface of the bone marrow, decrease the length of neutropenia after chemotherapy, inhibit the decrease in neutrophil counts from toxic chemotherapeutic agents, and stimulate certain immune cells, which serve to destroy tumor cells, viruses, and fungi

2. Uses
   a. Reduce the incidence and duration of infections
   b. In combination with chemotherapeutic agents, allow larger doses to be given in cancer
   c. Bone marrow transplants and radiation therapy
   d. Viral and fungal infections

3. Side effects (mild)
   a. CV: hypertension and edema
   b. GI: anorexia, nausea, vomiting, diarrhea
   c. Respiratory: cough, dyspnea, sore throat
   d. Hematologic: blood dyscrasias
   e. Comfort: headache, fever, bone pain

 WARNING!

Interactions may occur with antineoplastics.

4. Nursing implications
   a. Monitor BP and signs of edema
   b. Assess lung sounds, RR, productive or nonproductive cough
   c. Monitor CBC count
   d. Treat minor ailments with a nonopioid analgesic
   e. Assess for fatigue level
   f. Teach how to handle the syringes and needles, if taken at home

5. Common drugs
   a. Epoetin alfa (human recombinant erythropoietin) (Procrit or Epogen), increases hemoglobin level and hematocrit
   b. Filgrastim (Neupogen), increases neutrophil count
   c. Sargramostim (Leukine)

III. Drugs used to treat AIDS

A. Nucleoside inhibitors or reverse transcriptase inhibitors

1. Action: Inhibits reverse transcriptase, which is needed to convert RNA into DNA in HIV infection. HIV is a retrovirus, meaning that the genetic code is introduced opposite of a human gene (DNA → RNA).

2. Uses
   a. HIV infections, both early onset and advanced stages
   b. Lower transmission of HIV from mother to fetus

3. Side effects
   a. Toxicity: granulocytopenia and anemia
   b. Neurotoxicity: headache, insomnia, muscle pain, and nausea

   c. Overdose: anemia, fatigue, leukopenia, severe nausea, thrombocytopenia, vomiting, seizures

> ⚠ **WARNING!**
>
> Incidences have occurred in which these agents were taken in excess as a suicide attempt in HIV-infected individuals. Interactions can occur with other bone marrow depressants and certain antibiotics. Toxicity that occurs from the drugs may be difficult to distinguish from the symptoms of HIV infection.

   4. Nursing implications
      a. Monitor CBC count
      b. Perform a baseline neurologic assessment and check periodically thereafter
      c. Monitor the effectiveness of the drug and the amount taken
   5. Common drugs
      a. Zidovudine (Retrovir)
      b. Didanosine (Videx)
      c. Lamivudine (Epivir)
      d. Stavudine (Zerit)
      e. Zalcitabine (HIVID)
B. Nonnucleoside reverse transcriptase inhibitors
   1. Action: binds with the reverse transcriptase and inhibits the enzyme
   2. Uses: combination therapy with nucleoside inhibitors, reverse transcriptase inhibitors, or protease inhibitors
   3. Side effects
      a. GI: diarrhea, nausea
      b. Skin rashes
      c. Neurologic: headache

> ⚠ **WARNING!**
>
> Should be avoided in clients with impaired liver function. Interacts with benzodiazepines, calcium channel blockers, protease inhibitors, anticonvulsants, and cimetidine (Tagamet). The drug should *never* be used alone, because resistance develops rapidly.

   4. Nursing implications
      a. Administer antiemetic or antidiarrheal as needed
      b. Administer nonopioid analgesic as needed
      c. Assess liver function and liver enzymes before therapy
   5. Common drugs
      a. Delavirdine mesylate (Rescriptor)
      b. Efavirenz (Sustiva)

C. **Protease inhibitors**
   1. Action: inhibits the binding of the enzyme protease, which is needed for the HIV protein to mature. These agents act only during viral replication.
   2. Use: only for HIV infection, may be combined with nucleoside or reverse transcriptase inhibitors
   3. Side effects
      a. Kidney stones
      b. GI: abdominal pain, diarrhea, nausea, vomiting, altered sense of taste
      c. Neurologic: headache, insomnia, weakness

> ⚠ **WARNING!**
>
> Cautious use with clients having liver impairment. Interactions include toxicity of drugs activated by CYP3A4 (a liver enzyme). Should never be given at the same time as didanosine (Videx).

   4. Nursing implications
      a. Assess urine color, consistency, and ease in urinating
      b. Administer antiemetic, antidiarrheal as needed
      c. Implement safety measures in case of weakness
      d. Encourage sedatives and nonopoid analgesics as needed
   5. Common drugs
      a. Indinavir (Crixivan)
      b. Nelfinavir (Viracept)
      c. Ritonavir (Norvir)
      d. Saquinavir (Invirase)
D. **Antivirals (see Chapter 16, p. 269)**

WEB Resources

http://www.vaccines.com

http://dir.yahoo.com/Health/Medicine/Immunology/Immunizations/Vaccines/
   For a variety of choices.

http://www.cdc.gov/nip/publications/VIS/
   For a discussion of individual vaccines.

http://www.cdc.gov/health/diseases.htm
   About various diseases/immune system information.

http://www.cdc.gov/nip/recs/adult-schedule.pdf
   Adult immunization schedule (*Adobe* reader is needed for most items at CDC and can be downloaded from http://www.adobe.com).

http://www.cdc.gov/nip/recs/adult-schedule.pdf
   Childhood immunization schedule (*Adobe* reader is needed).

REVIEW QUESTIONS

1. A frantic mother calls the nurse at the physician's office. She states that her child is very sleepy, has a temperature of 100.4°F, and has a raised red area on his leg where he recently received the MMR (measles, mumps, rubella) injection. What should the nurse tell her?
   1. That these side effects are serious, so the child needs to be brought in to see the physician
   2. That these side effects are common, and she should call if the temperature goes above 102°F or if she cannot arouse the child
   3. That she is overreacting and should not panic
   4. That these side effects are common, so she should not be concerned at all

2. A client, age 22, accidentally falls into a hay baler while working on a farm. He has multiple deep wounds and requires surgery. A tetanus toxoid would be given based on which of these client responses in reference to the last tetanus shot?
   1. "I can't remember, but it was less than 5 years"
   2. "I can't remember, but it was less than 10 years"
   3. "I know I am up-to-date; I had an injection 2 years ago"
   4. "I think it was 3 years ago"

3. A client plans to become pregnant and wants to plan everything just right. She receives rubella as a prevention and calls the public health nurse to ask when she should begin trying to get pregnant. The nurse should suggest trying:
   1. No sooner than 3 months
   2. Whenever you feel like it
   3. No sooner than 2 months
   4. No sooner than 6 months

4. Blood work results on a 17-year-old client who had a stillbirth are normal. She is Rh-negative. The autopsy reveals the baby was Rh-positive. Which of these medications should she receive?
   1. Hepatitis B immune globulin (HBIG)
   2. *Haemophilus influenzae* vaccine (Hib)
   3. RhoD immune globulin (RhoGAM)
   4. Hepatitis B vaccine (Heptavax)

5. A client is concerned about having the current immunization schedule for a 13-month-old daughter. She calls the nurse at the health unit and asks which "shots" the daughter should have received by this time. What is the nurse's best answer?
   1. 3 DTP, 1 MMR, Tb, 3 HBV
   2. 2 DTP, Tb, 2 IPV, 3 HBV
   3. 3 DTP, 3 Hib, 2 IPV, 2 HBV
   4. 3 DTP, 3 Hib, Td, 2 IPV, 3 HBV

ANSWERS, RATIONALES, AND TEST-TAKING TIPS

Rationales	Test-Taking Tips

1. Correct answer: 2

These findings in the stem are common effects from MMR injection. Acetaminophen (Tylenol), rest, and normal movement of the leg are the best treatment. The information in option 1 is not correct and would panic an already frantic mother. Simple instructions would work best. Never tell a worried mother that she is overreacting. Concern is always warranted, but panic is unnecessary at this time.

Note that options 2 and 4 are similar. If trying to decide between the two options, be alerted to the clue in option 4: "not be concerned...at all." The inclusion of this absolute leads you to select option 2.

2. Correct answer: 2

With a multiple trauma or burns of more than 5 years ago, another injection is usually needed for prophylactic reasons. Injections are routinely given every 10 years. With an unknown or questionable date, injections are usually give for prophylactic reasons.

Write down for each of the options the length of time elapsed since the clients last tetanus shot. Option 1, less than 5 years; option 2, less than 10; option 3, 2 years ago; and option 4, 3 years ago. Therefore, select the longest time out. The question asks for the item to base your decision to give the shot.

3. Correct answer: 1

A 3-month wait from the time of the rubella immunization is recommended in the literature to prevent any complications to the fetus. Pregnancy too soon after injection could cause complications during the pregnancy or abnormalities in the baby. A 2-month wait is not long enough. A 6-month wait is too long.

Use the number approach if you have no idea of a correct answer. Eliminate option 2, which is known to be incorrect, since substances in vaccines, especially live forms, are teratogenic. Throw out the smallest and largest numbers, 2 and 6 months. Select 3 months in option 1.

4. Correct answer: 3

RhoD immune globulin provides temporary immunity from

Use common sense after rereading the stem. There is no information in the

Rationales	Test-Taking Tips

antibodies received from the child, and it protects the mother and the next baby from the incompatibility of the blood. It is passive-acquired immunity. In option 1, HBIG is to provide temporary immunity if there is contact with hepatitis B. It is passive-acquired immunity, the direct injection of antibodies in the form of an "immune globulin." Hib is to prevent infection from *Haemophilus influenzae*, which is serious in children and older adults. It is active-acquired immunity; the body has to actively produce its own antibodies within 2 to 3 weeks. Heptavax provides active-acquired immunity against hepatitis B. It is a series of 3 injections: the initial, then at 1 to 3 months from the first injection, and at 6 months from the initial dose.

stem about hepatitis or influenza, so the only possible answer is option 3.

5. Correct answer: 4

The schedule in option 4 is correct based on the child's age. The schedule in option 1 is incorrect for the child's age; the MMR is scheduled too soon. In option 2, for the child's age there should have been three DTP and three Hib injections. In option 3, for the child's age the HBV should be complete to a total of three; the Td is also needed.

The easiest way to remember the immunization injections for a 12-month-old is to list the numbers of option 4, which are 3, 3, 3, 2, 1. Then place the tests alphabetically to match the numbers DTP, HBV, HIB, IPV, and Td. These shots total 12 in number (add them up for yourself). Associate a 12-month-old with this group of injections, which total 12. Eliminate options 1 and 2 that have "Tb," which is not a type of immunization.

13

Drugs Affecting the Endocrine System

FAST FACTS

1. Evaluation of the effectiveness of these drugs is completed by clinical assessment for changes in the following (listed in order of priority):
   - LOC: irritability, agitation with hypoglycemia; drowsiness, confusion with hyperglycemia
   - HR, heart rhythm: increase or decrease, irregular or regular, palpitations
   - BP: hypotension or **HTN**
   - RR and respiratory depth: pattern, crackles
   - GU: Output greater than or less than intake; daily weight; urine positive for glucose level
   - GI: nausea, vomiting, anorexia, dry mouth, constipation
   - Laboratory tests: hormone and drug levels, CBC count, electrolytes (K, Mg, Na); creatinine, BUN, glucose levels
2. General: malaise, headache, faintness, skin turgor or rash, moon face, mood swings, tremors.
3. Insulin lispro (Humalog), an insulin analog, has an onset of 15 minutes, peaks in 40 to 60 minutes with a half-life of 46 minutes. It must be given 15 minutes before meals, so that the peak action coincides with the client's peak glucose level after the meal.

CONTENT REVIEW

OVERVIEW

I. Disorders of the endocrine system can result in:

   A. Hyperfunction of the endocrine system: where too much of a hormone is secreted or produced, or side effects are occurring from

medications for hypofunction. These are: thyrotoxicosis, hyperglycemia, hyperthyroidism, hyperparathyroidism.

B. **Hypofunction of the endocrine system:** where not enough of a hormone is secreted or produced or side effects are occurring from medications for hyperfunction. These are: Addison's disease, cretinism, hypoparathyroidism, hypoglycemia, hypothyroidism.

PITUITARY HORMONES

I. Anterior pituitary hormones (Box 13-1)

A. **Growth hormone**
   1. Action: increases cellular size and rate of growth
   2. Use: pituitary dwarfism
   3. Side effects
      a. Development of antibodies
      b. Gigantism, excessively rapid growth
      c. Hyperglycemia (diabetogenic effect)
      d. Sodium retention and edema

> **WARNING!**
>
> Contraindicated with concurrent use of glucocorticoids, which may hinder growth. Failure to grow may be from other factors, such as hypothyroidism, and should be treated if diagnosed.

   4. Nursing implications
      a. Monitor effects of the drug: height, weight, head circumference
      b. Give by injection only and mix with sterile water
      c. Assess glucose level; monitor for insulin resistance
      d. Monitor x-rays for bone development
      e. Monitor I&O and check for presence of generalized edema
   5. Common drugs
      a. Somatrem (Protropin)
      b. Somatropin (Humatrope, Nutropin)
      c. Octreotide acetate (Sandostatin)
      d. Bromocriptine (Parlodel)

Box 13-1
Anterior Pituitary Hormones

Somatotropin or growth hormone (GH)
Thyrotropin or thyroid-stimulating hormone (TSH)
Corticotropin or adrenocorticotropic hormone (ACTH)
Gonadotropins
   Follicle-stimulating hormone (FSH)
   Luteinizing hormone (LH), also called interstitial-stimulating hormone (ICSH)

B. **Corticotropin—ACTH (Acthar)**
1. Actions: controls cortisol release and assists in dealing with stress
2. Uses
    a. Diagnosis of adrenal insufficiency
    b. Myasthenia gravis
    c. Rheumatic disease
    d. Multiple sclerosis
3. Side effects
    a. Allergic reactions
    b. Acne
    c. CNS: mood swings, depression, euphoria, and nervousness
    d. Sodium retention, potassium loss, hyperglycemia
    e. Cushing's syndrome (from excess hormone)
    f. Suppression of immune system response

> ⚠ **WARNING!**
>
> These agents may cause muscle weakness in clients with myasthenia gravis. Any unusual bleeding or bruising should be reported.

4. Nursing implications
    a. Monitor for allergic response
    b. Promptly treat any signs of infection or fever of more than 99°F
    c. Monitor electrolyte and glucose levels
    d. Implement sensitivity testing before the first dose
    e. Inject these agents deeply into the gluteal muscle

C. **Thyroid-stimulating hormone (TSH)**
1. Actions
    a. Controls functional activity of the thyroid gland
    b. Increases production and release of the thyroid hormone
2. Use: diagnosing hypothyroidism
3. Side effects
    a. CV: cardiac arrhythmias, particularly atrial fibrillation, because thyroid hormones increase the cardiac contractility and heart rate
    b. Anaphylactic reactions, because of the cardiostimulant effect

> ⚠ **WARNING!**
>
> Contraindicated in clients with cardiac compromise and Addison's disease. There should be no physiologic response if the client has thyroid failure; a response occurs if there is pituitary failure and normal thyroid function.

4. Nursing implications
    a. Monitor cardiac status; ECG pattern, HR for increases or decreases, irregular rhythm
    b. Assess for allergic reaction: respiratory distress, itching, hives
    c. Give the first dose slowly and observe for complications

5. Common drugs
   a. Thyrotropin (Thytropar)
   b. Protirelin (Relefact TRH)

II. Posterior pituitary hormone (Box 13-2)

A. **Oxytocics: oxytocin**
   1. Actions
      a. Causes vasopressor activity
      b. Decreases urine output
      c. Increases water absorption
   2. Uses
      a. Diabetes insipidus
      b. GI bleeds
      c. Induction of labor for term babies
      d. Promotion of milk letdown and uterine involution
   3. Side effects
      a. CV: hypertension
      b. Water intoxication
      c. GI: nausea, vomiting
      d. Fetal complications during labor

   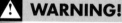 **WARNING!**

   Contraindicated in renal, CV disease, or severe toxemia.

   4. Nursing implications
      a. Monitor fetal activity: fetal heart tones (FHT), contractions, VS, especially for an increase in BP
      b. Monitor fluid status, I&O
      c. Administer antiemetics as needed if client is receiving nothing by mouth (NPO)
      d. Know that these drugs should never be given undiluted and should be maintained on an IV pump
   5. Common drugs
      a. Oxytocin (Pitocin, Syntocinon)
      b. Oxytocin citrate (Pitocin Citrate)

B. **Oxytocics: ergot alkaloids**
   1. Actions
      a. Contract smooth muscle, primarily on the uterus and blood vessels, with the greatest effect at term and postpartum
      b. Peripheral vasoconstriction

Box 13-2
Posterior Pituitary Hormones

Vasopressin or antidiuretic hormone (ADH)
Oxytocin

    c. Antihypertensive effect

    d. Alpha-adrenergic blockade

  2. Uses

    a. Production of uterine contractions

    b. Postpartal bleeding

    c. Migraine headaches

    d. Hypertension

  3. Side effects

    a. GI: nausea, vomiting, dry mouth from increased urinary output

    b. CV: increased BP

    c. **Ergotism**: cerebrospinal manifestations, such as spasms, cramps, dry gangrene

  4. Nursing implications

    a. Advise clients to take with or immediately after food

    b. Monitor I&O, encourage fluids

    c. Monitor VS and report increases in BP

    d. Monitor for spasms, headaches, cramps, dry gangrene; these indicate a need to reduce the dosage

  5. Common drugs

    a. Ergonovine maleate (Ergotrate Maleate)

    b. Ergotamine tartraye (Ergostat)

    c. Methylergonovine (Methergine)

C. Vasopressin: antidiuretic hormone (ADH)

  1. Action: maintains normal osmotic pressure and volume in the extracellular fluid (ECF) by regulating the amount of water absorbed at the renal distal tubule

  2. Uses

    a. Hormone replacement in diabetic clients

    b. Hemorrhage control

    c. Hypotension

    d. Diagnostically to determine the ability of the kidneys to concentrate urine

    e. Replacement therapy after head injury with diabetes insipidus

    f. Abdominal distention

  3. Side effects

    a. Comfort: irritation to tissue or vein, pain at injection site

    b. Fluid balance: water intoxication and hyponatremia

    c. CV: hypertension, anginal pain

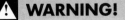 **⚠ WARNING!**

These agents are usually contraindicated in clients with severe cardiac conditions. Give with caution in elderly clients.

  4. Nursing implications

    a. Monitor VS for sustained rises in BP above 140/90 mm Hg; monitor ECG; assess for anginal pain

    b. Assess for weight changes; I&O

    c. Assess for signs of water intoxication; hyponatremia and decreased urine output

    d. Avoid extravasation of IV dosage forms; give deep IM. The IV forms must be rotated, gently shaken, and warmed completely to mix all the particles before administration. Note: may be given nasally, especially with long-term therapy.

  5. Common drugs

    a. Desmopressin acetate (DDAVP), usually nasally

    b. Vasopressin (Pitressin), may be given IM or IV

THYROID AND PARATHYROID HORMONES

I. Parathyroid hormone (Box 13-3)

A. Action: maintains calcium (Ca) levels in the blood by affecting the absorption of Ca from the gut and bone. Tip: The serum phosphate level changes in the opposite direction of the Ca level.

B. Agents for hypoparathyroidism: a deficiency of parathyroid hormone (PTH) that causes a low Ca level and high phosphate level (as in tetany, cardiac arrhythmias, neuromuscular irritability)

  1. Action: raises calcium and lowers phosphate

  2. Use: treat hypocalcemia

  3. Side effects

    a. Azotemia: excess nitrogenous waste in the blood with elevated serum BUN level

    b. Renal failure

    c. CV: hypotension and bradycardia

    d. Hypercalcemia

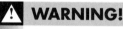 **WARNING!**

Check for allergies. Never mix calcium salts with bicarbonates, phosphates, or sulfates.

Box 13-3
Hormones Influencing Overall Function

Thyroid
    Thyroxine (T_3), triiodothyronine (T_4), calcitonin
Parathyroid
    Parathormone (PTH)
Pancreas
    Insulin, glucagon
Adrenals
    Mineralocorticoids, glucocorticoids

4. Nursing implications
   a. Monitor BUN for elevations over 20 mg/dl; creatinine levels over 1.2 mg/dl
   b. Monitor for signs of hypercalcemia: thirst, anorexia, polyuria, nausea, vomiting
   c. Monitor I&O
   d. Monitor BP for systolic readings below 90 mm Hg and ECG pattern for a drop in rate to less than 60 beats/min and symptoms of: dizziness, nausea, diaphoresis, blurred vision
5. Common drugs
   a. Calcium products
      (1) Calcium chloride
      (2) Calcium gluconate (Kalcinate)
   b. Vitamin D products
      (1) Ergocalciferol (Calciferol)
      (2) Calcifediol (Calderol)

C. **Agents for hyperparathyroidism: an excess of parathyroid hormone, which causes a high Ca level and low phosphate level**
   1. Action: lowers Ca and raises phosphate
   2. Use: treat hypercalcemia
   3. Side effects
      a. Flushing of the face
      b. Inflammation at site of injection
      c. GI: nausea, vomiting
      d. Hypocalcemia

> ⚠️ **WARNING!**
>
> Check for allergies. Nausea and vomiting may be a symptom of an overdose of antihyperparathyroidism agents.

4. Nursing implications
   a. Monitor for inflammation carefully
   b. Teach the client that nausea and vomiting usually occur with initial therapy and lessens as treatment continues
   c. Monitor for signs of hypocalcemia: tingling about the mouth or at fingertips, muscle twitching or spasms, tetany
5. Common drugs
   a. Calcitonin (Cibacalcin)
   b. Calcitonin-salmon (Calcimar)
   c. Etidronate disodium (Didronel)

II. Thyroid hormones (see Box 13-3)

A. **Thyroid agents for hypothyroidism**
   1. Action: replace missing thyroid hormones, synthetic or natural preparations of T_3 or T_4. Thyroid hormone is necessary for all cell metabolism.

2. Uses: treat decreased activity of the thyroid gland
    a. **Myxedema** (greater incidence in adults over age 50)
    b. Cretinism (congenital hypothyroidism)
3. Side effects
    a. CV: palpitations, tachycardia, angina
    b. CNS: nervousness, irritability, insomnia
    c. Weight loss
    d. Thyrotoxicosis **(or thyroid storm):** extreme hyperthyroidism or the sudden secretion of thyroid hormone in greater-than-normal amounts. In *hyper*thyroidism, in general, all body functions *increase,* except weight decreases.

> ⚠️ **WARNING!**
>
> Give dose carefully, usually small amounts in micrograms. Interactions: a decrease in the effectiveness of antidiabetic agents, increase in effectiveness of oral anticoagulants.

4. Nursing implications
    a. Encourage compliance with a single morning dose at breakfast to prevent sleep interferences
    b. Teach signs and symptoms of hypothyroidism and hyperthyroidism
    c. Hold if HR is more than 100 beats/min when taken for a full minute; take apical pulse
    d. Monitor HR, BP, and ECG
    e. Monitor weight and report loss in the absence of an attempt to reduce weight
5. Common drugs
    a. Levothyroxine sodium (Synthroid)
    b. Lithyronine (Cytomel)
    c. Liotrix (Thyrolar)
B. **Antithyroid agents for hyperthyroidism**
    1. Actions: lower the thyroid level by three mechanisms
        a. Interfere with the hormone production: iodine must be present in the body for thyroid hormone synthesis. A high dose of iodine **(iodism)** has a suppressant effect and causes a decrease in the production of thyroid hormone.
        b. Modify the response to the hormone by blocking the synthesis of thyroid hormone
        c. Destroy the gland: radioactive preparations destroy the thyroid tissue, thereby decreasing the production of thyroid hormone
    2. Uses: treat increased activity of the thyroid gland
        a. Hyperthyroidism (Grave's disease)
        b. Thyrotoxicosis, or thyroid storm

3. Side effects
   a. Granulocytopenia: decrease in number of granulocytes in the blood
   b. Hypersensitivity
   c. Iodism: excess iodine in the body manifested by increased thirst; burning, brassy taste in the mouth
   d. Weight gain
   e. Myxedema coma: severe hypothyroidism leads to coma or death
   f. In *hypo*thyroidism, in general, all body functions *decrease,* except weight increases

 WARNING!

These agents are contraindicated in pregnancy. Avoid OTC medications because they may contain iodine.

4. Nursing implications
   a. Dilute liquid iodine preparations in water and encourage use of a straw to prevent staining of the teeth
   b. Teach the client about hypothyroidism and hyperthyroidism. Thyroid storm is characterized by fever, tachycardia, CHF, and CNS changes.
   c. Monitor VS for sudden declines or elevations and body weight changes
   d. Teach client follow-up is needed to evaluate for hypothyroidism
5. Common drugs
   a. *Antithyroid drugs*: takes about 3 weeks for a desired response
      (1) Methimazole (Tapazole)
      (2) Propylthiouracil (PTU)
   b. *Iodides*
      (1) Strong iodine solution (Lugol's solution)
      (2) Potassium iodide solution (SSKI, Thyro-Block)
   c. *Radioactive iodine* (sodium iodide, iodine-^{131}I Iodotope) requires avoidance of extended contact with children, spouse, and coworkers for 1 week. Clients should refrain from coughing or expectoration for the first 24 hours, since the saliva and emesis are highly radioactive for the first 6 to 8 hours after the dose is taken. Fluids should be increased up to 3 to 4 L/day for the first 48 hours to help with the excretion of the agent. Clients should void frequently during this initial 48 hours to prevent a radiation effect on the gonads. Some authors suggest clients flush the toilet twice after each voiding. No restriction of the bathroom use is necessary for others in the family.
   d. *Beta-adrenergic blockers*: propranolol (Inderal) controls the symptoms of hyperthyroidism but does not lower T_3 and T_4 release.

ADRENAL HORMONES

I. Glucocorticoids (see Box 13-3, p. 216)

A. **Actions**
  1. Increase carbohydrate, protein, and fat metabolism
  2. Exhibit anti-inflammatory properties
  3. Suppress the normal immune response

B. **Uses**
  1. Topical and systemic inflammation
  2. Allergic disorders
  3. Collagen and rheumatic disorders
  4. Fractures, impaired healing
  5. Shock, cerebral edema
  6. Replacement in adrenal cortical insufficiency and Addison's disease
  7. Eye diseases
  8. Asthma
  9. Acute leukemia
  10. Skin disorders

C. **Side effects**
  1. Cushingoid findings
     a. Buffalo hump: accumulation of fat on the back of the neck from prolonged use of corticosteroids
     b. Moon face: rounded, puffy face from prolonged use of corticosteroids
     c. Cushingoid signs and symptoms: having the habitus and facies characteristic of Cushing's syndrome, which is characterized by excess cortisol
  2. Immunosuppressant effect: inability of the immune system to respond to antigenic stimulation from an inhibition of the cellular and humoral immunity
  3. Growth retardation, muscle wasting
  4. Hyperglycemia: blood glucose of more than 120 mg/dl
  5. Hypokalemia
  6. Mood swings
  7. Sterility
  8. CV: dysrhythmias, tachycardia (most common); HTN: blood pressure of 140/90 mm Hg or higher
  9. Inhibited protein synthesis

> ### ⚠ WARNING!
>
> Increased need for insulin or oral hypoglycemic agents may occur. Contraindicated in clients with TB or peptic ulcers (may worsen the disease).

D. **Nursing implications**
  1. Monitor for short-term use only; stress the severe side effects from long-term use

2. Teach that these drugs should not be abruptly withdrawn; taper off slowly over a 1- to 2-week period
3. Encourage a diet rich in protein and potassium
4. Schedule blood samples to be drawn at 7 AM and/or 4 PM to measure steroid level to determine hypofunction or hyperfunction of the adrenal gland
5. Monitor daily weight and teach client to weigh themselves because of the action of the drug. Report a weight gain of more than 5 pounds per day or week.
6. Advise client to wear a medical alert tag
7. Monitor and treat signs of inflammation immediately
8. Monitor HR and BP carefully; monitor ECG pattern
9. Monitor blood glucose, potassium, and protein levels at regular intervals

E. Common drugs
1. Hydrocortisone (Cortef, Hydrocortone)
2. Hydrocortisone sodium succinate (Solu-Cortef)
3. Cortisone acetate (Cortone)
4. Prednisone (Deltasone, Orasone)
5. Fludrocortisone (Florinef)
6. Betamethasone (Celestone)
7. Dexamethasone (Decadron)
8. Triamcinolone (Aristocort)

II. Mineralcorticoids

A. Actions: conserve the sodium stores in the body and affect fluid and electrolyte balance, thereby cause the reabsorption of sodium (Na) and excretion of potassium (K)

B. Uses
1. Addison's disease: a life-threatening condition caused by partial or complete failure of adrenocortical function
2. Adrenocortical insufficiency

C. Side effects
1. Electrolytes: hypokalemia, hypernatremia
2. Fluid balance: edema
3. CV: HTN

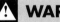 **WARNING!**

Explain to the client that these are lifelong medications and should not be withdrawn or stopped unless under a physician's supervision.

D. Nursing implications
1. Teach client to weigh daily; monitor for increases of greater than 2 to 5 pounds a week
2. Monitor BP for elevations greater than 20 mm Hg over the client's baseline
3. Encourage a diet rich in K; Na restriction

4. Monitor lab work: Na and K
5. Encourage the client to wear a medical alert tag
6. Recall tip: Addison's disease; note that the first three letters are "add," a clue that a hormone needs to be added because of the hypofunction.

E. **Common drug: fludrocortisone acetate (Florinef Acetate)**

DRUGS USED IN DIABETES MELLITUS

I. Hypoglycemic agents (see Box 13-3, p. 216)

A. **Actions: control carbohydrate metabolism and decrease glucose levels**

1. Oral agents stimulate the pancreas to secrete more insulin; not given in children or type I diabetics, in whom pancreatic beta cells do not function. Newer agents sensitize the body to the insulin that is present.
2. Insulin facilitates *inter*cellular movement of glucose from the extracellular space

B. **Uses: diabetes mellitus (DM), ketoacidosis, and coma associated with DM**

C. **Side effects**

1. Somogyi effect: hypoglycemia in the evening or night with rebound hyperglycemia in the early morning. The blood glucose level provides a good evaluation of the problem when samples are drawn around 3 am; the glucose level is typically low.
2. Hypoglycemia: weakness, hunger, sweating, nausea, blood glucose of less than 50 mg/dl
3. Local allergic reaction: itching, redness at the injection site
4. Dawn phenomenon: hyperglycemia in the early morning without previous hypoglycemia; increased plasma glucose concentration related to the growth hormone; treated by giving an extra dose of insulin

⚠ WARNING!

Assess for allergies to sulfa (some oral agents are contraindicated if sulfa allergies are present, because they are chemically related to beef or pork). Encourage the use of a medical alert tag. Only regular insulin can be given IV. Know whether or not the client has been using an air lock with SC injections.

D. **Nursing implications**

1. Know that insulin is available in various forms (Table 13-1, p. 224) for SC or IV administration. The GI tract digests insulin if given orally.
2. Schedule snacks around insulin's peak action time: the time when glucose level is lowest
3. Give insulin SC on a rotating basis; various SC sites have different absorption times—more rapid in the arms, less rapid in the abdomen, and the slowest in the thigh

4. Teach the client or family member how to give an injection and about the essential need to rotate sites

5. Teach all clients about foot care, exercise, and diet. Stress that *exercise decreases the need* for supplemental insulin, while most other factors increase the need for supplemental insulin.
   a. Hypoglycemia (blood glucose level less than 50 mg/dl): too much insulin, too little food, too much exercise
   b. Hyperglycemia (blood glucose level more than 120 mg/dl): too little insulin, too much food, too little exercise

6. Encourage compliance to prevent the complications of the disease process to the eye, the heart, and the kidneys. Complications are minimized when blood glucose level is controlled within normal parameters.

7. Teach how to self-monitor glucose level with the appropriate equipment

8. Know the onset and peak time for the type of insulin given

9. Know that insulin ordered to sliding scale is usually Regular. Sliding scale is additional insulin given intermittently for high blood glucose levels.

10. Do not shake, but gently rotate insulin bottle in the hands

11. Draw up regular insulin first when mixing agents

12. The open vial can be stored at room temperature. Once refrigerated, however, the vial should be kept in the refrigerator.

13. Monitor the glucose levels (fasting normal, 70–105 mg/dl). Check with physician for acceptable ranges for specific clients. With some clients, a serum glucose level below 150 mg/dl is sufficient.

E. Common drugs

1. See Table 13-1 for insulins, p. 224
   a. Insulin analog: insulin lispro (Humalog), rapid onset of action within 15 minutes; peaks within 40 to 60 minutes; duration 1 ½ hours; *must* be given 15 minutes before the meal
   b. Short-acting: Regular, Humulin-R, Semilente
   c. Intermediate-acting: NPH, Humulin-N, Lente
   d. Long-acting: Ultralente, rarely given
   e. Combinations: isophase human insulin plus human insulin, a combination of a percentage of rapid-acting insulin and a percentage of intermediate-acting insulin; written as 50/50 or 70/30, which indicates the percentage of each type of insulin.

2. Oral agents
   a. *Sulfonylureas*
      (1) Chlorpropamide (Diabinese)
      (2) Tolazamide (Tolinase)
      (3) Tolbutamide (Orinase)
      (4) Glipizide (Glucotrol)
      (5) Glyburide (Micronase, DiaBeta)
   b. *Biguanide:* metformin (Glucophage)

Text continues on p. 226

TABLE 13-1 Insulin Preparations

Classification	Type/Source	Description	Onset	Peak	Duration
				Pharmacokinetics	
Insulin analog Humalog, insulin lispro	Insulin analog *Rapid-acting*	Clear, fastest acting subcutaneous only *Must be given 15 min. before the meal to* *coincide with peak sugar level*	15 min.	40 to 60 min.	1½ hr.
Insulin injection (Regular or semilente) Novolin R Humulin R Regular Iletin I	*Short-acting* Human Beef/Pork	Clear solution containing no zinc or modifying agents; **IV only** or sub- cutaneous injection	SQ: ½ to 1 hr IV: 10 to 30 min.	2 to 4 hr 15 to 30 min.	6 to 8 hr 30 to 60 min.
Isophane insulin Suspension (NPH) Humulin N NPH Iletin I NPH-N	*Intermediate-acting* Human beef/pork purified pork	Cloudy suspension of insulin complex with protamine to slow absorption; subcutane- ous only	3 to 4 hr	6 to 12 hr	18 to 30 hr

Name	Source	Description	Onset	Peak	Duration
Intermediate-acting					
Insulin zinc Suspension (Lente) Humulin L Lente Iletin I Novolin L	Human beef/pork Human	Cloudy suspension containing 30% semilente insulin and 70% ultralente insulin; subcutaneous only	1 to 3 hr	8 to 12 hr	18 to 30 hr
Intermediate-acting (premixed)					
Isophane insulin Humulin 50/50 Humulin 70/30 Novolin 70/30 Recall tip: N comes before R alphabetically. Thus the 1st number is NPH and the second is Regular insulin	Human Human Human	Cloudy suspension of a percentage of insulin in the form of regular (rapid-acting), i.e. 30 represents 30% Regular and a percentage of insulin in the form of isophane insulin (intermediate-acting) i.e. 70 represents 70% NPH Note: 50/50 has equal parts of Regular and NPH Give subcutaneous only	30 to 60 min. for Regular 2 to 4 hours for NPH	4 to 8 hr	18 to 28 hr
Long-acting					
Extended insulin zinc suspension (Ultralente)	Human	Cloudy when well mixed; large complexes of insulin with zinc to slow absorption; no protein modifiers; subcutaneous only	4 to 6 hr	18 to 24 hr	36 hr or longer

Note: Insulins are packaged in vials, cartridges, and pens.

    c. *Alpha-glucosidase inhibitors*
       (1) Migitrol (Glyset)
       (2) Acarbose (Precose)
    d. *Glitazones*
       (1) Rosiglitazone (Avandia)
       (2) Pioglitazone (Actose)

II. Hyperglycemic agents (see Box 13-3, p. 216)

  A. Action: stimulate glucose synthesis to raise the glucose level and provide immediate glucose for use
  B. Use: severe hypoglycemic states
  C. Side effects
    1. Hyperglycemia: polydipsia, polyuria, polyphagia
    2. GI: nausea, vomiting with low glucose level
    3. CNS: coma

> ⚠ **WARNING!**
>
> Client and family should be taught how to use at home and always have available.

  D. Nursing implications
    1. Know that consciousness should return within 15 to 20 minutes after initial glucose injection; may repeat dose with dextrose, 50% solution, by IV route
    2. Glucagon should be used as soon as concentrated and given SC, IM, or IV
    3. Know that clients who do not lose complete consciousness can be *offered 4 ounces of regular soda (not diet)* instead of or in addition to glucagon. A syrup base is absorbed more rapidly than a juice base.
    4. Give dextrose, 50% solution, by slow IV push for unconscious clients
    5. Monitor glucose levels fasting, before meals, and at bedtime
  E. Common drugs
    1. Glucagon
    2. Dextrose, 50% solution
    3. Diazoxide (Proglycem)

WEB Resources

http://health.yahoo.com/health/Diseases_and_Conditions/Disease_Feed_Data/
   Insulin_dependent_diabetes_mellitus__IDDM_/
http://www.diabetes.org/mendosa/default.asp
http://www.diabetes.org/ada/c30c.asp
http://www.diabetes.org/publications/adasearch/
   QUERY.ASP?qu=medications&FreeText=&sc=%F&RankBase=1000&pg=2
   Diabetes.

http://www.endocrineweb.com/Diabetes/2insulin.html

http://www.diabetes.org/publications/adasearch/query.asp
Variety of reference links about diabetes medications and insulin information.

http://www.users.fast.net/~sttaylor/
http://www.endocrineweb.com/hyper4.html
http://www.endocrineweb.com/hypo2.html
Thyroid content about hyper- and hypo- types.

http://www.endocrineweb.com/osteoporosis/fosamax.html
http://www.druginfonet.com/deltason.htm
http://www.endocrineweb.com/sitesearch/
References for a variety of endocrine disorders.

REVIEW QUESTIONS

1. During preparation to administer Regular and NPH insulin, why would the nurse draw up the Regular first?
   1. It is easier to see the correct dose
   2. It avoids contamination of the solution in the regular insulin vial
   3. It avoids contamination of the solution in the NPH vial
   4. It is not as thick and therefore easier to draw up

2. A client is given the usual 7:30 AM dose of NPH insulin along with an added amount of regular insulin to scale because the glucose is 329 mg/dl. When would the first signs of insulin action be expected to occur?
   1. 10:30 AM
   2. 8:00 AM
   3. 9:00 AM
   4. 9:30 AM

3. A client self-monitors glucose levels at home and reports that every morning the level is extremely high. The glucose is within normal limits the rest of the day. The nurse would explain that this is called the
   1. Somogyi effect
   2. Peak time
   3. Dawn phenomenon
   4. Onset time

4. A client, age 16, is having difficulty doing insulin self-injections. The client wants to take the insulin in an oral form. How should the nurse respond?
   1. Insulin is better than the oral agents
   2. Oral agents are more expensive than insulin
   3. Insulin is not available orally because the GI tract would destroy it
   4. Oral agents can be destroyed by the GI tract

5. A client diagnosed with hyperthyroidism would most likely be prescribed which of these medications?
   1. Levothyroxine sodium (Synthroid)
   2. Thyroglobulin (Proloid)
   3. Calcitonin-human (Cibacalcin)
   4. Strong iodine solution (Lugol's solution)

ANSWERS, RATIONALES, AND TEST-TAKING TIPS

Rationales	Test-Taking Tips

1. Correct answer: 2

The NPH insulin is modified with a protein that can alter the regular insulin, which is unmodified and thereby contaminates the Regular insulin solution. The dose should be correct no matter which agent is drawn up first. The Regular insulin would not be harmful if some got into the NPH vial. The thickness of the solution is basically the same for both types of insulin.

Close your eyes and picture yourself drawing up the regular insulin and the NPH. Then think about what you saw in terms of common sense. The sequence of drawing up of one medication first and then the other in the same syringe is to prevent contamination of the first drug that was drawn up. Recall tip to picture the sequence: think of what you are in school for: to become an **RN**. Thus you draw up the **R**egular insulin before the **N**PH insulin to prevent contamination of the regular insulin.

2. Correct answer: 2

The onset time for Regular insulin is 30 minutes to 1 hour. Therefore, the Regular insulin, which should act first, could start between 8:00 and 8:30 AM. Option 3 would be too much time for the onset of Regular insulin. Options 1 and 4 would be the onset time for NPH, which is 2 to 4 hours.

Read carefully to note that the question is asking about "the first sign of insulin action," *not the peak action,* which has typically been asked throughout your educational process. Avoid knee-jerk thoughts. Also read carefully to acknowledge that the client received both Regular and NPH insulin. Thus, the focus of the question is about the Regular insulin.

3. Correct answer: 3

The dawn phenomenon is characterized by findings of a normally controlled glucose level throughout the day, except in the early morning, when it is high. The Somogyi effect is characterized by findings of hypoglycemia in the early morning, between 2:00 and 3:00 AM. The client might report waking up sweating in the

A helpful way to remember Somogyi effect is to make a story about a person called Somogyi. Somogyi had a work pattern on the night shift that was characterized by a slump at the middle of the night. Then, at the end of the shift, Somogyi had an overreaction when attempting to elevate his position in front of the supervisor when the morning checks were made. In

Rationales	Test-Taking Tips

middle of the night or waking up from nightmares, which are signs of hypoglycemia. Rebound hyperglycemia then occurs in the morning. For this problem, therapy may be directed at a decrease in the insulin dosage. In options 2 and 4, the peak or onset time of insulin depends on the type of insulin and when it was given. This information is not given in the stem, so eliminate these options.

contrast, a worker called Dawn coasted all night and, in the morning, reacted like Somogyi with an effort to impress the supervisor during morning checks. The work pattern indicates whether the glucose is high or low during the night and can be matched with the name of the employee.

4. Correct answer: 3

Insulin is not available orally, because gastric acid destroys it. Neither insulin nor oral agents are necessarily better than the other. Not all diabetics need insulin. The point in option 2 is not necessarily true and is irrelevant to the given question. Oral agents, such as Micronase, are not destroyed by the GI tract.

Careful reading is a must for questions like this. Note that the client asks about "insulin in an oral form." The only response that directly answers the question is option 3. Options 1, 2, and 4 can be clustered with the term "oral agents" and eliminated as the correct answer.

5. Correct answer: 4

Option 4 is an antithyroid agent used to lower thyroid levels. Options 1 and 2 are thyroid agents used to treat hypothyroidism. The agent in option 3 is used to treat hyperparathyroidism. It increases calcium deposited in the bone.

Eliminate options 1 and 2 by thinking about what you know. Each of these medications has a "thyro" in it. This clue hints that these drugs may supplement thyroid hormone. Think about what you know about option 3. Look at the beginning of the drug for the clue: *cal*citonin. Think calcium. This drug is associated with calcium, which is unrelated to thyroid therapy.

14

Drugs Affecting the Respiratory System

FAST FACTS

1. Evaluation of the effectiveness of these drugs is completed by clinical assessment for changes in the following (listed in order of priority):
   - RR: allergic reaction, respiratory arrest, wheezes, peak-flow meter
   - HR: increase or decrease, rhythm: irregular or regular, palpitations
   - BP: hypotension or HTN
   - GI: nausea, vomiting, anorexia, diarrhea
   - Laboratory results: peak/trough level; CBC count; ALT, AST, creatinine level, blood glucose levels
   - General: tremors, nervousness, headache, faintness, skin turgor or rash, mood swings, malaise, moon-shaped face
2. If the inhaler is not available, drinking two caffeinated colas will elicit the same response as medications used for asthma.
3. Know that inhalers can be used 20 minutes apart. If administered three times in one attack, seek medical attention.
4. The effectiveness of asthma therapy can be determined by use of a peak-flow meter before and after treatment and as a guide for the relief of symptoms.
5. Prophylactic asthmatic drugs, called nonsteroidal antiallergy agents, prevent the release of histamine. They have no effect in acute asthma attacks.

CONTENT REVIEW

BRONCHODILATORS

I. Groups of drugs

A. Sympathomimetics: beta-receptor agonists

B. Xanthine derivatives

II. Sympathomimetics: beta-receptor agonists

A. **Action: stimulate the production of cyclic adenosine monophosphate (CAMP), which relaxes smooth muscle**

B. **Uses**
1. Bronchospasms
2. Chronic pulmonary diseases
3. Asthma
4. Airway obstruction

C. **Side effects**
1. CNS: anxiety, restlessness, insomnia, tremors, headache
2. CV: palpitations, dysrhythmias
3. Respiratory: rebound bronchospasm
4. GU: urinary retention
5. GI: nausea, gastroesophageal reflux (esophageal burning)
6. Oral infections

⚠ WARNING!

Contraindicated in clients with HTN, dysrhythmias; increased cardiac effects with theophylline preparations. Clients should have these inhalers available at all times to use in an acute attack. Recommend that clients use the inhalers *before an activity that triggers an attack.* TIP: If the inhaler is not available, drinking two caffeinated colas will elicit the same response as these medications.

D. **Nursing implications**
1. Assess respiratory status, respiratory effort, RR, wheezing, dyspnea, and arterial blood gases
2. Instruct client on how to use an inhaler or respiratory apparatus at home (Figure 14-1). Placing the cannister of an inhaler in a bowl of water helps the client determine if the canister is empty (floats) or full (sinks).
3. Monitor ECG and cardiac status
4. Administer with meals if GI upset occurs
5. Emphasize compliance with dosage and schedule
6. Instruct clients to take these medications early in the evening if insomnia occurs
7. Suggest antacids if gastroesophageal reflux occurs. This may be severe with inhalers and require prescription medications.
8. Instruct client, especially children, to use the inhaler before brushing their teeth to decrease oral irritation, and to clean the inhaler mouthpiece with warm water once a week.
9. Recommend a spacer device with inhalers for children, since it helps to administer the full dose as well as decrease the taste of the medicine
10. Know that inhalers can be used 20 minutes apart. If administered three times in one attack, seek medical attention.

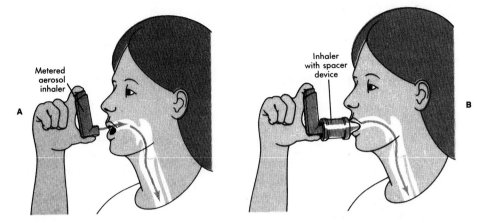

Figure 14-1 Metered-dose inhaler. **A.** Cannister without a spacer. **B.** Cannister with a spacer for clients with coordination difficulty. Spacer improves drug delivery deep into lungs. (From Clark J, Queener S, & Karb V: *Pharmacologic basis of nursing practice,* ed 6, St. Louis, 2000, Mosby.)

    11. Know that the effectiveness of therapy can be determined by use of a peak-flow meter before and after treatment as well as for the relief of symptoms

  E. Common drugs
    1. Epinephrine (Adrenalin, Sus-phrine, AsthmaHaler Mist, Bronkaid Suspension Mist)
    2. Isoproterenol hydrochloride (Isuprel)
    3. Isoetharine hydrochloride (Bronkosol)
    4. Albuterol (Proventil, Ventolin)
    5. Metaproterenol sulfate (Alupent)
    6. Terbutaline sulfate (Brethine)

III. Xanthine derivatives: methylxanthines

  A. Actions: inhibit phosphodiesterase, an enzyme responsible for breaking down CAMP. Because this enzyme is inhibited, more CAMP is available for bronchodilation. These agents also stimulate cardiac muscle and the CNS, increase cardiac output, produce diuresis, and decrease PVR.

  B. Uses
    1. Bronchospasm
    2. Asthma
    3. Wheezing and dyspnea associated with pulmonary diseases
    4. COPD or CAL

  C. Side effects
    1. CNS stimulation: tremors (a later sign of toxicity), nervousness, insomnia, agitation, convulsions

 2. CV stimulation: tachydysrhythmias, tachycardia, angina, hypotension, palpitations
 3. GI distress: nausea (a first sign of toxicity), vomiting, anorexia
 4. Toxicity

> ⚠ **WARNING!**
>
> Interactions include increased side effects with high intake of caffeine and chocolate and altered cardiac status with most of the cardiac drugs. Monitor blood levels of drug for toxicity: therapeutic blood level is 10 to 20 μg/ml; toxicity may occur with small increases of more than 20 μg/ml. Ingestion of peanuts may make breathing more difficult as a result of a substance in the peanut.

D. Nursing implications
 1. Give during the daytime to prevent insomnia
 2. Instruct client as follows:
    a. Reinforce the need for compliance with dosing, schedule, and blood work
    b. Do not crush or alter the dosage form
    c. Have clients take with milk or food if GI distress occurs
    d. Avoid smoking, because it increases metabolism of these agents
 3. Monitor for side effects and report the first sign of cardiac disturbances. The event of tachycardia does not warrant discontinuing the drug; instead, the dosage may need to be decreased.
 4. Monitor HR, BP, and ECG status for rhythm changes and watch for HR of over 120.

E. Common drugs
 1. Aminophylline (Aminophyllin, Somophyllin), available in PO and IV forms
 2. Oxtriphylline (Choledyl)
 3. Theophylline (Theolair)
 4. Anhydrous theophylline (Theodur)

DRUGS USED FOR ASTHMA

I. Prophylactic asthmatic drugs: nonsteroidal antiallergy agents

A. Action: prevent the release of histamine
B. Use: prevent acute attacks in asthma
C. Side effects
 1. CNS: headache
 2. Respiratory: bronchospasm
 3. GI: dry throat

> ⚠️ **WARNING!**
>
> These agents should not be mixed with bronchodilators when given by inhalation but should be mixed with saline. These drugs are not absorbed well by the oral route and therefore must be given by inhalation.

D. **Nursing implications**
   1. Teach client how to use inhaler or nebulizer
   2. Use humidifier if necessary
   3. Assess breath sounds frequently, before and after treatment
   4. Use cautiously in clients with severely compromised respiratory status

E. **Common drugs**
   1. Cromolyn sodium (Intal)
   2. Pirbuterol (Maxair)
   3. Nedocromil (Tilade)

II. Antiinflammatory agents: corticosteroids

A. **Actions: inhibit bronchoconstriction to enhance bronchodilation; decrease activity of inflammatory cells in the respiratory tract**

B. **Uses**
   1. Asthma
   2. Withdrawal from systemic corticosteroids
   3. Exacerbation of COPD or CAL

C. **Side effects**
   1. Oral and nasal irritation
   2. Fungal infections
   3. Death from adrenal insufficiency
   4. Delayed growth and development
   5. Gastroesophageal reflux

> ⚠️ **WARNING!**
>
> Use of this agent if the client has been on systemic corticosteroids requires slow withdrawal of the systemic agent while increasing use of the new agent. Instruct client that these drugs are not to be used in acute attacks or with status asthmaticus.

D. **Nursing implications**
   1. Carefully monitor client during stressful situations or when acute asthma attacks occur
   2. Assess oral cavity, encourage drinking of water after each inhalation
   3. Allow 1 to 2 minutes between inhalations
   4. Encourage client to use the inhaler before brushing the teeth to reduce oral infections and to wash the mouthpiece with warm water and dry thoroughly once per week

5. Recommend the use of a spacer device with inhalers for children
6. Monitor for signs of adrenal insufficiency: muscle pain, weakness, depression
7. Assess for allergies or prior complications with corticosteroid use
8. Monitor growth and development, especially in children
9. Administer antacid therapy as needed. If reflux (esophageal burning) becomes too excessive, medical attention should be sought.

E. Common drugs
1. Beclomethasone dipropionate (Vanceril, Beclovent)
2. Dexamethasone sodium phosphate (Decadron Phosphate)
3. Flunisolide (AeroBid)
4. Fluticasone propionate (Flovent)
5. Triamcinolone (Azmacort)

III. Leukotriene modifiers

A. Action: inhibition of leukotrienes at receptors in the smooth muscle of airways, which is triggered by inflammatory mediators

B. Uses: prophylactic treatment of mild to moderate persistent asthma or to replace corticosteroid therapy. These drugs are NOT effective in acute asthma attacks.

C. Side effects
1. Elevated liver enzymes: ALT, AST
2. CNS: headache, dizziness
3. GI: abdominal pain, gastroenteritis, dyspepsia, diarrhea, nausea
4. Respiratory: nasal congestion, cough, sinusitis

⚠ WARNING!

Contraindicated in status asthmaticus, severe liver disease, alcoholism, pregnancy, or in children less than age 6.

D. Nursing implications
1. Monitor liver enzymes as necessary
2. Notify the physician if rescue inhalers are required more often than usual while on these agents
3. Administer during evening hours for the most effectiveness

E. Common drugs
1. Montelukast (Singulair)
2. Zafirlukast (Accolate)
3. Zileuton (Zyflo)

UPPER RESPIRATORY SYSTEM DRUGS

I. Decongestants

A. Action: shrink nasal membranes by a vasoconstrictive mechanism

B. Uses: upper respiratory infection (URI), sinusitis

C. Side effects
1. CNS stimulation: nervousness, restlessness, insomnia
2. GI: nausea, vomiting
3. CV: palpitations, HTN
4. Rebound engorement: swelling and congestion of the nasal mucosa when the parasympathetic nervous system tries to equalize the effects of the sympathomimetic decongestant drugs

> ## ⚠ WARNING!
>
> Consult pharmacist before taking these products with diet pills. Consult physician before use if HTN is present.

D. Nursing implications
1. Instruct the client not to overuse the agent because it may be habit-forming with episodes of rebound engorement. Limit the number of days used.
2. Have clients limit caffeine intake
3. Advise clients to maintain a sitting position when they take these drugs
4. Suggest that clients take medication early in the morning or afternoon if insomnia occurs
5. Monitor VS; consult MD if HTN occurs
6. Have clients take drugs with or immediately after food if GI distress occurs

E. Common drugs
1. Oxymetazoline (Afrin, Dristan)
2. Phenylephrine (NeoSynephrine)
3. Pseudoephedrine plus chlorpheniramine plus dextromethorphan plus acetaminophen (Comtrex)
4. Pseudoephedrine hydrochloride (Sinutab, Sudafed)

II. Antihistamines
A. Action: compete for histamine (H_1) receptor sites
B. Uses
1. Rhinitis: inflammation of the mucous membranes of the nose accompanied by swelling of the mucosa and nasal discharge
2. Common cold
3. Allergic responses: itchy, watery eyes
4. Sinusitis

C. Side effects
1. Anticholinergic effects: dry mouth, urinary retention, dilated pupils, tachycardia, decreased GI motility
2. CNS: headache, sedation, dizziness; antihistamines cross the blood-brain barrier
3. CV: hypotension, palpitations

> ⚠️ **WARNING!**
>
> Caution older adults in particular about sedative and cardiac effects. Cautiously use in elderly clients. Repeated doses in children particularly may cause the opposite CNS effects: hyperactivity and insomnia.

D. Nursing implications

1. Advise clients to take at bedtime if possible to avoid sedation during the day
2. If taken during the day, caution the client about safety measures with driving, operating machinery, and ambulating. Sedation usually decreases with repeated doses.
3. Treat the anticholinergic effects as needed
4. Monitor vital signs

E. Common drugs

1. Diphenhydramine hydrochloride (Benadryl)
2. Terfenadine (Seldane)
3. Brompheniramine maleate (Dimetane)
4. Clemastine fumarate (Tavist)
5. Loratadine (Claritin)
6. Fexofenadine (Allegra)
7. Doxylamine succinate (Unisom)

DRUGS AFFECTING COUGH

I. Diluents

A. Sterile water

1. Action: liquefies mucus, which facilitates removal of secretions
2. Uses
   a. Helps remove secretions
   b. Decreases mucus plug formation
   c. Diluent given by ultrasonic nebulization
3. Nursing implications
   a. Know that if taken systemically, tap water acts as an expectorant
   b. Advise clients to consume 2 to 3 quarts of tap water per day to help eliminate secretions unless contraindicated by presence of congestive heart failure (CHF) or fluid restrictions

B. Sterile normal saline (sodium chloride)

1. Action: exerts osmotic pressure on plasma fluids, which results in hydration of respiratory secretions
2. Nursing implications: cautious use by clients with cardiac problems or when edematous states exist

II. Mucolytic drugs

A. **Actions: work directly on mucus to reduce thickness and make secretions less tenacious. Alters metabolism of acetaminophen to decrease injury to the liver in overdose.**

B. **Uses**
   1. Inhalation treatments
      a. Respiratory conditions with thick mucus
      b. Cystic fibrosis
   2. Orally: acetaminophen overdose

C. **Side effects**
   1. GI: nausea, vomiting (may be from rotten egg odor and foul taste during inhalation therapy)
   2. Respiratory: bronchospasm
   3. Burning in back of throat

⚠ WARNING!

Use cautiously in older adults or individuals with severe respiratory insufficiency (may cause bronchospasm).

D. **Nursing implications**
   1. Know that drugs may be given via nebulizer, IV, orally, or instilled in endotracheal tube
   2. Dilute with sterile water to ensure that all of drug is given
   3. Offer a face cloth after inhalation (drug leaves sticky coating on the face)
   4. Suction and encourage coughing after administration
   5. Assess lung sounds and respiratory status
   6. Administer by mouth, mixed with iced liquid, and have clients drink with a straw to minimize contact with the taste buds on the tongue, about 17 doses over a 4-day period in acetaminophen overdose
   7. Disguise odor of rotten eggs if given PO by mixing with 4 ounces of iced soft drink or juice and give with a straw

E. **Common drug: acetylcysteine (Mucomyst)**

III. Expectorants

A. **Actions: remove viscid secretions by reduction of the adhesiveness and surface tension. Iodide preparations act directly on bronchial tissue to increase the secretion of respiratory fluids and decrease the viscosity of mucus.**

B. **Uses**
   1. Respiratory difficulty in children
   2. Bronchitis
   3. Persistent coughs
   4. Mucus plugs
   5. Influenza
   6. Common cold

C. **Side effects: rare, may include GI upset (nausea)**

> ⚠ **WARNING!**
>
> Some of these products, especially OTC, may contain alcohol and sugar. Cautious use in the very young and elderly. Alcohol-free and sugar-free products are available.

D. Nursing implications
1. Assess lung sounds and secretions: color, consistency, amount
2. Offer 2 to 3 quarts of fluid per day unless contraindicated
3. Administer potassium iodide solution (SSKI) with juices to disguise taste; have client use a straw to decrease taste
4. Suggest that parents and older clients purchase the alcohol-free and sugar-free products

E. Common drugs
1. Potassium iodide solution (SSKI)
2. Guaifenesin (Robitussin, Glycotuss)
3. Dextromethorphan hydrobromide plus benzocaine (Vicks Formula 44D Cough Syrup)
4. Dextromethorphan hydrobromide plus guaifenesin plus phenylpropanolamine hydrochloride (Naldecon)

IV. Antitussives

A. Actions: suppress the cough reflex center in the medulla. Some formulas are peripherally acting and some are centrally acting.

B. Uses: suppress nonproductive cough and/or assist in nighttime sleep in children with productive cough. Can be combined with a narcotic or nonnarcotic agents.

C. Side effects
1. Respiratory: dry secretions
2. CNS: drowsiness without respiratory depression
3. GI: constipation
4. Narcotic abuse

> ⚠ **WARNING!**
>
> A synergistic effect can occur with alcohol and other CNS depressants.

D. Nursing implications
1. After taking the syrup, have clients wait 15 to 20 minutes before drinking any liquid
2. Monitor use because these are controlled substances
3. Suggest for clients to take the drug at bedtime
4. Monitor bowel elimination
5. Humidify air during sleep to improve effectiveness

E. Common drugs
1. Nonnarcotic
   a. Benzonatate (Tessalon Perles)
   b. Diphenhydramine hydrochloride (Benylin, Robitussin DM)

2. Narcotic
   a. Codeine sulfate
   b. Hydrocodone bitartrate (Hycodan)

WEB Resources

http://www.healthanswers.com/centers/disease/overview.asp?id=asthma&filename=757.htm
   Respiratory diseases and medications

http://search.health.yahoo.com/search/yhealth?p=asthma&R=disease
   Asthma information and answers.

REVIEW QUESTIONS

1. A client, age 4, with bronchitis, is producing a thick, yellow sputum, is febrile, and is not sleeping well at night. Dextromethorphan hydrobromide plus guaifenesin plus phenylpropanolamine hydrochloride (Naldecon), 1 teaspoon (5 ml) tid during waking hours, and dextromethorphan hydrobromide plus guaifenesin plus phenylpropanolamine hydrochloride plus codeine (Naldecon CX), 1 teaspoon (5 ml) at night, have been prescribed. What would the nurse explain to the client's mother?
   1. The Naldecon is better and therefore given more often
   2. There is no difference between the two; they both help him bring up the secretions
   3. The Naldecon helps him bring up the secretions during the day, and the Naldecon CX suppresses the cough at night
   4. The Naldecon is more potent in bringing up secretions

2. The active ingredient in most antitussives that makes them controlled substances is
   1. Codeine sulfate
   2. Phenobarbital sodium
   3. Meperidine hydrochloride
   4. Morphine sulfate

3. While making early morning rounds, the nurse notices a client's hands trembling. This client with chronic airway limitation (CAL) is receiving aminophylline through a continuous drip. The client says he feels fine but could not sleep last night. The nurse would be concerned about which of these items?
   1. CNS depression sometimes accompanying xanthine derivatives
   2. CNS stimulation often accompanying xanthine derivatives
   3. Anticholinergic effects of theophylline
   4. Cardiovascular depression accompanying aminophylline therapy

4. During an assessment for sinusitis and influenza, the client uses oxymetazoline (Afrin) nasal spray twice. When asked about the use of the agent, the client replies, "I can't seem to get my nose open no matter how much I use this stuff." The nurse would suspect which of these problems?
   1. CNS stimulation
   2. Improper administration
   3. Rebound engorgement
   4. Oxymetazoline toxicity

5. Instructions for a client with asthma who is learning to use an inhaler should include which of these actions?
   1. Hold the inhaler between the lips, activate the inhaler, and take a deep breath

2. Shake the inhaler while holding it between two fingers, exhale completely, activate the inhaler for as many puffs as the physician ordered as you inhale slowly and deeply, and hold breath for approximately 5 to 10 seconds
3. Hold the inhaler between two fingers, take a deep breath as you activate the inhaler for as many puffs as the physician ordered, and continue inhaling for 5 seconds
4. Shake the inhaler, then take several deep breaths while activating the inhaler

ANSWERS, RATIONALES, AND TEST-TAKING TIPS

Rationales	Test-Taking Tips

1. Correct answer: 3

The Naldecon helps to bring up the secretions during waking hours, and the codeine helps to suppress the cough. The Naldecon is not better but serves a different purpose during the day. Option 2 is partially true, but the difference is that the codeine in the Naldecon CX helps to suppress the cough. There is no truth to the statement in option 4.

Remember that codeine controls the cough to allow for rest. Note that it doesn't *eliminate* the cough reflex. It *suppresses* the cough reflex.

2. Correct answer: 1

Codeine is used in many prescription cough agents to suppress coughs. The agent in option 2 is not used in respiratory agents because of the CNS depressant effect. Meperidine would decrease respiratory rate and depth, which could worsen most respiratory problems. In general, morphine is not used for respiratory problems. It is used, however, specifically in acute pulmonary edema, not to affect the lung or the respiration or decrease pain, but to decrease severe anxiety, which in turn helps to get breathing under control.

Make an educated guess and eliminate options 2, 3, and 4. That leaves option 1. If you had no idea of the correct option, pair up options 3 and 4, since they are in the same classification, and eliminate them. Then "go with what you know": phenobarbital is more commonly used for seizure activity. Select option 1.

3. Correct answer: 2

Stimulation of the CNS creates nervousness and trembling and is a common side effect with xanthine derivatives. Theophylline products do not have anticholinergic effects.

Match the clues in the stem, "could not sleep" and "hands trembling," both of which reflect a stimulation of the body. Then look for an option with the word "stimulation" or something similar. Select option 2. Note that in options 1 and 4, the wording suggests a slowing.

4. Correct answer: 3

Frequent administration of oxymetazoline or any similar nasal sprays can cause rebound engorgement, which is the swelling and the congestion of the nasal mucosa when the parasympathetic nervous system tries to equalize the effects of the sympathomimetic decongestant drugs. The complaints by the client do not match the information in option 1, CNS stimulation. Administration, even if improper, would not cause these symptoms. This medication usually has no toxic effects.

Think about what clues you know from the stem and the options. Match ideas: "can't get my nose open" suggests "engorgement."

5. Correct answer: 2

This is the best explanation of the length of inhalation after activation of the inhaler; if a second dose is needed the client should wait 1 to 2 minutes. The explanation in option 1 is true but not clear enough. The client should exhale before activating the inhaler and taking a deep breath. Activation of the inhaler should be made slightly after initial inhalation.

As you read through each option, act the direction out. This takes no more time and will help clarify the information in terms of actions and sequence of actions. If you do this "acting out," it will be obvious that option 2, which has the most detail, is the correct answer.

15

Drugs Used To Treat Cancer

FAST FACTS

1. Evaluation of the effectiveness of these drugs is completed by clinical assessment for changes in (listed in order of priority) the following:
   - Relief of symptoms or selective toxicity without severe side effects of the agents
   - Laboratory: CBC count; BUN, creatinine, electrolyte levels
   - Decreased incidence of infection: stomatitis, cellulitis, thrombophlebitis
   - Management of nausea, vomiting, and diarrhea without weight loss
   - General: lack of malaise or fatigue, alopecia
2. Effectiveness of the drug depends on the number of cells in division.
3. Recovery periods are needed to allow normal cells to regenerate. Therefore, chemotherapy may be given for several months and then stopped for a time.
4. Combination therapy is often more effective than single-agent therapy.
5. Because the *bone marrow, hair follicles,* and cells of the *GI tract* have the highest growth fraction, these areas suffer the greatest toxicity.
6. Therefore, common side effects include **bone marrow depression, alopecia,** nausea and vomiting.
7. Nonvesicants should be given first.
8. Instruct the client to report infusions that feel different than previously (may be first sign of extravasation).
9. Perform a fresh venipuncture for administering these agents if possible.
10. Use a forearm rather than the dorsum of the hand; see preparation and handling.

CONTENT REVIEW

ANTINEOPLASTICS

I. General considerations

A. **Goal of treatment is to destroy cancer cells, while conserving normal cells, by interfering with cancer cell reproduction. These agents are used for the following:**
   1. Cure cancer
   2. Relieve symptoms
   3. Prevent complications
   4. Reduce tumor size before surgery

B. **Two types of** *chemotherapeutic agents*
   1. **Cell-cycle specific**: respond during a specific cycle of the cell; usually work best in multiple, repeated doses
   2. **Cell-cycle nonspecific**: respond during any phase, sometimes in more than one phase at a time. These agents are dose-dependent.

C. **Growth fraction: the number of proliferating cells in the system at a given moment. Because the bone marrow, hair follicles, and cells of the GI tract have the highest growth fraction, these areas suffer the greatest toxicity. Therefore, common side effects include** *bone marrow depression, alopecia,* **nausea and vomiting.**

D. **Principles of chemotherapy**
   1. Timing of dose around the cell cycle and in relation to other drugs is critical
   2. Combination therapy is often more effective
   3. Effectiveness of the drug relies on the number of cells in division at the time of therapy

E. **Recovery periods are needed to allow normal cells to regenerate. Therefore, chemotherapy may be given for several months and then stopped for a time.**

F. **Agents are classified according to tissue response if infiltration occurs**
   1. **Vesicant:** causes blisters, tissue sloughing, necrosis
   2. **Nonvesicant:** usually administered first, no severe tissue destruction
   3. **Irritant:** causes cellulitis, thrombophlebitis, possible necrosis

II. Preparation and administration

A. **Handling of chemotherapeutic agents**
   1. Use gloves, protective garment, mask
   2. Use laminar flow hood for preparation
   3. Prime the IV line with normal saline, then hang the chemotherapeutic agent bag. The IV line can also be primed under a laminar flow hood.
   4. Dispose of all materials used in the preparation and the administration into a container labeled "hazardous waste"

B. **Management during administration**
   1. After drawing up the medication, change the needle
   2. Check that the client has been informed of the benefits and the risks
   3. Choose an appropriate site (start distal and move to proximal sites; avoid sites over joints)
   4. Know drug compatibilities and the characteristics of the individual drug being administered
   5. Consider the sequence, the delivery, the vesicant properties
   6. Check for blood return in IV according to agency policy
   7. Avoid extravasation of IV; stabilize with splint if necessary during the infusion

III. Side effects and nursing implications

A. **Bone marrow depression: monitor CBC count for a drop in levels**
   1. Leukopenia: a decrease in the number of WBCs. Assess for infection. A body temperature of 99°F in the leukopenic client is of concern. Teach the client the signs of infection and that purulent drainage may not be present during infection.
   2. Thrombocytopenia: a decrease in the number of platelets. Assess for bleeding, such as petechiae (typically on the chest or upper arms).
   3. Anemia: a decrease in hemoglobin; monitor hemoglobin level and hematocrit. Assess for clinical findings: pallor of the skin, increased fatigue, or shortness of breath, especially with activity; suggest the use of iron preparations.

B. **Nausea, vomiting, and diarrhea: give antiemetics before symptoms develop and before therapy begins; offer antidiarrheals as needed; encourage small, frequent meals; monitor weight daily; avoid exposing client to strong odors; monitor electrolyte levels and teach the client the symptoms of electrolyte loss; teach the client to avoid enemas and rectal suppositories; discourage irritating foods and juices, such as fruit, fruit juices, spicy foods, raw vegetables, corn, and coffee; monitor for signs of dehydration**
   1. Chemotherapy agents stimulate the chemoreceptor trigger zone
   2. Nausea or vomiting may be psychogenic or anticipatory

⚠ WARNING!
Instruct the client to notify the physician if diarrhea or vomiting is severe or persists longer than 2 to 4 days.

C. **Stomatitis: inflammation of the mouth; assess oral cavity, offer good mouth care and topical antibiotics or analgesics**

D. **Alopecia: loss of hair; may be most distressing for clients. Suggest a wig, scarf, hat, or refer the client to resources for effective management of this problem; teach the client that alopecia may involve the eyebrows, eyelashes, nasal and pubic hair; instruct the client to wash remaining hair, even though it is sparse, every 2 to 4 days with a mild shampoo; cooling the head with cold compresses**

TABLE 15-1 Antineoplastic Agents: Classifications, Actions, Side Effects, Uses, and Considerations

Classification/Action	Side Effects						Uses	Considerations
	S	NS	BD	N-V	Alo	Sto		
Alkylating Agents Carboplatin (Paraplatin) Chlorambucil (Leukeran) **Cisplatin (Platinol)** *Mechlorethamine (Mustargen)* Ifosfamide (Ifex) with Mesna (Mesnex) to decrease side effects Cyclophosphamide (Cytoxan) Streptozocin (Zanosar) ▼Disrupt structure of DNA		*	++	+	+		Leukemia; Hodgkin's disease; lymphoma; cancers of the breast, ovaries, testes, prostate	Cause infertility problems Mustard only used as topical Carboplatin has less renal toxicity Contraindicated with some vaccines and corticosteroids
Antimetabolites Cytarabine (Cytosar, ARA-C) Floxuridine (FUDR) Flourouracil (5-FU) Methotrexate (Folex, Mexate) Methotrexate (MTX) ▼Inhibit DNA and RNA synthesis	*		++			+	Leukemia; cancers of the breast, GI tract, neck, cervix Effective in rapidly proliferating cancers	Can cause nephrotoxicity and liver dysfunction Monitor BUN, creatinine levels Encourage fluids Taking folic acid may increase protection of normal cells Some are irritants

Hormonal Agents
Androgens: nandrolone (Durabolin)
Progesterones
  Medroxyprogesterone (Depro-Provera)
Antiandrogens
  Goserelin (Zoladex)
			+		+		Cancers of prostate, breast, endometrium, renal system	Mostly palliative
								Teach about characteristics of opposite sex, decreased libido, and breast tenderness

Drug	*	NV	Alo	Sto	Uses	Concerns
Estrogens						
Estramustrine (Emcyt)						
▼Cytostatic; alter hormonal environment of tumor	*					
Antibiotics						
Doxorubicin (Adriamycin)					Hodgkin's disease, testicular carcinoma, breast and bladder cancers	All are vesicants except bleomycin is an irritant
Bleomycin (Blenoxane)						Severe tissue damage if extravasation
Plicamycin (Mithracin)		++	+			Teach about signs of infection
Idarubicin (Idamycin)				++		May cause hepatotoxicity
▼Bind with DNA; cytotoxic effect; antimicrobial activity	*					Avoid with live vaccines
Mitotic Inhibitors						
Paclitaxel (Taxol)					Breast carcinoma, lymphomas, leukemia	May cause hepatotoxicity
Vinblastine (Velban)			+	+	Wilm's tumor, sarcomas	Severe CNS and neuro side effects such as neuropathy and paresthesias
Etoposide (VP-16)		++				Mobility and ADLs need to be assessed
Vincristine (Oncovin)						
▼Inhibit cell mitosis	*					
Radioactive Drugs						
Sodium radioiodine (Idodotope)					Leukemia, thyroid cancer	Require protective isolation to prevent radiation contamination
Sodium radiophosphate				++		May cause radiation sickness
Radiogold (^{198}Au, ^{32}P)		++				
▼Emit radiation to destroy specific tissue	*					

*classified as:
S = Cell-cycle specific
NS = Cell-cycle nonspecific

Side effects:
NV = Nausea/vomiting
Alo = Alopecia
Sto = Stomatitis

+ = Frequently occurs
++ = Severe side affect

Bold = **vesicant**
Italics = *irritant*
▼ = Action of drug

before IV chemotherapy causes vasoconstriction and less of the agent reaches the scalp.

E. Extravasation and infiltration: cellulitis, thrombophlebitis, necrosis at IV site; monitor the IV site frequently for a strong blood return and signs of infiltration or leakage; if infiltration occurs apply ice to the site if agent is a vesicant or irritant to minimize the spread of the agent and change the IV site; give the agents according to their classification as vesicant, nonvesicant, or irritant; nonvesicants should be given first. Instruct the client to report infusions that feel different than previously (may be first sign of extravasation). Perform a fresh venipuncture for administering these agents if possible; use a forearm rather than the dorsum of the hand; see preparation and handling.

IV. Classification of agents (Table 15-1)
A. Alkylating agents
B. Antimetabolites
C. Antibiotics
D. Hormonal agents
E. Radioactive agents
F. Miscellaneous individual agents

V. General nursing implications
A. Recommend use of body surface area (BSA) to determine correct dosage
B. Avoid inhalation and contact with skin during the preparation, the administration, and the disposal of these agents
C. Know hospital protocol for administration of the agents
D. Stress the need for compliance

 WARNING!

These agents should not be administered to pregnant clients or by pregnant health care workers.

WEB Resources
http://health.yahoo.com/health/drugs_tree/medication_or_drug/
Use this site to get information on individual drugs.

REVIEW QUESTIONS

1. A client with cancer of the testes is receiving an antibiotic antineoplastic agent. The nurse would advise him to do which of these actions?
   1. Eat six small meals instead of three large ones
   2. Report a body temperature of 101°F or above, chills, and any discomfort
   3. Drink 2.4 L of fluids per day to prevent constipation
   4. Report signs of nephrotoxicity

2. Which of these problems might occur because of the effects of chemotherapeutic agents on cells with a high growth fraction?
   1. Headache
   2. Hypernatremia
   3. Diarrhea
   4. Constipation

3. Antimetabolites cause which severe side effect?
   1. Liver complications
   2. Infertility
   3. Differences in sex characteristics
   4. Ototoxicity

4. Before administration of a parenteral chemotherapeutic agent, the nurse would perform which nursing assessment?
   1. Assess bowel sounds
   2. Check the last CBC count for a high WBC count
   3. Assess for stomatitis
   4. Check for adequate blood return from the IV

5. A client has the signs of bone marrow depression and thrombocytopenia. The nurse would teach the client to observe daily for which finding?
   1. Infection
   2. Stomatitis
   3. Petechiae
   4. Diarrhea

6. Two chemotherapeutic agents are ordered: one is a vesicant, the other a nonvesicant. In what order would the nurse give them?
   1. Give the nonvesicant first because the vesicant may irritate the IV site
   2. Give the vesicant first to get the most difficult one infused first
   3. It should not matter
   4. Administer the agents together

ANSWERS, RATIONALES, AND TEST-TAKING TIPS

Rationales	Test-Taking Tips

1. Correct answer: 2

Bone marrow depression is the prime side effect and could cause leukopenia. If nausea is a problem, six small meals could help. Constipation and nephrotoxicity are not common side effects.

Think about what you know and then make an educated guess. Most chemotherapy for cancer has side effects of bone marrow depression. This results in a decreased WBC count with increased risk of infection. Thus, option 2 is best.

2. Correct answer: 3

Diarrhea is common because the cells of the GI tract multiply rapidly and the rapid-growing cells are more affected by antineoplastic agents, since tumors are typically fast-growing. A high growth fraction does not affect the brain. A high growth fraction has no effect on sodium level. Constipation is not a common side effect of these drugs.

Think of a high growth fraction as a magnet that attracts the antineoplastic drugs, which result in an irritability or toxicity of specific cells. Of the given options, only option 3 suggests irritability.

3. Correct answer: 1

Hepatotoxicity is a common severe side effect of these agents. Option 2 is not a side effect of these drugs. Option 3 is a major side effect of the hormonal antineoplastic agents. Complications in hearing are not common with chemotherapeutic agents.

The clue in the stem is the word "severe." It leads to option 1, since, of the given options, this option would be the most severe in any situation.

4. Correct answer: 4

A healthy IV line with adequate blood flow is necessary to prevent vascular complications. Many of the agents are irritating if extravasation occurs. Assessing bowel sounds may be advisable if nausea and diarrhea

Think about what you know in general about IV therapy. Before administration of an IV medication, the line must be patent, especially if the agent is caustic to the vein.

are present, but not before administration of the agent. Option 2 is not a necessary nursing action before these agents are given. Since many of the agents lower the WBC count and it is expected of the therapy, high WBC counts are not as common. Stomatitis is usually a side effect of the agents.

5. Correct answer: 3

Bleeding is a risk in the event of thrombocytopenia because of the decrease in platelets. Petechiae, especially on the anterior chest or upper arms, is an early sign of low platelets. Infection would be a concern if leukopenia were present. Stomatitis is not a complication arising from bone marrow depression. Option 4 is not a side effect of bone marrow depression but rather a side effect of selected drugs.

If you have no idea of a correct answer, cluster options 1, 2, and 4 under the umbrella of "involvement with inflammation." The only option that is different is option 3.

6. Correct answer: 1

If the vesicant were given first and caused irritation, the nonvesicant could not be given, unless a new line was started. The agent with the most irritating characteristics should be given last. Because of the possibility of complications from the vesicant, it does make a difference which agent is given first. Two agents should never be given at the same time because of the possible side effects and complications.

Use common sense to conclude that the least irritating agent is to be given first.

16

Drugs Used to Treat Infections

FAST FACTS

1. Obtain culture and sensitivity studies before the initial dose of antibiotics, then monitor any repeat culture and sensitivity studies.
2. Evaluation of the effectiveness of these drugs is completed by clinical assessment for changes in:
   - Infection: signs of recovery are decreased body temperature; less redness, warmth, swelling, exudate; lack of superinfections
   - RR: arrest, wheezes: allergic reaction
   - Laboratory: peak/trough levels; WBC and CBC count; BUN, creatinine, and glucose levels; ALT and AST levels
   - Comfort: pain
   - GI: lack of diarrhea, nausea, vomiting
3. Methicillin-resistant *Staphylococcus aureus* (MRSA) infection is often treated with vancomycin.
4. Aminoglycosides have the side effect of ototoxicity and nephrotoxicity.
5. Vancomycin is the only antibiotic used to treat antibiotic-induced colitis from *Clostridium difficile.*
6. Antivirals require around-the-clock administration.
7. Advise clients to protect themselves against exposure to sunlight with appropriate clothing, not sunscreens, which are usually ineffective when photosensitivity is a side effect of the antibiotic.

CONTENT REVIEW

ANTIBIOTICS

I. General information

A. **Agent classifications**

1. Narrow-spectrum: treat relatively limited number of organisms; less likely to disrupt the normal flora; used when an organism has been identified by a culture
2. Broad-spectrum: treat multiple organisms; more likely to disrupt the normal flora; used often when a specific causative organism is unknown

B. **General side effects**

1. Hypersensitivity
2. Toxicity to various organs: kidney, liver, skin, bone marrow
3. **Superinfection** caused by the disruption of the normal flora of the body. Symptoms include black, furry tongue; thrush (candidiasis); vaginal discharge from vaginitis

C. **Many microorganisms have become resistant to antibiotics. A culture and *sensitivity* study or Gram stain is preferred to specify the exact organism.**

D. **General nursing implications**

1. Assess for the results of the culture and sensitivity studies or ensure that the culture has been completed before starting a new antibiotic
2. Instruct the client to do the following:
   a. Take all of the medication, even after symptoms subside, to prevent recurrence of the infection

⚠ WARNING!

Resistance of organisms to antibiotics has become a serious problem. Failure to take the complete dosage of an antibiotic regimen fosters the development of resistance. Reinforce this fact to all clients.

   b. Use another type of contraception if the client is taking birth control pills. Many antibiotics will decrease the effectiveness of birth control pills.

⚠ WARNING!

During antibiotic therapy, this problem is often not communicated to clients and pregnancy does frequently occur in all age groups, since no protection beyond the birth control pills is used.

   c. Immediately report any signs of allergic reaction

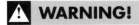

WARNING!

Anaphylaxis is not an uncommon reaction to these agents.

3. Monitor blood levels of the drug
   a. **Peak**: time of maximum effect, commonly measured immediately after the drug has been infused
   b. **Trough**: level before the next dose; sample should be drawn 10 to 30 minutes before the next dose is given or as specified in agency protocol
4. Monitor the CBC count, especially the WBC count and the differential to evaluate the effectiveness of the antibiotic; expect a WBC count decreased to within the normal range
5. If severe diarrhea occurs, instruct the client to take buttermilk or yogurt to replace the normal intestinal flora
6. Know the difference between the following:
   a. Bacteriostatic: restrains the reproduction of bacteria
   b. Bactericidal: destroys the bacteria

II. Penicillins
A. **Actions: interfere with cell wall synthesis and division of bacteria; bactericidal**
B. **Uses: prophylaxis**
   1. Gram-positive cocci, rods, and anaerobic bacteria
   2. Pharyngitis: inflammation of the pharynx
   3. Endocarditis: an abnormal, infectious condition that affects the endocardium and heart valves; the tricuspid valve is more commonly affected in IV drug abusers
   4. Pneumonia
   5. Meningitis
   6. STDs: syphilis, gonorrhea
   7. *Shigella* species: gram-negative organisms that cause gastroenteritis and bacterial dysentery
   8. *Salmonella* species: gram-negative, rod-shaped bacteria; affects the GI tract
   9. Upper respiratory infections (URI)
   10. Urinary tract infections (UTI)
   11. Otitis media
   12. Sinusitis
C. **Side effects**
   1. Rash with urticaria on abdomen, scalp, or arms: usually the first finding in an allergic reaction
   2. Anaphylaxis
   3. Serum sickness: an immunologic disorder that may occur 2 to 3 weeks after the administration of an antiserum
   4. Hematologic reactions: decreased hemoglobin, prolonged bleeding

5. GI: diarrhea, nausea, vomiting
6. Immunologic: superinfection, oral thrush (candidiasis)

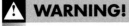

> ⚠ **WARNING!**
>
> These drugs are unique; allergy can develop after multiple use over time or at an initial use.

D. Nursing implications

1. Assess for known previous allergies
2. Discontinue immediately if signs of allergic reactions occur and notify the physician. Diphenhydramine hydrochloride (Benadryl) may be given for mild reactions.
3. Monitor for seizures in clients with renal disease
4. Know that penicillin G (Pentids) should be given with food
5. Instruct client to wear a medical alert bracelet
6. Assess for respiratory distress: wheezing, dyspnea, crowing sounds, respiratory arrest. Treat with epinephrine SC or IV.
7. Instruct clients to report signs of rash that occur 2 to 3 weeks after administration of the drug; thrush (candidiasis), vaginitis, or other infections
8. Monitor CBC count
9. Advise the consumption of yogurt or buttermilk to normalize GI flora if persistent diarrhea occurs
10. Know that the dose of injectable penicillins usually given for STDs is a large quantity, 8 to 10 ml, and is thick like liquid glue, so 16- or 18-gauge needles are used, the Z-track method is used, and the dose is divided into two injections of 4 to 5 ml each

E. Drug categories

1. Natural penicillins
   a. Penicillin G potassium (Pentids)
   b. Penicillin V (V-Cillin K)
2. Penicillinase-resistant penicillins
   a. Methicillin (Staphcillin)
   b. Nafcillin (Unipen)
3. Aminopenicillins
   a. Amoxicillin (Amoxil)
   b. Ampicillin (Polycillin)
4. Extended-spectrum penicillins
   a. Piperacillin (Pipracil)
   b. Carbenicillin (Geopen)
   c. Ticarcillin (Ticar)
5. Combination products
   a. Amoxicillin plus clavulanic acid (Augmentin)
   b. Ampicillin plus sulbactam (Unasyn)
   c. Ticarcillin plus clavulanic acid (Timentin)

III. Cephalosporins

A. **Actions: inhibit cell wall synthesis, thereby resemble penicillin action. Work especially well on rapidly growing organisms; they are bacteriostatic and bacteriocidal.**

B. **Uses**
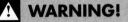
1. URI
2. UTI
3. MRSA: usually treated with vancomycin
4. Beta-hemolytic streptococci
5. *Klebsiella* species infections
6. Presurgical prophylaxis of infection

C. **Side effects**
1. Superinfections: thrush (candidiasis); vaginal discharge from vaginitis; black, furry tongue
2. More resistance to gram-positive organisms as spectrum broadens (third generation)
3. False-positive blood glucose values
4. Nephrotoxicity: toxicity to the kidney
5. Pain at injection site
6. GI: upset, nausea

> ⚠ **WARNING!**
>
> Assess for allergies; clients allergic to penicillin may not be able to take these agents either. Usually clients do not exhibit anaphylaxis, but may develop allergic reactions.

D. **Nursing implications**
1. Monitor renal status: I&O, serum creatinine level
2. Assess for superinfection and teach clients about the use of buttermilk and yogurt to minimize diarrhea
3. Monitor IV infusion closely for pain and irritation
4. Monitor glucose level if client is diabetic
5. Stop infusion and call physician if infiltration or phlebitis present
6. Advise clients to avoid alcohol because it increases sensitivity
7. Know that sometimes the antifungals for vaginitis are given simultaneously with antibiotics to prevent the vaginitis, especially in women who have a history of such infections

E. **Drug generations according to spectrum**
1. First generation: work best against gram-positive bacteria; often used in clients allergic to penicillin
    a. Used to treat infection from *Escherichia coli*, *Klebsiella* species, *Proteus* species, *Salmonella* species, *Shigella* species
    b. Common drugs
        (1) Cephalothin (Keflin)
        (2) Cephalexin (Keflex)
        (3) Cephapirin (Cefadyl)
        (4) Cephradine (Anspor)
        (5) Cefadroxil (Duricef)

2. Second generation: work best against gram-negative bacteria
   a. Uses: *Proteus* species, *E. coli, Haemophilus influenzae*
   b. Common drugs
      (1) Cefamandole (Mandol)
      (2) Cefoxitin (Mefoxin)
      (3) Cefaclor (Ceclor)
      (4) Cefotetan (Cefotan)
      (5) Loracarbef (Lorabid)
3. Third generation: work best against gram-negative bacteria
   a. Uses: *Serratia* species, *Pseudomonas aeruginosa*
   b. Common drugs
      (1) Cefotaxime (Claforan)
      (2) Cefoperazone (Cefobid)
      (3) Ceftriaxone (Rocephin)
      (4) Ceftazidime (Fortaz)
   c. Beta-lactam antibiotics: act similar to cephalosporins
      (1) Aztreonam (Azactam)
      (2) Imipenem-cilastatin (Primaxin)
      (3) Loracarbef (Lorabid)

IV. Tetracyclines (broad-spectrum)

A. **Actions: inhibit protein synthesis in the bacterial cell; bacteriostatic**
B. **Uses**
   1. Gram-positive and gram-negative bacteria
   2. Aerobic and anaerobic bacteria
   3. Lyme disease
C. **Side effects**
   1. Superinfection: black, furry tongue; thrush (candidiasis); vaginal discharge from vaginitis
   2. Interferes with normal calcification and may cause permanent gray or brownish discoloration of the teeth if given to children under age 8
   3. Photosensitivity: sunscreens alone do not seem to decrease photosensitivity
   4. GI disturbances: nausea, vomiting, diarrhea
   5. Hepatotoxicity: toxicity to the liver

> ⚠ **WARNING!**
>
> Contraindicated for use in children under age 8 because of permanent gray or brown discoloration of teeth while teeth are still in development stages. Teeth are fully developed at age 8. Decreased absorption if taken with iron, milk, and antacids containing aluminum, calcium, sodium, or magnesium. Culture and sensitivity studies should be obtained before administration of the agent the first time.

D. **Nursing implications**
  1. Have clients take on an empty stomach (for better absorption), unless GI disturbances occur. Can be taken with food but this may decrease absorption.
  2. Advise clients to use protection in direct sunlight; clothing rather than sunscreen
  3. Assess for signs of superinfection: oral cavity; thick, white vaginal discharge
  4. Monitor laboratory values for elevated ALT or AST levels

E. **Common drugs**
  1. Doxycycline (Vibramycin)
  2. Minocycline (Minocin)
  3. Oxytetracycline (Terramycin)

V. Aminoglycosides

A. **Actions: inhibit protein synthesis; bacteriostatic (low doses) and bacteriocidal (high doses)**

B. **Uses**
  1. Gram-negative bacilli
  2. Treatment of TB
  3. Enterococcal endocarditis
  4. Alternate treatment for MRSA

C. **Side effects**
  1. Ototoxicity: toxic to nerves or organs of hearing; results in hearing loss
  2. Nephrotoxicity
  3. CNS: dizziness, vertigo, ataxia
  4. Neurotoxicity: neuromuscular blockade, the inhibition of a muscular contraction activated by the nervous system, which results in weakness or paralysis

⚠ WARNING!

Interactions: inactivated when mixed with extended-spectrum penicillins; separate administration by at least 2 hours. Culture and sensitivity studies should be obtained before administration of the agent for the first time.

D. **Nursing implications**
  1. Use cautiously with anesthetics and muscle relaxants
  2. Caution the client about safety measures while driving, operating machinery, and walking, if weakness or paralysis of muscles occurs
  3. Monitor renal function: creatinine, I&O
  4. Monitor peak and trough levels
  5. Assess for hearing loss
  6. Give with a large amount of fluids: at least 2 L/day

E. Common drugs
1. Gentamicin (Garamycin)
2. Amikacin (Amikin)
3. Tobramycin (Nebcin, Tobrex)
4. Kanamycin (Kantrex)
5. Neomycin
6. Streptomycin

VI. Macrolides
A. Actions: bind to ribosomes to inhibit protein synthesis; bacteriostatic action
B. Uses
1. Gram-negative and gram-positive organisms
2. *S. aureus* infections
3. Pneumonia
4. Clients allergic to penicillin
C. Side effects
1. GI disturbances: diarrhea, nausea, vomiting
2. Hepatotoxicity
3. Immunologic: superinfections, vaginitis, thrush (candidiasis), secondary infections
4. Skin: rash

> ⚠️ **WARNING!**
>
> Culture and sensitivity studies should be obtained before administration of the agent for the first time. Do not administer with fruit juices or meals, which may decrease the absorption; however, if GI symptoms occur, giving the drug with a small amount of food could help the client tolerate these side effects better. May increase theophylline levels.

D. Nursing implications
1. Assess for frequency, amount, and color of diarrhea
2. Monitor weight loss, especially in children
3. Monitor for signs of hepatotoxicity (increases in ALT, AST levels)
4. Give with a full glass of water and on empty stomach unless there is GI distress. Giving with food will decrease absorption.
5. Monitor for secondary infections
E. Common drugs
1. Erythromycin ethylsuccinate (EES)
2. Clarithromycin (Biaxin)
3. Azithromycin (Zithromax)
4. Erythromycin base (E-Mycin)
5. Dirithromycin (Dynabac)

VII. Sulfonamides (broad-spectrum)

A. Action: interfere with para-aminobenzoic acid (PABA) to decrease synthesis of folic acid, which is needed for bacteria survival

B. Uses
1. Gram-negative and gram-positive organisms
2. UTI
3. Otitis media
4. Vaginal infections
5. Prostatitis: inflammation of the prostate gland

C. Side effects
1. Renal calculi
2. Hypersensitivity: severe nausea and vomiting
3. Nephrotoxicity
4. Hematologic: decrease in WBC count, hemolytic anemia
5. Photosensitivity
6. Immunologic: superinfections
7. GI: nausea and vomiting
8. Stevens-Johnson syndrome: fever, malaise, toxemia

> ⚠ **WARNING!**
>
> Hypersensitivity can occur with these agents; assess for prior or current allergies. Culture and sensitivity studies should be obtained before administration of the agent for the first time. Resistance to this drug class has become problematic.

D. Nursing implications
1. Encourage fluids up to 1.5 L/day
2. Monitor I&O, creatinine level
3. Monitor CBC count, WBC count
4. Advise clients to protect against sunlight with clothing, because sunscreens may not be effective
5. Have clients take on an empty stomach (for better absorption), unless GI disturbance occurs; then take with small amount of food
6. Monitor for superinfections and report abnormal drop in the WBC count

E. Common drugs
1. Trimethoprim plus sulfamethoxazole (Bactrim, Septra)
2. Sulfadiazine
3. Sulfisoxazole (Gantrisin)

VIII. Quinolones

A. Action: interrupt DNA synthesis, broad-spectrum, bactericidal

B. Uses
1. Infection from *E. coli*
2. Gram-negative organisms

      3. UTI, STDs

      4. Bronchitis

  C. Side effects

      1. Photosensitivity

      2. GI irritation: nausea

      3. Immunologic: superinfections

      4. Renal: worsening renal failure

      5. CNS toxicity: visual disturbances

> ⚠ **WARNING!**
>
> Avoid use of antacids containing aluminum or magnesium at the same time; there should be at least 1 to 2 hours between medication times. Obtain culture and sensitivity studies before administration of the agent for the first time.

  D. Nursing implications

      1. Advise clients to protect against sunlight with appropriate clothing, not sunscreens, which are ineffective

      2. Inform the client that urine may be colored brown or bright orange

      3. Monitor renal status (offer 1 to 2 L/day of fluids unless contraindicated), I&O, serum creatinine level for an increase

      4. Have clients take on an empty stomach, unless GI irritation occurs; then take with foods

      5. Know that foods may decrease absorption

  E. Common drugs

      1. Fluoroquinolones

        a. Ciprofloxacin (Cipro)

        b. Norfloxacin (Noroxin)

        c. Ofloxacin (Floxin)

        d. Levofloxacin (Levaquin)

      2. Antibiotics related to quinolones

        a. Cinoxacin (Cinobac)

        b. Nalidixic acid (NegGram)

  F. Phenazopyridine hydrochloride (Pyridium or Urogesic): a nonnarcotic analgesic that soothes the urinary mucosa and may be used in conjunction with the common drugs

IX. Penicillin substitutes

  A. Action: Similar to penicillins, inhibit cell wall synthesis, narrow-spectrum

  B. Uses

      1. Serious gram-positive infections: staphylococci or streptococci

      2. MRSA

      3. Clients allergic to cephalosporins and penicillins

      4. Antibiotic-induced colitis from *C. difficile* (vancomycin only)

C. **Side effects**
   1. Red neck syndrome, an allergic reaction to a rapid infusion of vacomycin only. It is characterized by flushing, pruritis, and erythema of the head, neck, and upper body due to histamine release. Other systemic allergic findings are hypotension, tachycardia, chills, fever.
   2. Toxicities: nephrotoxicity, ototoxicity
   3. Pseudomembranous colitis (clindamycin only)
   4. GI: nausea, vomiting, stomatitis

> ⚠ **WARNING!**
>
> Obtain culture and sensitivity studies before starting medication. Many incompatabilities exist with these drugs. They are usually prescribed IV to be administered without simultaneous administration of other medications: seek references if medications have to be mixed.

D. **Nursing implications**
   1. Infuse over 60 minutes IV with the use of a controller or pump
   2. Monitor peak and trough levels closely
   3. Instruct client to report tinnitus or persistent diarrhea
   4. Assess BUN and creatinine levels for 3 days

E. **Common drugs**
   1. Clindamycin (Cleocin)
   2. Vancomycin (Vancocin)
   3. Spectinomycin (Trobicin)

X. Chloramphenicol (Chloromycetin)

A. **Action: bactericidal in high doses, inhibits protein synthesis, broad-spectrum**

B. **Uses: (not used as frequently as previously)**
   1. *Salmonella* species
   2. Ampicillin-resistant strains of *H. influenzae*
   3. Fatal blood disorders

C. **Side effects**
   1. Gray-baby syndrome or gray syndrome, a toxic condition in neonates, especially premature infants. Caused by a reaction to this drug resulting in a characteristic ashen-gray cyanosis, abdominal distention, hypothermia, vomiting, respiratory distress, and vascular collapse. It is fatal if the drug is continued.
   2. Bone marrow toxicity

D. **Nursing implications**
   1. Monitor CBC count, particularly low platelet count, RBC count, and WBC count
   2. Give IV slowly
   3. Administer on empty stomach, if oral form is given

URINARY ANTISEPTIC AGENTS

I. Action: Work locally by concentrating in renal tubules. They do not exert a systemic effect

II. Use: UTI: from gram-positive or gram-negative organisms

III. Side effects: nausea, vomiting, diarrhea

IV. Nursing implications
A. Assess for resolution of UTI
B. Advise clients to take with food if GI disturbances occur

V. Common drugs
A. Nitrofurantoin (Furadantin, Macrobid)
B. Nitrofurantoin macrocrystals (Macrodantin)

ANTITUBERCULAR AGENTS

I. Actions: exert either a tuberculostatic or tuberculocidal effect by the inhibition of mycolic acid, a necessary metabolite of the organism *Mycobacterium tuberculosis*

II. Uses
A. Prevent or treat tuberculosis
B. Treat Hansen's disease (leprosy)
C. Treat persons with positive tuberculin tests or a known exposure to TB

III. Side effects
A. Hepatotoxicity, jaundice
B. CNS: headache, vertigo
C. Neuritis: inflammation of a nerve from vitamin B_6 deficiency: numbness, tingling in the fingers, hands, or feet; these findings are also called peripheral neuropathies or parasthesias
D. GI: nausea, vomiting, and diarrhea

⚠ WARNING!

Stress avoidance of alcohol because of the hepatotoxic effect and possible further impairment of the liver

IV. Nursing implications
A. Administer on empty stomach
B. Know that drugs are prescribed for extended periods (more than 6 months) because the organism may lie dormant in an individual

C.   Stress compliance in completing the prescription even though symptoms are gone
D.   Monitor liver status for elevated serum ALT and AST levels and jaundice, which may be noted initially in the sclera of the eye
E.   Monitor body weight
F.   Instruct client that rifampin (Rifadin) may color body fluids red-orange
G.   Recommend that the client eat foods high in vitamin B$_6$ (pyridoxine) to prevent or minimize the peripheral neuropathies

V. Common drugs
   A.   Tuberculosis
      1. Isoniazid (INH)
      2. Rifampin (Rifadin)
      3. Streptomycin
      4. Cycloserine (Seromycin)
      5. Capreomycin (Capastat)
   B.   Dapsone (DDS): used to treat Hansen's disease

ANTIVIRALS

I. Action: interfere with DNA replication of virus. This interference also can occur in the host cell.

II. Uses
   A.   Herpes simplex virus (HSV)
      1. HSV-1: oral herpes, herpes labialis, causes infections around face area
      2. HSV-2: herpes genitalis, causes infection in the genital region
   B.   Influenza A and B pneumonia of which respiratory syncytial virus (RSV or RS virus) is a more common cause in premature and normal infants
   C.   AIDS, retinitis in AIDS clients
   D.   Hepatitis C

III. Side effects
   A.   GI: nausea, vomiting, diarrhea
   B.   Renal: toxicity
   C.   CV: phlebitis

⚠ WARNING!
Use gloves, as some of the lesions are contagious. Use of condoms should be encouraged if HSV or HIV are present. Blood levels should be monitored and the agents should be given *around the clock* as prescribed.

IV. Nursing implications

A. Give with foods to decrease the side effects
B. Monitor IV carefully; prevent phlebitis, characterized by redness, irritation, swelling, heat, pain
C. Monitor I&O, BUN and creatinine levels

V. Common drugs

A. Herpes: acyclovir (Zovirax)
B. Respiratory syncytial virus: ribavirin (Virazole)
C. Influenza A: amantadine hydrochloride (Symmetrel)
D. Interferon alfa (Intron)
E. Valacyclovir (Valtrex)
F. For treatment of AIDS (see Chapter 12)
   1. Didanosine (Videx)
   2. Zidovudine (AZT)
   3. Amantadine (Symmetrel): retinitis in AIDS clients
   4. Ganciclovir (Cytovene): retinitis in AIDS clients

OTHER AGENTS

I. Antifungals

A. Action: alter the permeability of the cell membrane
B. Uses
   1. Systemic and topical fungal infections
   2. Histoplasmosis: an infection caused by inhalation of spores of the fungus *Histoplasma capsulatum*
   3. Thrush: candidiasis (caused by *Candida albicans*) of the tissue of the mouth
C. Side effects
   1. Renal: nephrotoxicity
   2. Immunologic: fever, chills
   3. Phlebitis
   4. GI: nausea, vomiting
   5. Hypokalemia: low potassium level (<3.5 mEq/L)
   6. Hypomagnesemia: low magnesium level (<1.5 mEq/L)

> ⚠ **WARNING!**
>
> These agents often must be used for 7 to 10 days for complete results to be obtained; instruct the client not to stop taking the agents because results are not seen immediately.

D. Nursing implications
   1. Monitor electrolytes, BUN and creatinine levels, CBC count
   2. Monitor I&O for signs of nephrotoxicity
   3. Assess VS and treat fever with acetaminophen
   4. Instruct client to report any abnormal symptoms

    5. Instruct client to swish nystatin (Mycostatin) around the mouth and then swallow; avoid drinking fluids for 1 hour

    6. Monitor IV site for redness, irritation, pain, warmth, or swelling

E. Common drugs

    1. Amphotericin B (Fungizone)

    2. Miconazole (Monistat): vaginitis

    3. Ketoconazole (Nizoral): vaginitis

    4. Nystatin (Mycostatin): thrush (candidiasis)

    5. Fluconazole (Diflucan)

II. Antihelmintic agents

A. Action: destroy parasitic helminths (worms) by affecting their nervous system

B. Uses: treat roundworms, tapeworms, flatworms, pinworms, flukes

C. Side effects

    1. Toxicity: medicine kills the helminth, which spills out its toxin

    2. GI distress: nausea, anorexia

    3. Hematologic: dehydration, anemia

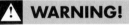 **WARNING!**

Assess for proper identification of the type of worm. Stress good handwashing, gloving, and proper disposal of feces and urine.

D. Nursing implications

    1. Suggest treatment of all members in the household who live with the infected client to prevent recurrence

    2. Encourage washing bed linen with hot water to destroy the parasites

    3. Instruct client to take the *entire* recommended dose

    4. Monitor CBC count

E. Common drugs

    1. For amebiasis: metronidazole (Flagyl)

    2. For roundworm/hookworm: mebendazole (Vermox)

    3. For pinworm: pyrantel pamoate (Pin-X)

    4. Chloroquine (Aralen)

III. Antimalarial agents

A. Action: kill the parasite

B. Use: malaria

C. Side effects

    1. GI distress: nausea

    2. Agranulocytosis

    3. CNS: headache, agitation, fatigue

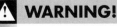 **WARNING!**

Instruct client to complete the entire course of therapy.

   D. Nursing implications
   1. Know that clients may begin taking these drugs 1 to 2 weeks before traveling to an endemic area
   2. Give with food to minimize GI distress
   3. Monitor WBC count for severe changes
   E. Common drugs
   1. Chloroquine (Aralen)
   2. Hydroxychloroquine sulfate (Plaquenil)
   3. Pyrimethamine (Daraprim)
   4. Quinine

WEB Resources

http://dir.yahoo.com/Health/Pharmacy/Drugs_and_Medications/Types/Antibiotics/
   Information on various antibiotics.

http://health.yahoo.com/health/drugs_tree/medication_or_drug/
   Allows for an opportunity to look up individual drugs.

http://dir.yahoo.com/Health/Pharmacy/Drugs_and_Medications/Types/Antivirals/
   Provides a source for information about antivirals.

REVIEW QUESTIONS

1. Nephrotoxicity and ototoxicity are major side effects with which of these drug groups?
1. Penicillin
2. Sulfonamides
3. Erythromycin
4. Aminoglycosides

2. Nursing implications for clients on antibiotics for an extended period would include which of these actions?
1. Take with a full glass of water or food
2. Take buttermilk or yogurt if diarrhea occurs
3. Watch for a decrease in urine production
4. Watch for an increase in urine production

3. A serious and dangerous side effect of penicillin is which of these problems?
1. Anaphylaxis
2. Nephrotoxicity
3. Hepatotoxicity
4. Neuromuscular blockade

4. The best antibiotic for a UTI is which of these groups?
1. Penicillin G (Pentids)
2. Tobramycin sulfate (Tobrex)
3. Trimethoprim plus sulfamethoxazole (Bactrim)
4. Erythromycin ethylsuccinate (EES)

5. Because a client's annual tuberculosis test result was positive, the nurse anticipates that which agent will be prescribed prophylactically?
1. Cloroquine (Aralen)
2. Mebendazole (Vermox)
3. Isoniazid (INH)
4. No agent; obtain a chest x-ray film

6. Which is the best agent for amebiasis?
1. Mebendazole (Vermox)
2. Metronidazole (Flagyl)
3. Pyrantel pamoate (Antiminth)
4. Chloroquine (Aralen)

ANSWERS, RATIONALES, AND TEST-TAKING TIPS

Rationales	Test-Taking Tips

1. Correct answer: 4

Both of these findings are major side effects of the aminoglycosides and should be monitored carefully. The most common side effect of penicillins is a rash with itching and is initially found on the abdomen or the scalp. Renal calculi from crystals is a major side effect of sulfonamides, especially if insufficient fluids are taken during therapy. GI disturbance, especially diarrhea, is a common side effect of erythromycin.

The clue in the stem is the word "major." The aminoglycosides: gentamicin, kanamycin, and streptomycin, can be thought of as the "mycin" family with "major" problems when given. These drugs are usually given IV and therefore affect the kidney more than the liver in terms of toxicity. The oral medications are more likely to cause toxicity of the liver, called hepatotoxicity.

2. Correct answer: 2

All antibiotics can destroy the normal flora in the intestines, and diarrhea can occur. Yeast, buttermilk, or yogurt can help replace the bacteria normally found here. Some of the agents require increased fluid intake for an overhydration effect because of their effect on the kidneys. Not all antibiotic agents are nephrotoxic. None of the antibiotic agents result in an increase in urine output.

The clue in the stem is the key word "extended." Think of superinfections or secondary infections as the result of the suppression of normal flora. In short-term therapy, this may be less likely.

3. Correct answer: 1

Severe allergic responses, such as anaphylaxis, are more common with the penicillin group. Aminoglycosides are particularly nephrotoxic. Tetracyclines are hepatotoxic. Aminoglycosides can produce a neuromuscular blockade effect.

The clues in the stem are the words "serious" and "dangerous." Read the options with these two words in mind. Then think of the worst result from each of the options. In option 1, if anaphylaxis occurs, the worst result is a quick death. Death may also be the end result of other conditions in the other options. However, it would take longer. Option 1 is the best answer.

4. Correct answer: 3

Sulfonamides are broad-spectrum antibiotics and work well on UTIs. Penicillins work best on gram-positive bacteria. Aminoglycosides, such as tobramycin, work best on gram-negative bacilli. Macrolides, such as erythromycin, work best on pneumonia or *S. aureus* infections.

Remember Bactrin is used for **B**ladder infections.

5. Correct answer: 3

Isoniazid is the recommended drug to treat a positive tuberculin skin test or the active disease. The agent in option 1 is recommended for malaria. The agent in option 2 is recommended for roundworms. The most current recommendation is to treat a client with a positive tuberculin test with 6 months of isoniazid, whether the chest x-ray result is positive or not.

Eliminate option 4 since it does not answer the question of which agent. Then think about what you know. Most likely, isoniazid is a more familiar drug to you than the other listed drugs. Select the drug you know and avoid selection of an option just because you don't know about it. Eliminate the action and thought of "I'll select this because I haven't heard of it, so it must be the correct answer."

6. Correct answer: 2

Metronidazole (Flagyl) is the drug of choice for amebiasis. Mebendazole is the drug of choice for roundworms. Pyrantel pamoate (Antiminth) is the drug of choice for pinworms. Chloroquine (Vermox) is the drug of choice for malaria.

For this type of difficult question, select an answer and go on. Keep your emotional reaction to a minimum, so you can think about the questions that remain. This would be a good time for a few deep breaths with your eyes closed to clear your thoughts and relax your muscles.

17

Dermatologic Agents

FAST FACTS

1. Evaluation of the effectiveness of these drugs is completed by clinical assessment for changes in the skin: rash, irritation, dryness, itching.
2. Calamine plus diphenhydramine hydrochloride (Caladryl) is *not* recommended for children with chicken pox; it will slow the recovery. Use oatmeal baths to minimize itching.
3. Special considerations for silver sulfadiazine (Silvadene): it stains clothing or skin a gray color.
4. Client may need to acquire new clothing or shoes if treated for athlete's foot without positive results; for example, persistent findings of athlete's foot, even though therapy has been given for 3 weeks.
5. Excess absorption from leaving the application on for longer than recommended can enhance systemic absorption and toxicity during the therapy for lice.

CONTENT REVIEW

I. Antiseptics and disinfectants

A. Actions: denature protein, reduce surface tension, or interfere with the metabolic processes of cell growth. Includes alcohols, halogens, aldehydes, phenolic compounds, biguanides, surface-active agents, and oxidizing agents

B. Uses
1. Slows microorganisms that cause infection: bacteria, fungi, viruses, and spores
2. Cleaning wounds
3. Douches
4. Irrigants
5. Preparation of the skin for treatment or surgery

6. Astringent
7. Cleaning equipment

C. Side effects
1. Hypersensitivity: mostly skin irritation, burns on skin and mucous membranes
2. Teratogenic effects on fetus
3. Nephrotoxicity

⚠ **Warning!**
Use gloves to apply.

D. Nursing implications
1. Know the proper use of the agent; some can be used to pack wounds and some cannot
2. Watch for signs of hypersensitivity: rash, itching, redness, drying of skin
3. Know the proper dilution, if dilution is required
4. Know the organism on the skin and the agent sensitive to that organism. Some of these agents are not effective against spores.

E. Common drugs (see Table 17-1)

II. Baths
A. Uses
1. Cleanse
2. Soothe pruritis
3. Medicate
4. Reduce fever
5. Lubricate skin

B. Nursing implications
1. Know that these agents can cause drying of the skin
2. Use only tepid water, without alcohol, to lower body temperature of children or adults

C. Common drugs
1. Oatmeal (Aveeno)
2. Starch
3. Gelatin
4. Alpha-Keri lotion

III. Soaps and cleansers
A. Soaps
1. Uses: for cleaning the skin and in enemas to stimulate peristalsis; antimicrobial action
2. Nursing implications
   a. Advise that soaps may irritate mucous membranes
   b. Know that soaps may have glycerin or medication added
3. Common soaps (OTC): Safeguard, Zest, Dial, castile

TABLE 17-1 Antiseptics and Disinfectants: Chemical Categories

Agents	Antiseptic	Disinfectant
Acids		
Acetic	X	X
Benzoic	X	
Boric	X	
Lactic	X	
Alcohols		
Ethanol	X	X
Isopropanol	X	X
Aldehydes		
Formaldehyde		X
Glutaraldehyde		X
Dyes		
Gentian violet	X	
Carbol-fuchsin	X	
Halogens		
Chlorine compounds		
Sodium hypochlorite	X	X
Halazone		X
Iodine compounds		
Iodine (tincture and solution)	X	X
Iodophors (povidone)	X	
Mercurials		
Merbromin	X	
Thimerosal	X	
Yellow mercuric oxide	X	
Silver		
Silver nitrate	X	
Oxidizing Agents		
Benzoyl peroxide	X	
Hydrogen peroxide	X	X
Potassium permanganate	X	
Phenolic Compounds		
Cresol		X
Hexachlorophene	X	
Hexylresorcinol	X	
Resorcinol	X	
Surface-Active Agents		
Benzalkonium chloride	X	
Cetylpyridinium chloride	X	
Biguanides		
Chlorhexidine gluconate	X	
Nitrofurazone	X	

From Lilly L, Aucker R: *Pharmacology and the nursing process,* ed 2, St Louis, 1999, Mosby.

B. **Cleansers: soap-free or modified soap products; may include an emollient**
   1. Uses: persons with sensitive or irritated skin or those with previous reactions to soap products; do not have antimicrobial action
   2. Common cleansers
      a. Phisoderm
      b. Oatmeal (Aveeno bar)
      c. Dove, Caress, Neutrogena, Ivory
      d. Acne Aide
      e. Nivea skin cleansers

IV. Emollients
A. **Actions: fatty or oily substances that soften or soothe irritated skin and mucous membranes; often used as vehicles for other medications**
B. **Uses**
   1. Treat diaper rash
   2. Lubricate
   3. Soothe
   4. Insertion of tubes and catheters
C. **Common emollients**
   1. Petrolatum (Vaseline)
   2. Vitamin A & D ointment (Clocream, Desitin)
   3. Lubriderm lotion
   4. Nivea skin products, excluding cleansers
   5. Lanolin products
   6. Glycerin (Corn Husker's Lotion)
   7. K-Y products (liquid and jelly)

V. Solutions and lotions
A. **Actions**
   1. Treat inflammation
   2. Protect and heal skin
   3. Decrease itching
B. **Uses**
   1. Insect bites
   2. Diaper rash
   3. Prickly heat
   4. Poison ivy
   5. Acne
   6. Chicken pox
   7. Infections
   8. Wet dressings
C. **Common drugs**
   1. Calamine lotion: shake well before application; good for relieving itching
   2. Diphenhydramine hydrochloride (Benadryl)

3. Boric acid solution
4. Aluminum acetate solution (Burrow's solution)
5. Aluminum sulfate (Domeboro)

D. Calamine plus diphenhydramine hydrochloride (Caladryl) is *not* recommended for children with chicken pox, because it will slow the recovery. Use oatmeal baths to minimize itching.

VI. Astringents

A. Actions: provide comfort because of the tightening properties and an ability to decrease inflammation and exudate
B. Uses: acne, hemorrhoids
C. Common agents
1. Aluminum sulfate (Domeboro)
2. Tucks

VII. Skin protectants

A. Actions: protect or coat minor skin irritations
B. Uses: ulcers, wounds, protection of skin
C. Nursing implications
1. Advise clients that physical sunscreens are thick and offer the best protection but must be applied heavily
2. Know that chemical sunscreens are absorbing and the most appealing
3. Know that sun protection factors (SPF) range from 2 to 45 and should be chosen based on the climate and type of skin. The higher the number, the greater the protection.
D. Common drugs
1. Benzoin
2. Kerodex
3. **PABA** (sunscreen products)
4. Liquid petrolatum (mineral oil)

VIII. Rubs and liniments

A. Actions
1. Analgesic
2. Antiinflammatory
3. Local anesthetic
4. Antiseptic
B. Uses
1. Muscle aches
2. Neuralgia
3. Rheumatoid arthritis
4. Sprains
C. Common drugs
1. BenGay
2. Vaporub
3. Aspercreme

IX. Protectives

A. **Actions: soothe, cool, and form film on skin. The film aids healing and decreases odors.**

B. **Uses: wounds or minor abrasions**

C. **Nursing implications: may have to be peeled off because the powder sticks to wet surfaces only**

D. **Common drugs**
   1. Collodion
   2. Zinc oxide
   3. Talcum powder

X. Topical antiinfectives

A. **Antibacterials**
   1. Actions: inhibit or destroy microorganisms by interfering with metabolic activity; also retard growth of bacteria
   2. Uses
      a. Wounds, minor abrasions
      b. Acne
      c. Burns
      d. *Streptococcus* and *Staphylococcus* species infections
   3. Side effects and nursing implications
      a. Be alert to the fact that hypersensitivity may cause burning, itching, and blistering; use cautiously in children and elders
      b. Systemic absorption: monitor for renal insufficiency

> ⚠️ **Warning!**
>
> Apply with gloves or some type of applicator, such as a tongue blade. Special considerations for silver sulfadiazine (Silvadene): stains clothing or skin a gray color

   4. Common drugs
      a. Bacitracin (Baciguent)
      b. Neomycin sulfate (Myciguent)
      c. Silver sulfadiazine (Silvadene Cream)
      d. Mupirocin (Bactroban)
      e. Calcium mupirocin (Bactroban Nasal)
      f. Benzoyl peroxide
      g. Erythromycin (EryDerm, Erygel)
      h. Tretinoin (retinoic acid)
      i. Isotretinoin (Accutane)

B. **Antivirals**
   1. Actions: inhibit viral replication, decrease pain, and increase healing of skin lesions
   2. Uses: treat HSV infection, varicella zoster

3. Side effects
   a. Skin reactions: stinging, itching, and rash
4. Common drugs
   a. Acyclovir (Zovirax)
   b. Penciclovir

C. Antifungals
1. Actions: offer fungistatic and fungicidal properties
2. Uses
   a. Superficial fungal infections
   b. Athlete's foot
   c. Jock itch
   d. Ringworm
   e. *Candida albicans* infection, including candidiasis

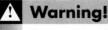 **Warning!**

Client may need to acquire new clothing or shoes if treated without positive results; for example, recurrent or persistent findings of athlete's foot, even though therapy has been given for 3 weeks.

3. Side effects
   a. Skin: local irritation, pruritis, burning, scaling
4. Common drugs
   a. Clotrimazole (Lotrimin)
   b. Tolnaftate (Tinactin)
   c. Nystatin (Mycostatin)
   d. Amphotericin B (Fungizone)
   e. Butoconazole (Femstat)
   f. Ketoconazole (Nizoral)

XI. Antiinflammatory agents
A. Actions
1. Alleviate inflammation response
2. Antipruritic
3. Vasoconstrictive
4. Reduce itching, redness, and swelling associated with an allergic response

B. Uses
1. Psoriasis
2. Dermatitis
3. Minor skin irritations
4. Allergic responses

⚠ Warning!

Do not use with an antifungal. Do not use on broken skin, since increased absorption results.

  C. **Side effects**

    1. Skin: acne eruptions, allergic contact dermatitis, burning, dryness, itching, hirsutism, alopecia

    2. Overgrowth of bacteria, fungi, or virus

  D. **Nursing implications**

    1. Application of a dressing increases absorption on thick lesions

    2. Use gloves or an applicator such as a tongue blade for application to the site

  E. **Common drugs**

    1. Hydrocortisone (Cortaid)

    2. Betamethasone valerate (Valisone)

    3. Desoximetasone (Topicort)

    4. Fluocinonide (Lidex)

    5. Flurandrenolide (Cordran)

XII. Antiparasitic agents

  A. **Groups**

    1. Scabicides: eradicate scabies

    2. Pediculicides: eradicate lice

  B. **Actions: cause paralysis and death of parasites by blocking their nerve impulse transmission**

  C. **Side effects**

    1. Systemic effect, which can cause toxicity to kidneys, heart, and CNS

    2. Seizures

    3. Renal complications

    4. Drying out of hair and skin

    5. Irritation to skin: itching, stinging

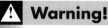 **Warning!**

> Gloves should be used if the nurse applies the medication. All members of the household who live with the client may need to be treated. Excess absorption or leaving application on for longer than recommended can enhance systemic absorption and toxicity, especially neurologic findings. Use by elders should be with caution due to toxic effects.

  D. **Nursing implications**

    1. Encourage client to read the instructions well on the medication

    2. Know that instructions about application techniques vary

      a. Some agents require a repeat application in 7 to 10 days, others require a one-time dose

      b. Shampoos are left on 4 to 10 minutes. Instructions indicate whether hair is shampooed wet or dry.

      c. Lotion may need to be re-applied in 24 hours, followed by a shower

      d. Bedding and clothing should be washed with hot water and bleach if possible

E. **Common drugs**
   1. Lindane lotion and shampoo (Kwell)
   2. Pyrethrins with piperonyl butoxide (RID)
   3. Permethrin (NIX)
   4. Malathion (Ovide)
   5. Crotamiton (Eurax)

XIII. Keratolytics

A. **Action: softens and loosens the outer, horny layer of thickened skin by removing excess keratin**
B. **Uses**
   1. Acne
   2. Warts
   3. Psoriasis
   4. Corns and calluses
C. **Side effects: evaluate the affected area of these clients for disruption of skin integrity**

⚠ Warning!

Advise client to be careful when scraping the softened, thickened skin to prevent abrasions or cutting the skin underneath the callus.

D. **Nursing implications: repeat application and apply dressings**
E. **Common drugs**
   1. Salicylic acid (Occlusal)
   2. Sulfur (Sebulex)

XIV. Debriding agents—Proteolytic preparations

A. **Actions: digest or liquefy necrotic tissue and purulent exudate**
B. **Uses: debride decubiti, burns, severe wounds**
C. **Side effects**
   1. Allergic response
   2. Pain at the site
   3. Bleeding at the site
D. **Nursing implications**
   1. Use a tongue depressor to apply
   2. Avoid excess heat
   3. Protect the healthy skin
   4. Clean the area, if needed, before application
E. **Common drugs—Proteolytic enzymes**
   1. Fibrinolysin plus desoxyribonuclease (Elase)
   2. Trypsin plus Peru balsam plus castor oil (Granulex)
   3. Sutilains (Travase)
   4. Collagenase (Santyl)

F. Common drugs—Nonenzyme forms

1. Absorptive beads: dextranomer (Debrisan) is poured into the wound and acts by physical absorption of wound
2. Duo-Derm or op site: dressings used for decubitus and stasis ulcers. Duoderm has moisture-reactive particles that create a soft gel over the wound. Liquefied material resembling pus is evident when the duoderm is removed. Both dressings should be changed every 7 days.
3. Metronidazole (Flagyl): used investigationally to treat grade 3 and 4 decubitus ulcers that are infected.

WEB Resources

http://www.medscape.com/server-java/SearchClinical?QueryText=Psoriasis
  Psoriasis (Medscape requires a registration that is free).

http://www.woundcarenet.com/awcdbcat5.htm#Cat2
  Debriding agents (choose individual category).

http://tray.dematology.uiowa.edu/ImageBase.html
  Site has information and pictures of dermatological conditions with treatments.

http://www.dermis.net/biddb/index_c.htm (be sure and choose the English version)
  Site has many pictures of dermatological conditions for identification and treatment.

REVIEW QUESTIONS

1. A common side effect of silver sulfadiazine (Silvadene) cream used on burns is which of these findings?
   1. Hives
   2. Drying of the skin
   3. Graying of the skin
   4. Burning on the skin

2. A client, age 32, has athlete's foot with itching and discomfort. The nurse would recommend which of these products?
   1. Acyclovir (Zovirax)
   2. Hydrocortisone
   3. Clotrimazole (Lotrimin)
   4. Ketoconazole (Nizoral)

3. A frantic mother calls because her infant has excessively dry skin that is beginning to look cracked. The mother states that she has been washing the baby with Irish Spring soap. The nurse might recommend which of these substances?
   1. Safeguard soap
   2. Oatmeal (Aveeno) cleansing bar
   3. Calamine lotion after the bath
   4. Dove bar

4. The nurse's aide reports that a client has red, bleeding, irritated buttocks from frequent diarrheal stools. The nurse should begin to use which preparation for protection of the skin?
   1. Lubriderm
   2. Zinc oxide
   3. Glycerine (Corn Husker's solution)
   4. Silver sulfadiazine (Silvadene)

5. Instructions for a mother to treat her child's chicken pox would be the use which of these products?
   1. Oatmeal (Aveeno) baths for soothing and calamine lotion
   2. Oatmeal (Aveeno) baths for healing and diphenhydramine hydrochloride plus calamine (Caladryl Lotion)
   3. Oatmeal (Aveeno) cleansing bar and calamine lotion
   4. Alpha-Keri lotion in her bath water

ANSWERS, RATIONALES, AND TEST-TAKING TIPS

Rationales	Test-Taking Tips

1. Correct answer: 3

The ingredients in the agent cause graying of the clothing and the skin. Silver sulfadiazine (Silvadene) does not commonly result in irritation and hives. It dries the wound but not the skin. It helps the healing process of burns and does not cause a burning or stinging sensation unless an allergic reaction has occurred.

Think of what information is given in the stem as you read the options: a drug is applied topically for burns. Eliminate options 1 and 2, since they are unlikely to appear on burned skin. Use an educated guess to eliminate option 4, which is a common reaction to any substance to which the skin is sensitive. Select option 3.

2. Correct answer: 3

This is an antifungal and used to treat athlete's foot. Acyclovir (Zovirax) is used primarily for herpes simplex virus, such as fever blisters. Hydrocortisone is used primarily for inflammation. Ketoconazole (Nizoral) is used for seborrheic dermatitis.

On these types of questions when you may have no idea of the correct answer, make a selection. Go to the next question only after you have done a relaxation exercise, such as a few slow, deep breaths. Keep your tiredness or tenseness to a minimum so you can better answer the questions that remain. Remember there will be a few questions that have unfamiliar content.

3. Correct answer: 4

Dove is gentle and does not dry the skin. Safeguard, an antibacterial or antimicrobial soap, is harsh for an infant and will dry the skin. The oatmeal could soothe but the continued use of Irish Spring would continue to dry the skin. A deodorant soap is antimicrobial and therefore dries the skin out. Calamine lotion would further dry the skin.

The best action on these types of questions is to use your common knowledge of soaps and eliminate those substances known to dry, such as calamine lotion, which is used in events of poison ivy allergies to dry the area affected.

4. Correct answer: 2

Zinc protects the skin, assists in the healing process, and coats the skin to provide a barrier from

The clue in the stem is to "protect" the skin. Of the given substances, associate zinc oxide with use in the

the stool. Lubriderm would not heal broken, irritated skin. Glycerine would soften skin and may irritate open, broken skin. Silvadene does heal the skin, but in this case the priority is the protection from the diarrhea.

summertime as a skin protectant from the sun: recall those white-nosed children on the beach. Thus, select option 2.

5. Correct answer: 1

These agents in option 1 together offer the most relief from itching or urticaria. Caladryl should not be used because it prolongs the healing time and dries the skin. The approach in option 3 is not inappropriate, but rubbing the skin with a washcloth to use the oatmeal bar soap may not be tolerated well by the child. Alpha-Keri would not soothe the itching.

Test tip: It is important to identify the difference between "calamine" and "Caladryl. " Remember that Caladryl has a d in it and has a greater drying effect than calamine.

18

Drugs Affecting the Gastrointestinal System

FAST FACTS

1. Evaluation of the effectiveness of these drugs is completed by clinical assessment for changes in the following:
   - GI: nausea, vomiting, anorexia, diarrhea, constipation, blood present in stool or emesis
   - Relief of pain
   - CV: HR, heart rhythm, BP
   - Laboratory: CBC count, electrolytes
   - General: headache, drowsiness, confusion
2. Have clients take antacid drugs 1 hour after eating and *do not have them take other medications within 1 to 2 hours of taking the antacid.*
3. Shake most liquid antacids well and follow with a full glass of water unless instructed otherwise.
4. Inform clients that they may experience better relief from antacid liquids than tablets.
5. If digestants are taken on an empty stomach, the result may be enzyme action on the mucosa when no food is present and bleeding may result.
6. Never give ipecac syrup with or after activated charcoal; if needed, give it before the activated charcoal.
7. Never give ipecac syrup to clients who accidentally ingested a caustic substance.
8. Give ipecac *syrup;* 100% pure ipecac is 14 times stronger and can result in death.

CONTENT REVIEW

DRUGS USED TO TREAT PEPTIC ULCER DISEASE AND GASTRIC HYPERACIDITY

I. Antacids

A. Actions: neutralize gastric acid and raise the pH of the stomach, thereby relieving heartburn and the pain associated with gastric disorders

B. Uses
1. Indigestion
2. Reflux esophagitis: esophageal irritation and inflammation resulting from reflux of the stomach contents into the esophagus
3. Peptic ulcers: treatment and prevention
4. Decrease high serum phosohate levels in renal failure; the aluminum antacids (Amphogel, Basogel)

C. Side effects
1. GI: rebound hyperacidity: an excessive amount of acidity in the stomach
2. GI disturbances
   a. Constipation (aluminum and calcium)
   b. Diarrhea (magnesium)
   3. Electrolyte disturbances mOm-, moala
   a. Hypermagnesemia: hypotension, nausea, vomiting, ECG changes (magnesium-containing antacids)
   b. Hypophosphatemia: anorexia, malaise, muscle weakness (aluminum-containing antacids)
   c. Hypernatremia

> ⚠ **Warning!**
>
> Instruct clients to inquire about interactions with any new medications and OTC preparations. Interactions are too numerous to name within this text. Of special importance is the decrease in absorption of medications when these agents are given, especially with digoxin and antibiotics. Give sodium products cautiously in CV or renal disease to avoid the risk of complications from sodium retention.

D. Nursing implications
1. Assess the effectiveness of the medication
2. Monitor for signs of electrolyte disturbances
3. Advise clients to avoid other medications that lower the stomach pH or increase hyperacidity, such as caffeine and acetylsalicylic acid (aspirin)
4. Have clients take drugs 1 hour after eating and *do not have them take other medications within 1 to 2 hours of taking the antacid*
5. Shake most liquids well and follow with a full glass of water

unless instructed otherwise
6. Inform clients that they may experience better relief from liquids than tablets
7. Monitor for constipation and diarrhea. Medication or dose may need to be changed.

E. Common drugs
1. Aluminum hydroxide (AlternaGel, Amphojel)
2. Magnesium hydroxide (Milk of Magnesia)
3. Calcium carbonate (Alka-Mints, Tums)
4. Sodium bicarbonate ($NaHCO_3$)
5. Aluminum-magnesium complex (Maalox, Riopan, Riopan Plus)
6. Magnesium-hydroxide plus aluminum hydroxide with simethicone (Maalox TC, Mylanta II)
7. Bismuth subsalicylate (Pepto-Bismol)

II. H_2 histamine receptor antagonists and gastric protectants

A. Actions: inhibits the release of histamine at histamine (H_2) receptor sites and decreases gastric acidity; forms a complex that adheres to ulcer site

B. Uses
1. Treatment of ulcers
2. Prevention of stress ulcers
3. Hyperacidity
4. GI bleeding
5. Prevention of allergic responses
6. Gastroesophageal reflux associated with inhalation therapy

C. Side effects
1. CNS: confusion, especially in elderly clients
2. GI: nausea, diarrhea, abdominal pain
3. Hematologic: anemia, blood dyscrasias
4. CV: severe bradycardia after IV administration

⚠ Warning!

Interactions include increased action of many of the cardiac drugs and anticoagulants. Misoprostol (Cytotec) can cause uterine contractions and miscarriages.

D. Nursing implications
1. Instruct client to limit caffeine intake
2. Should administer before meals (ac) and at bedtime (hs)
3. Do not administer at the same time as antacids
4. Assess pulse rate and LOC before, during, and after administration of IV forms, especially in older clients

E. Common drugs
1. Histamine₂ or H_2 receptor antagonists
   a. Cimetidine (Tagamet)

       b. Ranitidine (Zantac)

       c. Famotidine (Pepcid)

       d. Nizatidine (Axid)

  2. Gastric mucosa protectants

       a. Sucralfate (Carafate) forms a barrier at the ulcer site, prevents NSAID-induced gastric ulcers and absorbs pepsin. It must be taken on an empty stomach for the best effect.

       b. Misoprostol (Cytotec) is used with peptic ulcers.

III. Proton (acid) pump inhibitors

A. Action: block the enzyme that secretes hydrogen ion (or proton) into the parietal cells of the stomach. More potent than H_2 receptor antagonists.

B. Uses

  1. Severe erosive esophagitis, not responsive to H_2 receptor antagonist therapy

  2. Short-term treatment of active peptic ulcer disease

  3. Gastric hypersecretion disorders

C. Side effects

  1. Long-term: overproduction of gastrin, which can cause tumors

  2. CNS: headache, dizziness, fatigue

  3. GI: abdominal pain, nausea, diarrhea

  4. GU: hematuria, proteinuria

⚠ Warning!

Interactions with oral anticoagulants, diazepam, and phenytoin; most often exhibited by toxic blood levels.

D. Nursing implications

  1. Know that antacids may be administered together with these agents

  2. Need to report any changes in urinary elimination or diarrhea

E. Common drugs

  1. Lansoprazole (Prevacid)

  2. Omeprazole (Prilosec)

IV. Anticholinergic agents (antispasmodics)

A. Actions

  1. Reduce gastric acid secretion

  2. Decrease smooth muscle motility

  3. Delay gastric emptying time

B. Uses

  1. Adjuncts to peptic ulcer disease

  2. Spasms and cramping associated with irritable bowel syndrome

  3. Colic in children

C. Side effects

  1. CV: tachycardia

2. GI: dry mouth, constipation
3. GU: urinary retention
4. CNS: sedation (may be a preferred side effect)

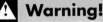 **Warning!**

> Tachycardia may occur with even small doses and HR should be monitored carefully.

D. **Nursing implications**
   1. Know that many of these agents come from belladonna plants and are termed belladonna alkaloids. Many others contain atropine sulfate (the prototype).
   2. Monitor bowel elimination and offer assistance as needed
   3. Monitor HR for rates over 100 beats/min
   4. Monitor I&O ratio: offer gum or hard candy for dry mouth or lemon glycerine swabs for sedated clients
   5. Assess for urinary retention: distention, frequent voiding of small amounts

E. **Common drugs**
   1. Atropine sulfate
      a. Clidinium bromide (Quarzan)
      b. Glycopyrrolate (Robinul)
      c. Propantheline bromide (Pro-Banthine)
   2. Belladonna alkaloids
      a. Hyoscyamine sulfate (Levsin, Anaspaz)
   3. Other: dicyclomine hydrochloride (Bentyl)

V. Antimicrobials

A. **Action: effective against *Helicobacter pylori*, the major cause of peptic ulcers. These agents are often used in combination for *H. pylori*. (See individual drug groups in Chapter 16 p. 257.)**
B. **Common drugs**
   1. Amoxicillin (Amoxil, Trimox)
   2. Clarithromycin (Biaxin)
   3. Metronidazole (Flagyl)
   4. Amoxicillin and clavulanate potassium (Augmentin), especially in children

OTHER GASTROINTESTINAL AGENTS

I. Gastrointestinal stimulants

A. **Action: Act directly or indirectly to stimulate the muscarinic receptors in the nervous system that control motility in the intestine; parasympathomimetics; serotonin antagonists; dopamine antagonists; acetylcholinesterase inhibitors**
B. **Uses**
   1. Gastroesophageal reflux

2. Stimulate atonic bladder and GI tract, particularly post-surgery
3. Diabetic gastroparesis
4. Antiemetic for chemotherapy

C. Side effects
1. GI: diarrhea, abdominal cramping, nausea, and belching
2. CNS: headache, fatigue
3. General: salivation, flushing of the skin, sweating

> ⚠ **Warning!**
>
> Contraindicated in clients with GI hemorrhage, mechanical bowel obstruction, or bowel perforation. Interaction with anticholinergic or ganglionic blockers.

D. Nursing implications
1. Assess for bowel sounds, distention of bladder, patency of catheters
2. Monitor elimination status: urinary and bowel

E. Common drugs
1. Bethanechol chloride (Duvoid, Urecholine), mainly for GU tract
2. Metoclopramide (Reglan), mainly for GI tract
3. Neostigmine methysulfate (Prostigmin)

II. Digestants

A. Action: work in various ways to aid in digestion by replacing missing substances that naturally digest food

B. Uses
1. Malabsorptive syndromes: a complex of symptoms that result from disorders in the intestinal absorption of nutrients
2. Achlorhydria: absence of hydrochloric acid in the gastric juice
3. Hypochlorhydria: a deficiency of hydrochloric acid in the gastric juice
4. Cystic fibrosis
5. Chronic pancreatitis

C. Side effects: few side effects occur; are usually mild, and vary with each drug

> ⚠ **Warning!**
>
> If taken on an empty stomach, may result in enzyme action on the mucosa when no food is present; bleeding may result.

D. Nursing implications
1. Instruct clients to take with or immediately after meals
2. Advise client to drink a full glass of water with each dose

E. Common drugs
1. Hydrochloric acid
2. Pancreatin (Dizymes)
3. Famotidine (Pepsin)

III. Antiflatulent agents

A. **Action: aids in breaking up gas bubbles trapped in the intestines**

B. **Uses**

   1. Postoperatively
   2. Children with colic

C. **Side effect: constipation**

⚠ Warning!

Avoid routine daily use.

D. **Nursing implications**

   1. Instruct client to drink plenty of water
   2. Treat the constipation as needed

E. **Common drug: simethicone (Mylicon)**

IV. Antiemetics

A. **Drug groups**

   1. Phenothiazines
   2. Antihistamines
   3. Anticholinergics
   4. Antiserotonergic antiemetics (HT_3 antagonists)
   5. Other individual drugs

B. **Actions: varies with the group used**

   1. Phenothiazines decrease the response of the chemoreceptor trigger zone by inhibiting the dopaminergic receptors
   2. Antihistamines block the H_1 receptors
   3. Anticholinergics prevent motion sickness by decreasing GI motility and secretions
   4. Antiserotonergic antiemetics (HT_3 antagonists) block serotonin, which is a major neurotransmitter for emesis. These agents block serotonin at the 5-HT_3 receptor located on the vagal nerve.

C. **Uses**

   1. Severe nausea
   2. Vomiting
   3. Before, during, or after chemotherapy
   4. Motion sickness

D. **Side effects are group-related, but may include the following**

   1. Anticholinergic effects: dry mouth, constipation, urinary retention, tachycardia, photophobia
   2. CNS: drowsiness
   3. Extrapyramidal findings with phenothiazines: tardive dyskinesia, chorea, athetosis, parkinsonianism
   4. Hypersensitivity

> ⚠️ **Warning!**
>
> Tissue sloughing is common with many of these drugs after IM administration; the Z-track method should always be used and documented.

E. Nursing implications

1. Advise clients that for motion sickness they need to take the drug 30 minutes to 1 hour before the activity that causes nausea
2. Implement safety measures; caution the client about the sedative properties
3. Assess for dry mouth, constipation, urinary retention, and tachycardia; monitor I&O

F. Common drugs

1. *Phenothiazines*
   a. Chlorpromazine hydrochloride (Thorazine)
   b. Prochlorperazine maleate (Compazine)
   c. Trimethobenzamide hydrochloride (Tigan)
2. *Anticholinergic*
   a. Scopolamine hydrobromide (Triptone)
3. *Antihistamine*
   a. Diphenhydramine hydrochloride (Benadryl)
   b. Promethazine (Phenergan)
   c. Dimenhydrinate (Dramamine)
   d. Hydroxyzine pamoate (Vistaril)
   e. Meclizine hydrochloride (Antivert)
4. *Antiserotonergic antiemetics (5-HT$_3$ antagonists)*
   a. Ondansetron (Zofran)
   b. Granisetron (Kytril)
   c. Dolasetron (Anzemet)
5. *Cholinergics*
   a. Metoclopramide hydrochloride (Reglan)

V. Emetics

A. Actions: irritate the stomach and stimulate the vomiting center in the brain

B. Uses

1. Overdose of drugs
2. Accidental poisoning with noncaustic substances

C. Side effects

1. Toxicity
2. Abuse by bulemic clients

> ### ⚠ **Warning!**
>
> Interactions occur with alcohol and CNS depressants. Never administer to semicomatose or comatose clients. Never give with or after activated charcoal. If needed, give before the activated charcoal. Never give to clients who accidentally ingest a caustic substance. Give ipecac *syrup;* pure ipecac is 14 times stronger and can result in death.

D. Nursing implications

1. Instruct clients to have a bottle of ipecac syrup, not pure ipecac, at home in case of accidental ingestion, especially with children. Note expiration date.
2. Warn clients that it can be very messy and difficult for a child to ingest
3. Administer an ipecac syrup dose of 10 ml followed by a glass of water in children under age 1; 15 ml, followed by a glass of water, for children over age 1; and 15 to 30 ml, followed by several glasses of water, for adults
4. May repeat ipecac syrup dose in 30 minutes, if first dose does not produce emesis

E. Common drugs: Ipecac syrup

VI. Laxatives (cathartics)

A. Actions: specific to the group (Table 18-1)

B. Side effects

1. Dehydration, electrolyte depletion
2. GI: straining; irritation of hemorrhoids
3. Abuse: misuse of the agents

> ### ⚠ **Warning!**
>
> These agents may be habit-forming. Contraindicated in clients with CV problems, increased ICP, or elders with fecal impaction.

C. General nursing implications

1. Monitor electrolyte levels and I&O ratio, poor skin turgor, increased thirst, dry mucous membranes
2. Assess bowel elimination pattern, GI discomforts
3. Discontinue if diarrhea persists; do not give if obstruction is suspected
4. Teach clients that proper diet and exercise aids in regular elimination
5. Know that clients who should avoid straining may benefit from a lubricant laxative. Mineral oil enemas work well without causing severe strain in clients who have had a recent heart attack, clients with increased ICP, or older clients with fecal impaction; they also work well when saline is contraindicated.

TABLE 18-1 Laxatives—Actions and Concerns

Name	Mechanism of Action	Nursing Considerations
Stimulants		
Senna (Senokot) Phenolphthalein (Ex-Lax) Cascara sagrada (Cascara) Castor oil Senna concentrate (Senna-Gen)	Irritant to bowel; peristalsis is stimulated Used in preparation for surgery, acute constipation, obstructions that are not complete	Not recommended for children; highly abused Avoid in pregnancy Should obtain results in 6 to 12 hr
Salines/Osmotics		
Normal saline solution Magnesium citrate (Citrate of Magnesia) Epsom salts Magnesium salts (MOM) Sodium biphosphate (Fleet) Glycerin suppositories (Senokot) Lactulose (Chronulac)	Act by drawing water into the bowel and increasing peristalsis Used for elimination of poisons, before procedures, removal of parasites, mild constipation	Electrolyte imbalance and dehydration can occur Fleet enemas are given rectally and come in an oil-retention form that is good for older clients
Bulk-Forming		
Psyllium hydrophilic muciloid (Metamucil) Methylcellulose (Maltsupex, Citrucel) Polycarbophil (Fibercon)	Act by forming a soft, bulky mass from absorbing water Used for chronic constipation, in infants suffering from continuous constipation, in pregnant females	May take up to 24 hours to work Monitor elimination Take with a full glass of water
Stool Softeners		
Mineral oil Docusate sodium (Colace) Docusate calcium (Surfak) Docusate potassium (Dialose)	Coat the fecal mass with oil to help lubricate for easier elimination or reduce surface tension of feces Used in older adults when straining is prohibited (MI, eye surgery)	Assess electrolyte levels Offer candy or juice to disguise the taste Monitor electrolytes May take 1-2 days to work

6. Monitor the amount and frequency of laxatives taken especially for clients at risk for bulemia and anorexia

VII. Antidiarrheals

A. **Groups**
   1. Absorbents
   2. Opiates
   3. Anticholinergics

B. **Actions: relieve symptoms or work against the cause of the diarrhea. Absorbents bind with bacteria or toxins.**

C. **Uses**
   1. Short-term diarrhea
   2. Irritable bowel syndrome
   3. Overdose

D. **Side effects**
   1. GI: constipation
   2. Abuse potential
   3. Anticholinergic effects: dry mouth, decreased secretions

> ## ⚠ Warning!
>
> Instruct the client that these agents relieve symptoms but do not cure the problem; notify the physician if diarrhea persists longer than 48 hours. If food poisoning is suspected, antidiarrheals should be avoided. The toxic substance needs to exit the GI tract. Advise clients to drink plenty of fluids, such as water or electrolyte replacements (Gatorade, Pedialyte). In these situations, advise clients to notify the physician if diarrhea for suspected food poisoning lasts longer than 48 hours or if the client has symptoms of severe dehydration or electrolyte imbalance, such as dizziness, persistent severe cramping, very dry mucous membranes, feeling of exhaustion, and severe weakness.

E. **Nursing implications**
   1. Know how to administer properly. Some of the agents can be given after each diarrhea stool.
   2. Assess elimination, dehydration, and the results obtained
   3. Monitor the amount and frequency of use of these agents
   4. Know that activated charcoal is a powder that must be mixed with water to administer; it is also used for overdose of caustic chemicals

F. **Common drugs**
   1. *Absorbents*
      a. Bismuth subsalicylate (Pepto-Bismol)
      b. Activated charcoal (Charcocaps)
      c. Kaolin and pectin (Kapectolin)
   2. *Opiates*
      a. Paregoric (camphorated opium tincture), used commonly for infants with colic

b. Synthetic opiates
   (1) Diphenoxylate hydrochloride plus atropine sulfate (Lomotil)
   (2) Loperamide (Imodium)
3. Anticholinergics: combination of alcohol, kaolin, atropine, hyoscyamine sulfate, and scopolamine hydrobromide (Donnagel suspension)
4. Octreotide (Sandostatin)

VIII. Flora modifiers

  A. **Action: replace normal flora**
  B. **Use: excessive diarrhea, usually from antibiotic use**
  C. **Side effects: overgrowth, since preparation contains *Lactobacillus* species organisms**
  D. **Common drug: Lactinex**

WEB Resources

Internet access for additional resources:

http://www.discoveryhealth.com/DH/
  ihtIH?t=8451&c=186999&p=~br,DSC|~st,8270|~r,WSDSC000|~b,*|#treat
  Information on gastroesophageal reflux disease (GERD)

http://www.discoveryhealth.com/DH/
  ihtIH?t=10915&p=~br,DSC|~st,20812|~r,WSDSC000|~b,*|#treat
  Provides content about various ulcers

REVIEW QUESTIONS

1. With an aluminum antacid, which of these findings would be expected?
1. Hyperkalemia
2. Hyponatremia
3. Hypophosphatemia
4. Hypercalcemia

2. A client is taking an antacid 1 hour after a meal and at bedtime and tetracycline every 6 hours. The best times to schedule each would be which of these?
1. Antacid 9 AM, 1 PM, 5 PM, 9 PM; tetracycline 8 AM, 2 PM, 8 PM, 2 AM
2. Antacid 8 AM, 12 PM, 4 PM, 9 PM; tetracycline 9 AM, 4 PM, 9 PM, 4 AM
3. Schedule both together
4. Antacid 7:30 AM, 11 AM, 4 PM, 9 AM; tetracycline 8 AM, 2 PM, 8 PM, 2 AM

3. An OTC medication that mothers can use for infants with excess flatus is which drug?
1. Hyoscyamine sulfate (Levsin)
2. Simethicone (Mylicon)
3. Famotidine (Pepcid)
4. Diphenoxylate hydrochloride plus atropine sulfate (Lomotil)

4. In preparing for a jet flight to Hawaii, a client plans to take dimenhydrinate (Dramamine) to relieve the motion sickness. When should the client take it?
1. Once the plane has taken off
2. At least 2 hours before departure
3. When she becomes nauseated
4. About 30 minutes before boarding

5. The best laxative for a client, age 63, who has had a heart attack and severe constipation would be which of these drugs?
1. 1 L normal saline with castile soap enema
2. Psyllium hydrophilic muciloid (Metamucil), 1 tsp tid
3. Oil-retention Fleet enema, holding for 15 to 30 minutes if possible
4. Senna (Senokot), 2 tsp bid

6. The best absorbent for accidental poisoning with a caustic substance would be which of these drugs?
1. Bismuth subsalicylate (Pepto-Bismol)
2. Syrup of ipecac
3. Activated charcoal
4. Dimercaprol (BAL)

ANSWERS, RATIONALES, AND TEST-TAKING TIPS

Rationales	Test-Taking Tips

1. Correct answer: 3

Low phosphorous levels are common with the aluminum-containing antacids. Thus, these antacids are used in renal failure to decrease the high phosphate levels. Antacids usually do not affect the potassium level. Sodium and magnesium levels may be raised with various antacids. High calcium levels may be evident in calcium-containing antacids.

Remember that the two major categories for antacids are magnesium and aluminum. The two electrolytes affected are magnesium and phosphorus. Match magnesium antacids with magnesium and the other type, aluminum antacids, binds phosphorus to lower its serum levels.

2. Correct answer: 1

This schedule separates the antacid and tetracycline by 1 hour and follows the usual mealtimes for the antacid. The antacid is ordered 1 hour after meals. Medications should not be scheduled at the same time as antacids, since the absorption can be diminished.

Make the question easy. Tetracycline is one of the drugs that needs to be taken on an empty stomach. Think about this as you read through the options by first looking at only the first time for each drug. You compare in option 1 antacid (A) 9 AM and tetracycline (T) 8AM, in option 2 A 8 AM, T 9 AM, option 4 A 7:30 AM, T 8AM. By this technique, it is evident that option 1 is correct, since the antibiotic is given first and the antacid after a meal and 1 hour from the antibiotic.

3. Correct answer: 2

Mylicon, available without a prescription, relieves excess gas associated with colic. Levsin will decrease flatus but must be prescribed by the physician. Pepcid in option 3 is used to treat ulcers and hyperacidity. Option 4, Lomotil, is an antidiarrheal agent that decreases peristalsis.

Eliminate options based on what you know. **L**omotil may cause drowsiness when given to **L**imit stools. **P**epcid is for **P**eptic ulcers. To decide between options 1 and 2, select the more familiar drug, Mylicon.

4. Correct answer: 4

Thirty minutes before the flight allows for absorption of the agent and a peak effect during the flight. The Dramamine may not be absorbed enough to relieve the motion sickness if the plane has already taken off. Two hours before would be too long, and the agent may not relieve the motion sickness. Option 3 would involve too long of a wait.

Recall the basic knowledge of drug administration by route and time of effect: PO = 30 minutes; IM = 15 minutes; IV = within 5 minutes; rectal suppository = 15 minutes; SL = within 5 to 10 minutes. Think basics. Now is a good time to stop and review other basic information such as traction care, positioning, and abbreviations. Be prepared. Avoid missing basic questions simply because of unfamiliar words or drugs.

5. Correct answer: 3

An oil retention enema would provide the relief needed without the strain on the CV system. Saline is not recommended for a cardiac client. Metamucil may not provide the immediate relief needed but would probably be a good *preventive* approach. Senna would not provide the immediate relief needed.

The clue in the stem is that the client is already constipated. The need is to help the stool slip out without straining. Thus, the oil retention enema is the best choice.

6. Correct answer: 3

Activated charcoal binds with the caustic agent to decrease the effects on the body. Pepto-Bismol would not be effective enough for a caustic agent. Vomiting is not recommended for a caustic substance. BAL is an antidote for heavy metal poisoning. It is given deep IM, since it is an oil-based medication. It is also used in arsenic, gold, mercury, and lead poisoning; administration is frequent, with the initial series of doses usually given daily for up to 10 days.

If you have no idea of the correct option, "go with what you know": that **a**ctivated charcoal is used to **a**bsorb.

19

Drugs Affecting the Ear and Eye

FAST FACTS

1. Evaluation of the effectiveness of these drugs is completed by clinical assessment for changes in the following:
   - Eyes: pupil reaction, sclera for redness, photophobia, and clarity of vision
   - Ear: presence of pain, drainage, hearing loss, and balance
   - General: dizziness
2. Handwashing before and after eyedrop administration is essential.
3. When beta-blocker eye drops are used, monitor VS, especially HR and BP, since systemic effects may occur.
4. Apply pressure to the lacrimal sac for 1 to 2 minutes to prevent systemic absorption of any eye drop.
5. Teach client not to put anything into the ear canal if itching occurs and not to try to remove the wax.

CONTENT REVIEW

AGENTS USED IN THE EYE

I. Mydriatics and cycloplegics

   A. **Actions**
      1. Mydriatics exert a sympathetic nervous system response and cause dilatation of the pupil by contraction of the pupil's dilator muscle
      2. Cycloplegics paralyze the fine-focusing muscle (accommodative muscle) by blocking cholinergic stimulation of the muscle of the iris; clients have trouble focusing the near and the far vision

B. **Groups of drugs**
   1. Sympathomimetic
   2. Anticholinergic agents
   3. Prostaglandin inhibitors
   4. Adrenergic drugs
   5. Alpha-adrenergic blockers

C. **Uses**
   1. Intraocular examinations
   2. Before and after eye surgery to prevent miosis or treat inflammation
   3. Iris refraction in children

D. **Side effects**
   1. Eye: local irritation, burning
   2. Vision: blurred near vision; photophobia
   3. Systemic reactions: dry mucous membranes, hypotension, ↑ or ↓ HR

> ⚠ **Warning!**
>
> These agents are contraindicated in closed-angle glaucoma. Some of these agents can increase IOP, causing ocular congestion.

E. **Nursing implications**
   1. Instruct the client to wear dark sunglasses until clear vision resumes
   2. Teach the client proper instillation (Figure 19-1)
   3. Hold pressure on lacrimal sac for 1 to 2 minutes after administration

F. **Common drugs**
   1. *Sympathomimetic*
      a. Epinephrine hydrochloride (Epifrin)
      b. Naphazoline hydrochloride (Naphcon)
      c. Phenylephrine hydrochloride (Neo-Synephrine)
      d. Tetrahydrozoline hydrochloride (Murine Plus)
      e. Oxymetazoline (OcuClear)
   2. *Anticholinergic*
      a. Atropine sulfate (Isopto Atropine)
      b. Cyclopentolate hydrochloride (Cyclogyl)
      c. Scopolamine hydrobromide (Isopto Hyoscine)
      d. Homatropine hydrobromide (AK-Homatropine)
   3. *Prostaglandin inhibitors*
      a. Diclofenac (Voltaren)
      b. Flurbiprofen sodium (Ocufen)
   4. *Adrenergic drugs:* phenylephrine hydrochloride (AK-Dilate)
   5. *Alpha-adrenergic blocker:* Dapiprazole hydrochloride (Rev-Eyes) counteracts mydriasis induced by the adrenergic drugs

II. Miotics

A. **Actions: exert a parasympathetic response that results in the constriction of the pupil, contraction of the accommodative muscle,**

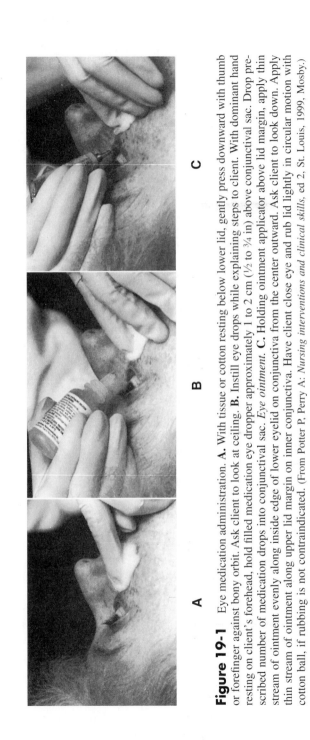

Figure 19-1 Eye medication administration. **A.** With tissue or cotton resting below lower lid, gently press downward with thumb or forefinger against bony orbit. Ask client to look at ceiling. **B.** Instill eye drops while explaining steps to client. With dominant hand resting on client's forehead, hold filled medication eye dropper approximately 1 to 2 cm (½ to ¾ in) above conjunctival sac. Drop prescribed number of medication drops into conjunctival sac. *Eye ointment.* **C.** Holding ointment applicator above lid margin, apply thin stream of ointment evenly along inside edge of lower eyelid on conjunctiva from the center outward. Ask client to look down. Apply thin stream of ointment along upper lid margin on inner conjunctiva. Have client close eye and rub lid lightly in circular motion with cotton ball, if rubbing is not contraindicated. (From Potter P, Perry A: *Nursing interventions and clinical skills*, ed 2, St. Louis, 1999, Mosby.)

and decreased resistance to outflow of aqueous humor for the end result of the following:

1. A decrease IOP: the internal pressure of the eye, regulated by resistance to the flow of aqueous humor
2. An increase outflow of aqueous humor

B. Groups of drugs
1. Direct-acting cholinergics (cholinomimetic drugs)
2. Prostaglandin analog

C. Uses: treatment of glaucoma and esotropia ("crossed eyes")

D. Side effects
1. Blurred vision and local irritation
2. Systemic absorption

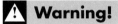 **Warning!**

Handwashing before and after instillation is essential.

E. Nursing implications
1. Administer at bedtime to decrease blurring of vision
2. Avoid if inflammation is present
3. Teach the client how to administer
4. Hold pressure at the lacrimal sac for 1 to 2 minutes to decrease systemic absorption

F. Common drugs
1. Direct-acting cholinergics (cholinomimetic drugs: strong and weak miotics)
   a. Pilocarpine hydrochloride (Pilocar)
   b. Carbachol (Isopto Carbachol)
   c. Physostigmine salicylate (Isopto Eserine)
   d. Isoflurophate (Floropryl)
   e. Demecarium bromide (Humorsol)
2. Prostaglandin analog: iatanoprost (Xalatan)

III. Other drugs used to lower IOP

A. Actions
1. Carbonic anhydrase inhibitors (CAI) reduce the amount of aqueous humor produced and thereby lower IOP
2. Beta-adrenergic blocking agents decrease the production of aqueous humor and thereby lower IOP
3. Osmotic agents increase plasma osmolarity and thereby lower IOP
4. Adrenergic drugs produce a vasoconstrictive effect, which decreases the production of aqueous humor and decreases IOP; often given with a CAI agent

B. Use
1. Open- and closed-angle glaucoma
2. Before and after eye surgery

C. Side effects
1. Bradycardia
2. Headache

3. Fatigue
4. Stinging when administered
5. Fluid imbalance

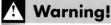 **Warning!**

CAI and osmotics are diuretics and increase urine production. Monitor electrolyte levels and advise client to instill early in the morning. Proper handwashing before and after eyedrop is administered is essential.

D. Nursing implications
1. Beta blockers: monitor VS, especially for decreases in HR and BP, since systemic effects may occur
2. Teach client how to administer and that stinging is not normal; client should not rub eye afterwards

E. Common drugs
1. *CAI*
   a. Acetazolamide (Diamox)
   b. Dichlorphenamide (Daranide)
   c. Methazolamide (Neptazane)
2. *Osmotics*
   a. Glycerin anhydrous (Opthalgan)
   b. Isosorbide (Ismotic)
   c. Mannitol (Osmitrol)
3. *Beta blockers*
   a. Timolol maleate (Timoptic)
   b. Levobunolol hydrochloride (Betagan)
   c. Carteolol hydrochloride (Ocupress)
   d. Betaxolol hydrochloride (Betoptic)
4. *Adrenergic drugs*
   a. Dipivefrin hydrochloride (Propine)
   b. Epinephrine borate or hydrochloride (Epinal, Epifrin)

IV. Anesthetic agents

A. Action: anesthetize the corneal surface
B. Uses
1. An aid to instruments that measure IOP or the removal of foreign bodies
2. Suture removal
3. Conjunctival scraping
4. Manipulation of lacrimal canal

C. Side effects
1. Stimulation of the CNS: syncope, nausea, and seizures
2. Hypotension
3. Transient eye pain, blurred vision, redness

D. Nursing implications
1. Provide protective eye patch while eye is anesthetized
2. Instruct client not to rub the eye to prevent corneal abrasions
3. Apply pressure to the lacrimal sac for 1 to 2 minutes to prevent systemic absorption

    E. **Common drugs**
       1. Proparacaine hydrochloride (Ophthaine)
       2. Tetracaine hydrochloride (Pontocaine Hydrochloride)

V. Antiinflammatory agents

    A. **Actions: decrease edema, redness, scarring, and exudate**
    B. **Groups of drugs**
       1. Corticosteroids
       2. Nonsteroidal agents
    C. **Uses: inflammatory disorders, hypersensitivity conditions**
    D. **Side effects**
       1. Increased IOP
       2. Optic nerve damage
       3. Decreased visual activity
       4. Cataracts

> ⚠️ **Warning!**
>
> Good handwashing is essential before and after eye drug instillation. Report to physician in 48 hours if original findings do not diminish.

    E. **Nursing implications**
       1. Instruct in proper administration
       2. Monitor for use on short-term basis only
       3. Instruct client not to rub eye
    F. **Common drugs**
       1. Dexaminationethasone (Maxidex)
       2. Prednisolone sodium phosphate (Ak-Pred)
       3. Diclofenac sodium (Voltaren)—nonsteroidal agent

VI. Antiinfectives

    A. **Actions: interfere or destroy microorganisms that cause these infections: *Staphylococcus, Streptococcus, Pseudomonas,* and *Klebsiella* species; *Escherichia coli, Neisseria gonorrhoeae***
    B. **Groups of drugs**
       1. Antibiotics
       2. Antifungals
       3. Antivirals
    C. **Uses**
       1. Infections: bacterial, fungal, and viral
       2. Pinkeye
       3. HSV-1 infection
       4. Conjunctivitis
    D. **Side effects**
       1. Local irritation
       2. Overgrowth of microorganism

> ### ⚠ Warning!
> Proper handwashing is essential. Report to physician in 48 hours if original findings do not diminish.

E. **Nursing implications**
   1. Teach proper administration
   2. Instruct client to notify physician if edema, redness, or pain does not decrease

F. **Common drugs**
   1. Antibiotics
      a. Bacitracin ophthalmic (AK-Tracin)
      b. Gentamicin sulfate (Garamycin Ophthalmic)
      c. Tobramycin (Tobrex)
      d. Sulfacetamide sodium 15% (Sulfair-15 Ophthalmic)
      e. Neomycin, polymyxin B sulfate, and bacitracin (Mycitracin)
      f. Chloramphenicol (Chloroptic)
   2. Antifungal: natamycin (Natacyn)
   3. Antiviral: trifluridine (Viroptic); idoxuridine (Herplex), vidarabine (Vira-A)

AGENTS USED IN THE EAR

I. Antiinfective agents

A. **Actions: inhibit or destroy gram-negative or gram-positive microorganisms that cause infection in the ear**

B. **Uses: treat external auditory canal infections (otitis externa) and middle ear infections (otitis media)**

C. **Side effects**
   1. Superinfections
   2. Hypersensitivity

> ### ⚠ Warning!
> Teach client to report ringing in the ear (tinnitus) and any decrease in hearing.

D. **Nursing implications**
   1. Assess for hypersensitivity; assess for culture and sensitivity before administration of the initial dose
   2. Teach the client how to instill the drops (Figure 19-2)
   3. Instruct the client to take all the medication prescribed

E. **Common drugs**
   1. *Topical*
      a. Chloramphenicol (Chloromycetin Otic)
      b. Neosporin
   2. *Oral*
      a. Ampicillin (Polycillin)
      b. Trimethoprim plus sulfamethoxazole (Septra)
      c. Penicillin VK (V-Cillin K)

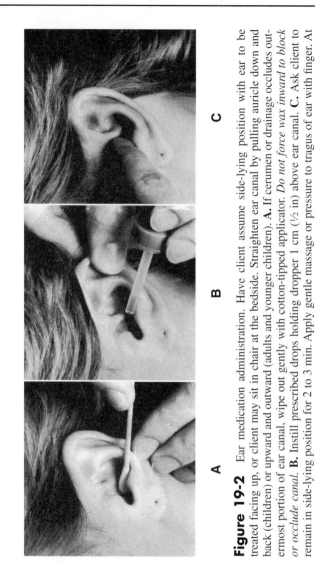

Figure 19-2 Ear medication administration. Have client assume side-lying position with ear to be treated facing up, or client may sit in chair at the bedside. Straighten ear canal by pulling auricle down and back (children) or upward and outward (adults and younger children). **A.** If cerumen or drainage occludes outermost portion of ear canal, wipe out gently with cotton-tipped applicator. *Do not force wax inward to block or occlude canal.* **B.** Instill prescribed drops holding dropper 1 cm (½ in) above ear canal. **C.** Ask client to remain in side-lying position for 2 to 3 min. Apply gentle massage or pressure to tragus of ear with finger. At times, physician may order the insertion of portion of cotton ball into outermost part of canal. Do not press cotton into canal. Remove cotton after 15 min. (From Potter P, Perry A: *Nursing interventions and clinical skills,* ed 2, St. Louis, 1999, Mosby.)

    d. Amoxicillin (Amoxil)
    e. Cefaclor (Ceclor)
    f. Amphotericin B (Fungizone)
    g. Amoxicillin plus clavulanic acid (Augmentin)

II. Antiinflammatory agents

  A. **Actions: inhibit edema and fibrin deposition to decrease inflammation of the ear**
  B. **Use: decrease inflammation in the external ear canal**
  C. **Side effects: mask underlying otic infections**

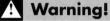 **Warning!**

    Do not administer if tympanic membrane is ruptured.
  D. **Nursing implications: Teach client not to put anything into the ear canal if itching occurs and not to try to remove the wax**
  E. **Common drugs**
    1. Dexamethasone sodium phosphate (Ak-dex)
    2. Hydrocortisone acetate (Coly-Mycin S Otic)

III. Anesthetic agents

  A. **Action: block nerve conduction**
  B. **Use: relieve ear pain temporarily**

⚠ Warning!

    Do not administer if tympanic membrane is ruptured.
  C. **Common drug: benzocaine (Auralgan Otic)**

IV. Ceruminolytic agents

  A. **Actions: emulsify hardened or impacted cerumen or prevent accumulation of cerumen**
  B. **Side effect: local irritation**
  C. **Nursing implications: instruct the client to irrigate the ear for 15 minutes after use and not to use cotton swabs**
  D. **Common drugs**
    1. Carbamide peroxide (Debrox)
    2. Triethanolamine polypeptide oleate-condensate (Cerumenex)

WEB Resources

http://health.yahoo.com/health/Diseases_and_Conditions/Disease_Feed_Data/Glaucoma/
  #Treatment
  Information for the care of glaucoma.

REVIEW QUESTIONS

1. Instructions to a parent for the instillation of ear drops in a 2-year-old would be which of these actions?
    1. Pull the auricle downward and slightly backward
    2. Pull the auricle upward and backward
    3. Pull the auricle downward and slightly forward
    4. Lay the child flat and do not pull the ear in any direction

2. After an eye examination, the nurse would instruct the client to do which of these actions?
    1. Expect burning and itching
    2. Wear sunglasses and avoid driving
    3. Expect blurred vision for several days
    4. Avoid reading for several days

3. If given with Timoptic drops, which of these medications would warrant careful monitoring of the cardiovascular system?
    1. Dexamethasone
    2. Neptazane
    3. Diamox
    4. Digoxin

4. To prevent systemic absorption of eye medications, the nurse should do which action?
    1. Put pressure on the tragus
    2. Hold slight pressure on the lacrimal sac for 5 minutes
    3. Hold slight pressure on the lacrimal sac for 1 to 3 minutes
    4. Gently rub the eye for 1 to 2 minutes

5. Medications, such as a carbonic anhydrase inhibitor (CAI), work in glaucoma in which manner?
    1. Increases the formation of aqueous humor
    2. Decreases the formation of aqueous humor
    3. Increases the outflow of aqueous humor
    4. Decreases the outflow of aqueous humor

ANSWERS, RATIONALES, AND TEST-TAKING TIPS

Rationales	Test-Taking Tips

1. Correct answer: 1

This action helps straighten the ear canal in children. The action in option 2 applies to adults. The action in option 3 does not assist with eardrop administration. A flat position is too vague to be a good choice for an answer.

Remember that adults grow "up"; therefore the instillation of ear medication is to pull back and "up." The child is the opposite: pull back and down for children age 5 or younger.

2. Correct answer: 2

The pupils are often dilated for an eye examination. Therefore the sunlight makes vision difficult since the dilated pupil results in photophobia. Driving could be dangerous if the vision is blurred from the dilatation. Clients would be able to see in the distance with close vision being very blurred. Burning and itching may signal an allergic reaction to any agent used. The blurred vision should subside within a few hours after the examination and should be reported if present 24 hours later. Reading may be difficult if the vision is blurred, but only for a few hours.

As you read the options look for clues. The words "several days" is the clue that options 3 and 4 are not reasonable choices. Between the remaining options, use basic knowledge that any substance put into the eye or on the skin that results in burning is inappropriate. Select option 2.

3. Correct answer: 4

Both of these agents, digoxin and timoptic, have the potential for lowering the heart rate. Therefore, VS should be monitored closely. Timoptic has similar properties to the oral beta blockers. The agents in options 1, 2, and 3 do not interact with Timoptic.

Think about what you know and then go with it. The most familiar drug listed is digoxin, and the question is asking about CV effects. Select option 4.

Rationales	Test-Taking Tips

4. Correct answer: 3

The action in option 3 is to avoid pressure on the tear duct and to prevent the medication from entering the sinuses. Pressure on the ear, option 1, does not affect eye drops. Option 2 is too long to hold pressure. Rubbing and excessive blinking should be avoided after application of eye drops or ointment.

"Go with what you know" if you have no clue of the correct answer. Eliminate options 1 and 4, which have nothing to do with systemic absorption. Or maybe you can eliminate option 1 because you cannot remember what it is. Avoid the selection of an answer that you don't know. To decide between options 2 and 3, think realistically and use common sense to select 1 to 3 minutes.

5. Correct answer: 2

Decreasing the aqueous humor is necessary in glaucoma to decrease the IOP. Options 1 and 4 would worsen the glaucoma. The formation, not the outflow, of aqueous humor is affected by these drops.

Miotic drops constrict the pupil and facilitate the outflow of the aqueous humor from the eye. In CAIs, the key word to remember is "inhibitors," which can be associated with a decrease in humor production.

20

Drugs Affecting Sexuality and Reproduction

FAST FACTS

1. Evaluation of the effectiveness of these drugs is completed by clinical assessment for changes in (listed in order of priority) the following:
   - General: weight gain, breast tenderness, changes in menses or libido
   - CV and respiratory: tenderness of calves; sudden shortness of breath is classic for pulmonary embolus; HR and BP for increase or decrease; rhythm for irregularity
   - LOC: mood swings, irritability
   - GI: nausea, vomiting, anorexia, abdominal pain, or cramping
   - Laboratory: PT and aPTT; CBC count; AST and ALT levels
2. Spermicides (creams, gels, and foams) are applied vaginally 10 to 15 minutes before penetration and ejaculation. Instruct clients not to douche for 6 to 8 hours afterwards.
3. Instruct the client that missing a dose of the oral contraceptive could result in pregnancy.
4. Contraceptive sponge: contains a spermicide that absorbs the semen; it can be left in for 24 hours.
5. If estrogen is prescribed, warn against cigarette smoking, since side effects are increased, especially in women over age 35 who smoke.
6. If started on antibiotics, alternate birth control actions are needed throughout the course of antibiotic therapy.

CONTENT REVIEW

FEMALE AND MALE SEX HORMONES

I. Estrogens

A. Actions: bind with receptors to produce the same effect as naturally occurring estrogen. Estrogen is necessary for the following:

1. Female reproductive organs
2. Secondary sex characteristics
   a. Fullness of breasts
   b. Appropriate distribution of body fat
   c. Soft skin texture
   d. Female growth and distribution of body hair
   e. Female voice
3. Maintenance of menstrual cycle
4. Growth of the ducts and nipples of the mammary glands

B. Uses

1. Menopausal symptoms: hot flashes, night sweats, somatic complaints, fatigue, insomnia, nervousness, headache, memory loss
2. Osteoporosis
3. Menstrual disturbances: abnormal uterine bleeding, premenstrual symptoms, dysmenorrhea
4. Breast cancer treatment in women
5. Oral contraceptives
6. Postcoital contraception
7. Lactation suppressant
8. Acne in females
9. Prostate cancer treatment in men

C. Side effects

1. GI: nausea, vomiting, loss of appetite
2. Fluid: salt and water retention, weight gain
3. Breast tenderness
4. Comfort: headache
5. Thromboembolic disorders
6. CV: hypertension

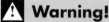 **Warning!**

Warn against cigarette smoking; side effects are increased in women over age 35 who smoke. Interactions occur with antihyperglycemic and anticoagulant drugs (increased dose may be needed).

D. Nursing implications

1. Monitor BP on a monthly basis because of hypertension risk
2. Instruct client to report any breakthrough bleeding between cycles of regular menses
3. Inform male clients receiving estrogen therapy that the female characteristics usually disappear when the therapy is complete and the drug is discontinued

    4. Offer instruction on how to use the form ordered: oral, intravaginal, transdermal

    5. Know that estrogens may alter certain laboratory test results

    6. Monitor for Homan's sign, complaints of pain in calves, which signals thrombophlebitis

    7. Monitor for weight gain and signs of edema

    8. Emphasize compliance

E. Common drugs

    1. Chlorotrianisene (Tace)

    2. Conjugated estrogenic substances (Premarin)

    3. Diethylstilbestrol (DES)

    4. Esterified estrogens (Estrace, Climara)

    5. Estropipate (Ogen)

II. Progestins

A. Actions: replace the missing progesterone by modifying the progesterone molecule from inactivation by the liver. Needed for the following:

    1. Preparation of the uterus and maintenance of the pregnancy

    2. Development of mammary gland duct during pregnancy

    3. Reduction of spontaneous contractions

B. Uses

    1. Dysmenorrhea: pain associated with menstruation

    2. Endometriosis: ectopic growth and function of endometrial tissue

    3. Functional uterine bleeding

    4. Prevention of abortion

    5. **Premenstrual syndrome** (PMS)

    6. Infertility: inability or difficulty in becoming pregnant

    7. Contraception

    8. With estrogen replacement therapy in women who have not had a hysterectomy to reduce the risk of uterine cancer

C. Side effects

    1. GI: nausea, vomiting

    2. Weight gain

    3. CNS: dizziness, headache

    4. Decreased libido

    5. Vascular: thrombolytic disease

⚠ Warning!

Contraindicated in clients with epilepsy, migraine headaches, cardiac disorders, and asthma.

D. Nursing implications

    1. Monitor Homan's sign and complaints of pain in the calf

    2. Monitor weight, I&O, dietary changes

    3. Assess for decreased libido

E. **Common drugs**
   1. Medroxyprogesterone acetate (Provera, Depro-provera)
   2. Progesterone (Progestasert)
   3. Norethindrone (Norlutin)
   4. Megestrol (Megace)
   5. Hydroxyprogesterone (Hylutin)
   6. Levonorgestrel (Norplant)

III. Oral contraceptives: birth control pills

A. **Actions: block** *follicle-stimulating hormone* **(FSH) and** *luteinizing hormone* **(LH), which decreases the release of the ovum and alters the viscosity of the mucus of the cervix, thereby hindering the fertilized ovum from proper implantation**

B. **Combinations**
   1. Fixed dose of estrogen and progestin
   2. Fixed estrogen dose (beginning of cycle after menses) followed by varying progestin dose (increasing in strength until day 21 of cycle) (low level dosage, then high level in cycle)
   3. Varying amounts of progestin and estrogen

C. **Side effects**
   1. Early signs of pregnancy: nausea, breast fullness, weight gain, dizziness, fatigue, depression, irregular bleeding
   2. Amenorrhea: the absence of menstruation
   3. CV: thromboembolic disorders
   4. Carcinogenesis and tumors

> ### ⚠ **Warning!**
>
> Interactions are numerous: antibiotics, anticonvulsants, anticoagulants, antihypertensive agents, caffeine, corticosteroids, analgesics.

D. **Nursing implications**
   1. Teach the client how to take the medications: begin on day 5 of the cycle and take 1 pill every day until day 21; then take the 7 pills containing no hormones during the menstrual cycle
   2. Instruct the client that missing a dose of the hormone could result in pregnancy
   3. Instruct the client to do breast self-examinations monthly along with monitoring of the monthly cycle to report any abnormalities
   4. Monitor Homan's sign and symptoms of clots in the lower extremities
   5. Encourage clients to stop smoking; cessation decreases the risk of thromboembolic disorders

E. **Common drugs** (Table 20-1)

IV. Contraceptives: other devices

A. Spermicides (creams, gels, and foams) are applied vaginally 10 to 15 minutes before penetration and ejaculation. Instruct clients not to douche for 6 to 8 hours afterwards.

B. Contraceptive sponge: contains a spermicide that absorbs the semen; it can be left in for 24 hours

C. Intrauterine devices (IUD): contains a reservoir of progesterone, which must be replaced every year

D. Subdermal implant: the Norplant system, which slowly releases progestin over 5 years

E. Morning-after pill (the estrogen hormone DES): used in rape, incest, or pregnancy when it threatens the woman's mental well-being. Must be taken within 72 hours of intercourse.

V. Androgens

A. Action: replacement therapy of testosterone given orally, subcutaneously, or intramuscularly. Testosterone is needed for the following:
   1. Male sex characteristics
   2. Normal development of male sex organs and structures (penis, prostate, seminal vesicles)
   3. Synthesis of sperm

B. Uses
   1. Hypogonadism: a deficiency in the secretory activity of the ovary or testes
   2. Delayed puberty
   3. Palliative management of metastatic breast cancer in postmenopausal women
   4. Endometriosis
   5. Impotence: inability to achieve penile erection
   6. Oligospermia: insufficient spermatozoa in the semen
   7. Cryptorchidism: failure of one or both testicles to descend
   8. Weight gain in debilitated clients

C. Side effects
   1. Signs of masculinization in females: hirsutism, acne, deepening of the voice, clitoral enlargement, menstrual irregularities, regression of the breasts
   2. Fluid: water and sodium retention, edema
   3. Increased libido

⚠ Warning!

Advise to avoid the use of **anabolic steroids** without a physician's guidance. Athletes and weight builders often misuse them.

D. Nursing implications
   1. Monitor weight gain
   2. Emphasize compliance

TABLE 20-1 Oral Contraceptives

Progestin:Estrogen	Progestin:Estrogen	Trade Name	Dose‡
Desogestrel: ethinyl estradiol	0.15 mg:30 µg	Desogen, Marvelon,† Ortho-Cept*	Monophasic: 21 days of active agent, then 7 days with placebo or no drug.
	0.15 mg:20 µg (21 tablets) and no progestin: 10 µg	Mircette	Biphasic: 21 days of 0.15 mg:20 µg tablets, then 2 days placebo, followed by 5 days of 10 µg ethinyl estradiol tablets.
Ethynodiol diacetate: ethinyl estradiol	1.0 mg:50 µg	Demulen 1/50, Zovia 1/50 E; Demulen 50†	Monophasic: 21 days of active agent, then 7 days with placebo or no drug.
	1.0 mg:35 µg	Demulen 1/35, Zovia 1/35E	
	2.0 mg:30 µg	Demulen 30†	
Levonorgestrel: ethinyl estradiol	0.1 mg:20 µg	Alesse, Levlite	Monophasic: 21 days of active agent, then 7 days with placebo or no drug.
	0.15 mg:30 µg	Levlen, Levora 0.15/30, Min-Ovral†, Nordette	
	0.05 mg:30 µg (6 tablets), and 0.075 mg:40 µg (5 tablets), and 0.125 mg:30 µg (10 tablets)	Tri-Levlen, Triphasil*, Triquilar†, Trivora	Triphasic: 0.05 µg:30 µg tablets are taken on the first 6 days of the cycle, 0.075 mg:40 µg tablets the next 5 days and the 0.125 mg:30 µg tablets the next 10 days, followed by 7 days of placebo or no drug.
Norethindrone	0.35 mg	Micronor*, Nor-QD	Continuous.
Norethindrone acetate: ethinyl estradiol	1 mg:20 µg	Loestrin 1/20, Loestrin Fe 1/20, Minestrin 1/20†	Monophasic: 21 days of active agent, then 7 days with placebo, 75 mg ferrous fumarate (Loestrin Fe), or no drug.
	1.5 mg:30 µg	Loestrin 1.5/30,* Loestrin Fe 1.5/30	
	1 mg:20 µg (5 tablets), and 1 mg:30 µg (7 tablets), and 1 mg:35 µg (9 tablets)	Estrostep	Triphasic: 1 mg:20 µg tablets are taken on the first 5 days of the cycle, 1 mg:30 µg tablets the next 7 days, and 1 mg:35 µg tablets the next 9 days, followed by 7 days of placebo or no drug.

Norethindrone: ethinyl estradiol	0.4 mg:35 μg 0.5 mg:35 μg	Ovcon-35 Brevicon,* Genora 0.5/35, Intercon 0.5/35, ModiCon, Necon 0.5/35, Nelova 0.5/35	Monophasic: 21 days of active agent, then 7 days with placebo or no drug.
	1 mg:35 μg	Brevicon 1/35,‡ Genora 1/35, Intercon 1/35, Necon 1/35, N.E.E. 1/35, Nelova 1/35, Norethin 1/35, Norinyl 1+35, Ortho-Novum 1/35	
	0.5 mg:35 μg (10 tablets), and 1 mg:35 μg (11 tablets)	Necon 10/11, Nelova 10/11, Ortho-Novum 10-11 Symphasic†	Biphasic: 0.5 mg:35 μg tablets are taken on the first 10 days of the cycle, the 1 mg:35 μg tablets the next 11 days, then 7 days with placebo or no drug.
	0.5 mg:35 μg (7 tablets), and 1 mg:35 μg (14 tablets)	Jenest	Biphasic: 0.5 mg:35 μg tablets are taken on the first 7 days of the cycle, the 1 mg:35 μg tablets the next 14 days, then 7 days with placebo or no drug.
	0.5 mg:35 μg (7 tablets), and 1 mg:35 μg (9 tablets), and 0.5 mg:35 μg (5 tablets)	Tri-Norinyl	Triphasic: 0.5 mg:35 μg tablets are taken on the first 7 days of the cycle, the 1 mg:35 μg tablets the next 9 days, the 0.5 mg:35 μg tablets the next 5 days, then 7 days with placebo or no drug.
	0.5 mg:35 μg (7 tablets), and 0.75 mg:35 μg (7 tablets), and 1 mg:35 μg 7 (tablets)	Ortho-Novum 7/7/7, Ortho 7/7/7†	Triphasic: 0.5 mg:35 μg tablets are taken on the first 7 days of the cycle, the 0.75 mg:35 μg tablets the next 7 days, the 1 mg:35 μg tablets the next 7 days, then 7 days with placebo or no drug.

*Available in Canada and the United States.

†Available in Canada only.

‡All oral contraceptives are FDA pregnancy category X.

TABLE 20-1 Oral Contraceptives—cont'd

Progestin:Estrogen	Progestin:Estrogen	Trade Name	Dose[†]
Norethindrone: Mestranol	1 mg:50 μg	Genora 1/50, Intercon 1/50 Necon 1/50, Nelova 1/50M Norethin 1/50M, Norinyl 1/50,[†] Ortho-Novum 1/50*	Monophasic: 21 days of active agent, then 7 days with placebo or no drug.
Norgestimate: ethinyl estradiol	0.25 mg:35 μg	Cyclen[†], Ortho-Cyclen	Monophasic: 21 days of active agent, then 7 days with placebo or no drug.
	0.18 mg:35 μg (7 tablets), and 0.215 mg:35 μg (7 tablets), and 0.25 mg:35 μg (7 tablets)	Ortho Tri-Cyclen, Tri-Cyclen[†]	Triphasic: 0.18 mg:35 μg tablets are taken on the first 7 days of the cycle, the 0.215 mg:35 μg tablets the next 7 days, the 0.25 mg:35 μg tablets the next 7 days, then 7 days with placebo or no drug.
Norgestrel: ethinyl estradiol	0.3 mg:30 μg 0.5 mg:50 μg	Lo/Ovral Ovral*	Monophasic: 21 days of active agent, then 7 days with placebo or no drug.
Norgestrel	75 μg	Ovrette	Continuous.

*Available in Canada and the United States.
[†]Available in Canada only.
From Clark JB, Queener SF, Karb VB: *Pharmacologic basis of nursing practice*, ed 6, St. Louis, 2000, Mosby.

    3. Teach the female client about potential side effects
    4. Recommend use of nonhormonal contraception
E. **Common drugs**
    1. Fluoxymesterone (Halotestin)
    2. Testosterone
    3. Testosterone cypionate (Depo-Testosterone)
    4. Danazol (Danocrine)
    5. Anabolic steroids
        a. Nandrolone phenopropionate (Durabolin)
        b. Nandrolone deconoate (Deca-Durabolin)
        c. Oxymetholone (Anadrol)

VI. Ovulation stimulants

A. **Actions: stimulate the growth and maturation of ovum and increase the release of gonadotropins**
B. **Use:** *infertility*
C. **Side effects**
    1. Multiple births
    2. Cysts on ovaries
    3. Breast tenderness
    4. Hot flashes, diaphoresis

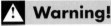 **Warning!**

These drugs are usually recommended for 3 months only.

D. **Nursing implications**
    1. Monitor compliance carefully because follow-up visits to the physician are necessary
    2. Instruct the client to report any symptoms
    3. Instruct the client to report any abdominal or side pain, which may indicate an ectopic pregnancy
E. **Common drugs**
    1. Clomiphene citrate (Clomid): first choice
    2. Menotropins (Pergonal)
    3. Bromocriptine mesylate (Parlodel)
    4. Danazol (Danocrine)
    5. Leuprolide (Lupron)

DRUGS USED DURING PREGNANCY

I. Uterine stimulants

A. **Action: stimulate the uterine smooth muscle**
B. **Groups**
    1. Oxytocin
    2. Ergot derivatives
    3. Prostaglandins

C. **Uses**
   1. Inducing more rapid deliveries
   2. Hemorrhages
   3. After cesarean section
   4. Abortions
D. **Side effects**
   1. GI: nausea, vomiting, diarrhea
   2. CV: postpartal hemorrhage
   3. CV: hypertension
   4. Tetany or uterine contractions

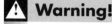 **Warning!**

Live births from abortion are possible.

E. **Nursing implications**
   1. Monitor VS, noting BP over 140/90 mm Hg or an increase of 20 mm Hg in systolic pressure from client's baseline
   2. Assess uterine contractions, hemorrhage; increased HR is the first sign
   3. Be aware that a live birth from an abortion is possible
   4. Have magnesium sulfate available for IV administration to counteract severe contractions
   5. Assess fetal heart tones (FHTs)
   6. Know that clients may complain of increased pain and cramping after administration, and analgesics may not totally relieve their pain
F. **Common drugs**
   1. Oxytocin (Pitocin)
   2. Ergot alkaloids
      a. Ergonovine maleate (Ergotrate)
      b. Methylergonovine maleate (Methergine)
   3. Prostaglandins: dinoprostone (PGF_2), a vaginal suppository or gel

II. Uterine depressants

A. **Action: most act on the beta$_2$ adrenergic receptors to inhibit uterine contractions by relaxation of smooth muscles in the uterus**
B. **Uses: uncomplicated premature labor, threatened miscarriage**
C. **Side effects**
   1. CV: hypertension and tachycardia in the mother
   2. Hyperglycemia
   3. Respiratory: pulmonary edema in the mother

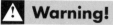 **Warning!**

Monitor IV closely and have the infusion on a pump; stop if complications occur.

D. **Nursing implications**
   1. Monitor the VS in the mother
   2. Place client on her left side

    3. Monitor FHTs
    4. Monitor blood glucose values
    5. Monitor lung sounds for crackles, edema in extremities; monitor I&O
  E. **Common drugs**
    1. Ritodrine hydrochloride (Yutopar)
    2. Isoxsuprine (Vasodilan)
    3. Terbutaline (Bricanyl or Brethine)
    4. Magnesium sulfate and Procardia plus Motrin are being used as uterine depressants. They are not FDA approved at this time.

III. Lactation suppressants
  A. **Action: prohibit prolactin secretion**
  B. **Use: suppress lactation after delivery**
  C. **Side effects are rare**
  D. **Nursing implications: give the agent 1 to 5 days after delivery**
  E. **Common drug: bromocriptine mesylate (Parlodel)**

WEB Resources

http://www.meriter.com/meriter/living/library/women/hormone/index.htm
   Gives information on hormone replacement therapy.

http://darkwing.uoregon.edu/~uoshc/oralcontracept.html
   Discusses oral contraceptives.

REVIEW QUESTIONS

1. A client who is taking tetracycline for her bronchitis asks the nurse about continuing with her birth control pills. She is in college and does not want to become pregnant. What should the nurse tell her?
1. Continue taking the prescribed birth control pills
2. Take a double dose for it to be effective
3. Use an additional form of protection, such as a spermicide
4. Continue the birth control pills because they will remain effective

2. A client, age 57, is having hot flashes, irritability, and extreme fatigue. The doctor determines that she has perimenopausal symptoms. The nurse anticipates that the physician will prescribe which hormone?
1. Androgen
2. Estrogen
3. Progesterone
4. Testosterone

3. When a middle-aged female enters the hospital, why should the nurse ask about estrogen therapy during the history taking section on the admission record?
1. It could be useful information
2. Estrogen therapy affects many laboratory tests
3. Clients on estrogen should be monitored for hypotension
4. Estrogen therapy should not be abruptly withdrawn

4. A client who has been trying to get pregnant has had no success for the past year. If test results indicate that she is infertile, the first drug of choice would be which of these?
1. Clomiphene citrate (Clomid)
2. Menotropins (Pergonal)
3. Bromocriptine mesylate (Parlodel)
4. Danazol (Danocrine)

5. A client's husband is transferred to the United States from France during her seventh month of pregnancy. During the stress of moving and a 10-hour flight, she begins to have severe labor pains. The nurse anticipates that, when this woman arrives at the maternity unit, she would most likely be placed on which drug IV drip?
1. Bromocriptine mesylate (Parlodel)
2. Ergotrate
3. Ritodrine (Yutopar)
4. Clomiphene citrate (Clomid)

ANSWERS, RATIONALES, AND TEST-TAKING TIPS

Rationales	Test-Taking Tips

1. Correct answer: 3

An additional contraceptive such as a spermicide or condom is recommended. The antibiotic can possibly cause the birth control pills to be less effective. Doubling a dose of medication is rarely a correct action and is not advisable. Option 4 is an incorrect statement, since there is no guarantee that the birth control pills will remain effective.

As you read the options think about the clue in the stem: the client does not want to become pregnant. Thus, if you can't recall any information about antibiotics and oral contraceptives, select option 3. Additional protection increases the odds that a pregnancy won't happen. This is a fact that you do know is true: the use of two methods is better than one. Avoid the selection of answers when you are unsure about the interactions or information.

2. Correct answer: 2

Exogenous estrogens act by exerting the same effect as naturally occurring estrogen. A client's internal estrogen levels decrease and are responsible for the symptoms of perimenopause, which may last from 1 to 10 years. Androgens are not recommended for menopausal symptoms. Progesterones are more commonly used for menstrual and pre-menstrual symptoms. Testosterone's action is the same as androgen's and it may be used to treat some forms of cancer.

Think of menopause as early older age and that estrogen needs to be replaced.

3. Correct answer: 2

Laboratory test results can be altered by estrogen. All home medications should be documented on the client's entrance into the hospital, but this is not one of the choices. Option 1 is too general to be

Be cautious: if you read, in option 3, "hypertension" instead of what is there, you had a problem with the hyper/hypo words. To eliminate this test error, when you see any hyper/hypo words, add an additional step. Write down on paper what you

Rationales	Test-Taking Tips

correct. Hypertension, not hypotension, is a common side effect, partly from the water retention and weight gain. There are no severe complications if the therapy is stopped.

think you are reading. Then go back to the specific word to see if it is the same. This prevents you from missing those easy questions. Thus you can immediately eliminate option 3. Then eliminate option 1, since it is too general for a specific question about a specific drug. Then reread the question, which has the focus of in-hospital care concerns. Option 4 introduces new information into the situation, suggesting that estrogen will be stopped. Option 2 is directly related to in-hospital care and is the best answer.

4. Correct answer: 1

Clomid is usually tried first for infertility problems. Pergonal is used for infertility but only after successive tries with Clomid. Parlodel is an ovulation stimulant but is not the first-line choice. Danocrine is usually not the first-line drug.

Remember that Clomid is first alphabetically, so associate that it is a first drug of choice for infertility.

5. Correct answer: 3

Yutopar inhibits uterine contractions and could decrease the chances of premature labor. Parlodel would not stop the possible premature labor. Ergotrate is a uterine stimulant and could induce premature labor. Clomid does not stop premature labor. Other drugs that might be used are Brethine, IV or PO, and magnesium sulfate, IV.

For these types of questions for which you have no idea of the correct answer, select an option and go on to the next question. Keep your emotional reactions and your tiredness to a minimum by taking three S-L-O-W deep breaths. Do this before reading the next question, so that you will have your clearest perception and thinking ability. Remember that you will have some questions with unfamiliar content area and will have to make an educated guess or use a test-taking skill.

21

Essential Odds and Ends

ANTICONVULSANTS

I. Oxazolidinediones: no longer commonly used
A. **Actions: decrease seizures in cortex, basal ganglia; decrease synoptic stimulation to low-frequency impulses**
B. **Use: most effective against absence seizures**
C. **Side effects**
   1. Extremely toxic
   2. Limited use because of toxicity
D. **Nursing implications**
   1. Monitor blood studies, CBC count, hepatic and renal function
   2. Teach that drug may take 1 to 4 weeks to work
   3. Teach that if rash develops, notify physician promptly
E. **Common drugs: trimethadone (Tridione), paramethadione (Paradione)**

II. Felbamate (Felbatol)
A. **Action: related to the anxiolytic agents, not fully understood, may reduce seizure spread and increase seizure threshold. Has weak inhibitory effects on GABA.**
B. **Uses: adjunctive therapy for partial seizures with and without generalization in adults**

⚠ Warning!

Not recommended as second-line therapy because of the severe risk of developing aplastic anemia. Should be used only when epilepsy is so severe that it is worth the risk of developing aplastic anemia. Used in children with *Lennox-Gastaut syndrome*.

C. **Side effects**
1. Aplastic anemia
2. Acute liver failure
3. Neurologic: insomnia, somnolence, dizziness, tremors, abnormal gait
4. Depression
5. Paresthesia, ataxia, stupor
6. Aggressive reactions, hallucinations, suicide attempts
7. Agranulocytosis
8. **Stevens-Johnson syndrome**
D. **Nursing implications**
1. Monitor laboratory work: CBC count, liver and renal function studies
2. Teach client and family about severe side effects
3. Institute and teach about safety measures
4. Do not abruptly discontinue

HERBAL PREPARATIONS

I. Ginkgo biloba
A. **Researchers have reported that ginkgo biloba (an OTC herbal preparation) and warfarin (Coumadin) should not be used together**
1. Evidence of increased PT
2. Evidence of intracranial bleed
3. Ginkgo biloba has antiplatelet properties
B. **Other agents also possess antiplatelet properties, such as Vitamin E.**

II. Other uses for OTC herbal products
A. **Green tea: antioxidant and anticancer activity**
B. **Valerian: sedative**
C. **Kava-kava: CNS depressant**
D. **St. John's Wort: useful in mild to moderate depression**
E. **Metabolife: May increased CNS effects especially if caffeine is not limited.**

NEUROLEPTIC MALIGNANT SYNDROME

I. A potentially fatal syndrome that can occur at any time during neuroleptic therapy

II. Signs and symptoms: convulsions, difficult or fast breathing, tachycardia, irregular pulse rate, excessive weakness, fatigue, altered LOC
A. Severe extrapyramidial effects can occur
B. Severe elevation of WBC count

III. Treatment
A. Supportive therapy on intensive care unit
B. Dantrolene and/or bromocriptine (experimental)

TOXICOLOGY AND POISONING

I. Initial steps
A. Be sure an airway has been established
B. Find out the substance name, route, how long ago, how much
C. Find out the name of the person, phone number, age

II. Treatment
A. Initiate gastric lavage when the client:
  1. Has taken a sedative or might aspirate
  2. Is unconscious
B. Initiate activated charcoal administration when
  1. Poison control centers list this as the treatment for the problem
     a. If unconscious person has been lavaged
     b. If client is conscious
  2. One hour after the final emesis, if *ipecac syrup* was administered
  3. If a corrosive substance was ingested
C. Give *ipecac syrup* when
  1. The client is conscious
  2. Poison control centers list this treatment
D. For a list of common antidotes, see Table 21-1; for a list of commonly abused drugs, see Table 21-2

WEB Resources
http://www.mothernature.com
  Resource site for a list of herbals, their properties, and interactions with prescription drugs.

TABLE 21-1	Specific Antidotes, Poisons, and Concerns		
Antidote	**Poison**	**Administration/Dosage**	**Comments**
Cholinergic Poisoning			
Atropine	Anticholinesterase Organophosphates Physostigmine	INTRAVENOUS: *Children*–0.02 mg/kg; *Adults*–1-2 mg. This is initial dose. Repeat every 20 min until copious secretions are controlled.	Blocks muscarinic receptors to prevent peripheral actions of excessive concentrations of neurotransmitter, acetylcholine. Muscarinic symptoms for which atropine is given include nausea, vomiting, diarrhea, sweat, increased bronchial and salivary secretions, and slow heart rate (bradycardia).
Pralidoxime chloride (PAM)	Anticholinesterase Organophosphates	*Organophosphate poisoning:* BY INFUSION in 100 ml saline over 15-30 min: *Children*–20-40 mg/kg; *adults*–1-2 g initially. A second dose can be given in 1 hr. *Carbamate (neostigmine, pyridostigmine) poisoning:* INTRA-VENOUS: *Adults*–1-2 g initially, followed by 250 mg every 5 min as necessary to reverse cholinergic crisis.	Reactivates enzyme acetylcholinesterase after inactivation by irreversible anticholinesterases or organophosphates. This allows acetylcholine to be degraded and relieves paralysis (overstimulation) caused by accumulated acetylcholine. Pralidoxime acts mainly outside CNS. In organophosphate poisoning, pralidoxime is given to restore neuromuscular function, especially to relieve paralysis of respiratory muscles. Atropine is given concurrently (see above) to relieve depression of respiratory center and to reverse muscarinic stimulation. In overdose by carbamate anticholinesterases (neostigmine, pyridostigmine and ambenonium, drugs for myasthenia gravis), pralidoxime antagonizes effects of these drugs on neuromuscular junction.

Physostigmine salicylate (Antilirium)	Antimuscarinic anticholinergic	INTRAVENOUS OR INTRAMUSCULAR: *Adults*—0.5-2 mg. INTRAVENOUS: *Children*—0.5 mg by slow (1 min) infusion. Repeat if needed at 5- to 10-min intervals until desired effect, or 2 mg total dose, is reached.	Reversible anticholinesterase that increases concentration of acetylcholine at its receptor sites. Reverses both CNS and peripheral anticholinergic effects. Useful for reversing toxic anticholinergic effects caused by overdose of atropine and other belladonna alkaloids, tricyclic antidepressants, phenothiazines, and antihistamines. Central anticholinergic effects include anxiety, delirium, disorientation, hallucinations, hyperactivity, seizures, and in extreme cases, coma, medullary paralysis, and death. Peripheral anticholinergic toxic effects include fast heart rate (tachycardia), fever, mydriasis (dilated pupils), vasodilation, urinary retention, decreased secretions, and decreased gastrointestinal motility.

Sedative-Hypnotic/Opioid Poisoning

Ethanol	Methanol Ethylene glycol	INTRAVENOUS: *Adults*—0.6 g/kg + 7-10 g over 1 hr; then 10 g/hr maintenance; *children*—0.6 g/kg + 4-5 g over 1 hr; 5 g/hr maintenance.	All three alcohols are metabolized by aldehyde dehydrogenase. Ethanol is preferred substrate and thereby blocks metabolism of methanol and ethylene glycol to toxins formaldehyde and formic acid (both alcohols) and oxylate (ethylene glycol). Ethanol is given in additional loading dose to achieve blood level of 100 mg/dl.

Continued

CNS, central nervous system.
Data from Clark JB, Queener SF, Karb VB: *Pharmacologic basis of nursing practice*, ed 6, St. Louis, 2000, Mosby.

TABLE 21-1	Specific Antidotes, Poisons, and Concerns—cont'd		
Antidote	**Poison**	**Administration/Dosage**	**Comments**
Sedative-Hypnotic/Opioid Poisoning—cont'd			
Flumazenil (Mazicon)	Benzodiazepines	INTRAVENOUS: *Adults*—initially 0.2 mg administered over 30 sec; if desired level of consciousness is not obtained, a further dose of 0.3 mg may be administered over another 30 sec. Additional doses of 0.5 mg may be administered over 30 sec at 1-min intervals to a cumulative dose of 3 mg. If client relapses, repeat doses at 20-min intervals as needed, but no more than 1 mg at a time and no more than 3 mg per hour.	Reversible antagonist of benzodiazepine receptor. Reverses cognitive, psychomotor, hypnogenic, and electroencephalographic effects of benzodiazepines. Because flumazenil increases level of consciousness in cases of benzodiazepine overdose even in presence of alcohol intoxication, flumazenil helps in diagnosis. Symptoms of poisoning with barbiturates, alcohol, and phenothiazines are not affected. However, flumazenil may worsen toxicity of tricyclic antidepressants. Flumazenil is also used to improve recovery from surgical sedation with benzodiazepines.
Fomepizole (Antizol)	Ethylene glycol	INTRAVENOUS: *Adult*—15 mg/kg body weight initially, followed by 10 mg/kg body weight every 12 hr for 4 doses, then 15 mg/kg body weight every 12 hr until ethylene glycol concentration decreases to less than 20 mg/dl.	Reversible inhibitor of alcohol dehydrogenase to decrease formation of toxic metabolites. The metabolite oxalate is toxic to the kidneys. Each dose of fomepizole should be administered over 30 min.

Naloxone (Narcan)	Narcotics (opioids), including pentazocine, propoxyphene, diphenoxylate	INTRAVENOUS (May also give intramuscularly or subcutaneously): *Adults*–0.4-2 mg. Additional doses are repeated at 2- to 3-min intervals until client responds or until 10 mg is given. *Children*–0.01 mg/kg with 0.1 mg/kg as subsequent dose.	Reversible antagonist of opioid receptor. Useful for reversing narcotic depression, including respiratory depression. Naloxone is preferred because it is pure opioid antagonist and causes no respiratory depression of its own. Naloxone is effective within 2 min and has duration of action of 1-4 hr. Because most opioids have a longer duration of action, effects of naloxone may wear off and client may relapse, requiring additional naloxone.

Specific Metabolic Poisons

Acetylcysteine (Mucomyst)	acetaminophen	ORAL: 140 mg/kg as 5% solution mixed with soda, water, or grapefruit juice. Follow with 17 maintenance doses of 70 mg/kg every 4 hr.	Acetylcysteine restores sulfhydryl groups depleted by acetaminophen metabolism. This prevents toxicity to liver produced by metabolites of acetaminophen. Acetylcysteine should not be given with activated charcoal because charcoal absorbs it.
Amyl nitrite Sodium nitrite sodium thiosulfate (Cyanide Antidote Package)	cyanide	*Amyl nitrite:* Crush ampule on gauze and have client inhale vapor. *Sodium nitrite:* Inject 10 ml of 3% solution after IV line is established. *Sodium thiosulfate:* Inject 50 ml of 25% solution after administration of sodium nitrite.	Cyanide has almond odor. Toxicity of cyanide is caused by its blockage of enzymes using oxygen in mitochondria (cytochrome oxidase), thereby depressing cellular respiration. Inhibition of cytochrome oxidase depends on binding of cyanide to ferric iron in cytochrome oxidase. Nitrite converts ferrous iron in hemoglobin to ferric iron, producing methemoglobin. This large pool of ferric iron in blood competes with cytochrome oxidase for cyanide, thereby restoring cellular respiration. Thiosulfate accelerates conversion of cyanide to relatively nontoxic thiocyanate, which is readily excreted in urine.

Continued

Data from Clark JB, Queener SF, Karb VB: *Pharmacologic basis of nursing practice*, ed 6, St. Louis, 2000, Mosby.

TABLE 21-1 Specific Antidotes, Poisons, and Concerns—cont'd

Antidote	Poison	Administration/Dosage	Comments
Metal Poisoning			
Deferoxamine mesylate (Desferal)	iron	INTRAMUSCULAR, CONTINUOUS SUBCUTANEOUS, OR SLOW INTRA-VENOUS: *Adults*—1 g initially, 0.5 g at 4 and 8 hr. Additional doses if needed, up to 6 g daily. For IV, do not give at rate greater than 15 mg/kg/hr. Administer IM if possible. *Children*—50 mg/kg IM or IV every 6 hr up to 15 mg/kg/hr by continuous IV. Maximum dosage: 6 g/24 hr or 2 g/dose.	Chelates iron and thereby prevents iron from entering cells and inhibiting chemical reactions. Chelate of iron and deferoxamine is rapidly excreted in urine, removing iron from body.
Dimercaprol (BAL)	arsenic gold mercury lead	INTRAMUSCULAR: Because dimer-caprol is oil, give deep intra-muscularly only. *Mild arsenic or gold poisoning:* 2.5 mg/kg 4 times daily, 2 days; 2 times, day 3; once daily, 10 days. *Severe arsenic or gold poisoning:* 3 mg/kg 4 hr for 2 days, 4 times day 3; twice daily 10 days. *Mercury poisoning:* 5 mg/kg ini-tially; 2.5 mg/kg 1.2 times daily for 10 days.	Dimercaprol is a sulfhydryl compound that chelates lead, arsenic, gold, and mercury and promotes their excretion in urine. Dimer-caprol also reactivates affected sulfhydryl enzymes. Peak plasma concentrations occur 30-60 min after administration. Excretion is complete in 4 hr. Dimercaprol is not very effective for poisoning caused by antimony and bismuth. It is contraindicated in iron, cadmium, and selenium poisoning because chelates are more toxic, especially to kidney, than metal alone. Alkalinization of urine protects kidney from breakdown of dimercaprol-metal complex in acid urine. Common side effects of dimercaprol are rise in blood pressure with tachycardia (fast heart rate) and burning sensation of lips, mouth, and throat.

Edetate calcium disodium (calcium disodium versenate)	lead	*Acute lead poisoning:* 4 mg/kg alone initially, then at 4-hr intervals with calcium disodium edetate (administered at separate site). Maintain for 2-7 days. INTRAVENOUS: 50-75 mg/kg/day in 3-6 doses, each dose administered over at least 1 hr. Can continue for up to 5 days. Wait 2 days before resuming therapy for additional 5 days. INTRAMUSCULAR: Preferred route for children. Give 35 mg/kg twice daily. After 3-5 days, discontinue for 4 days or more.	Calcium-bound to EDTA is displaced by lead and resulting chelate is excreted in urine (50% in 1 hr: 95% in 24 hr). EDTA can produce toxic effects, including renal damage and irregularities in cardiac rhythm. Doses must be carefully monitored.
Penicillamine (Cuprimine, Depen)	copper lead zinc mercury	ORAL.: *Adults—*1-1.5 g daily in 4 divided doses on empty stomach for 1-2 mo; *children—*30-40 mg/kg daily or 600-750 mg/m² daily for 1-6 mo.	Penicillamine chelates copper, lead, zinc, or mercury, promoting their excretion in urine. Side effects include allergic reactions (principally rashes) and loss of sweet and salt tastes. Severe side effects include bone marrow depression and renal toxicity.

Data from Clark JB, Queener SF, Karb VB: *Pharmacologic basis of nursing practice,* ed 6, St. Louis, 2000, Mosby.

TABLE 21-2   Selected Drugs Commonly Abused and Symptoms of Abuse

Drug Category	Street Names	Methods of Use	Symptoms of Use	Hazards of Use
Marijuana/ Hashish	Pot, grass, reefer, weed, Colombian, hash, hash oil, sinsemilla, joint	Most often smoked; can also be swallowed in solid form	Sweet, burnt odor Neglect of appearance Loss of interest, motivation Possible weight loss	Impaired memory, perception Interference with psychologic maturation Possible damage to lungs, heart, and reproduction and immune systems Psychological dependence
Alcohol	Booze, hooch, juice, brew	Swallowed in liquid form	Impaired muscle coordination, judgment	Heart and liver damage Death from overdose Death from car accidents Addiction
Stimulants				
Amphetamines* Amphetamine Dextroamphetamine Methamphetamine	Speed, uppers, pep pills Bennies Dexies Meth, crystal Black beauties	Swallowed in pill or capsule form, or injected into veins	Excess activity Irritability; nervousness Mood swings Needle marks	Loss of appetite Hallucinations; paranoia Convulsions; coma Brain damage Death from overdose
Cocaine	Coke, snow, toot, white lady, crack, ready rock	Most often inhaled (snorted); also injected or swallowed in powder form, smoked	Restlessness, anxiety Intense, short-term high followed by dysphoria	Intense psychologic dependence Sleeplessness; anxiety Nasal passage damage Lung damage Death from overdose

Nicotine	Coffin nail, butt, smoke	Smoked in cigarettes, cigars and pipes, snuff, chewing tobacco	Smell of tobacco High carbon monoxide blood levels Stained teeth	Cancers of the lung, throat, mouth, esophagus Heart disease, emphysema
Depressants				
Barbiturates Pentobarbital Secobarbital Amobarbital	Barbs, downers Yellow jackets Red devils Blue devils	Swallowed in pill form or injected into veins	Drowsiness Confusion Impaired judgment Slurred speech Needle marks Constricted pupils	Infection after parenteral use Addiction with severe life-threatening withdrawal symptoms Loss of appetite Death from overdose Nausea
Opioids Dilaudid, Percodan Demerol, Methadone		Swallowed in pill or liquid form, injected	Drowsiness Lethargy	Addiction with severe withdrawal symptoms Loss of appetite Death from overdose
Morphine	Dreamer, junk	Injected into veins, smoked	Needle marks	
Heroin Codeine	Smack, horse School boy	Swallowed in pill or liquid form		
Hallucinogens				
PCP (phencyclidine)	Angel dust, killer weed, supergrass, hog, PeaCe pill	Most often smoked; can also be inhaled (snorted), injected or swallowed in tablets	Slurred speech; blurred vision, uncoordination Confusion, agitation Aggression	Anxiety, depression Impaired memory, perception Death from accidents Death from overdose

*Includes lookalike drugs resembling amphetamines that contain caffeine, phenylpropanolamine (PPA), and ephedrine.

Continued

TABLE 21-2 Selected Drugs Commonly Abused and Symptoms of Abuse—cont'd

Drug Category	Street Names	Methods of Use	Symptoms of Use	Hazards of Use
LSD	Acid, cubes, purple haze	Injected or swallowed in tablets	Dilated pupils	Breaks from reality
Mescaline	Mesc, cactus	Usually ingested in their natural form	Delusions; hallucinations	Emotional breakdown
Psilocybin	Magic mushrooms		Mood swings	Flashback
Inhalants				
Gasoline		Inhaled or sniffed, often with use of paper or plastic bag or rag	Poor motor coordination	High risk of sudden death
Airplane glue			Impaired vision, memory and thought processes	Drastic weight loss
Paint thinner				Brain, liver, and bone marrow damage
			Abusive, violent behavior	
Nitrites	Poppers, locker room, rush, snappers	Inhaled or sniffed from gauze or ampules	Slowed thought	Anemia, death by anoxia
Amyl			Headache	
Butyl				

Data from McKenry L & Salerno E: *Pharmacology in nursing*, ed 20, St. Louis, Mosby, pp. 144-145.

Glossary

Activated partial thromboplastin time (aPTT) A test for detecting coagulation defects of the intrinsic system; used to monitor heparin activity.

Adrenergic agonists Also called sympathomimetic. Drugs that cause an adrenergic response from the body.

Adrenergic or sympathetic Pertaining to the sympathetic nerve fibers that use the neurotransmitters, epinephrine, or epinephrine-like substances.

Adrenergic receptor Two types: Alpha receptor—stimulation of results in an excitatory response. Beta receptor—stimulation of results in an inhibitory response.

Adrenergic response A sympathetic-like response, such as increased heart rate, peripheral vasoconstriction, and increased serum glucose.

Afterload The resistance against which the left ventricle must eject its volume of blood during contraction. The resistance is produced by the volume of blood already in the vascular system plus the diameter of the vessel walls. Left ventricular afterload: referred to as *peripheral* vascular resistance (PVR); right ventricular afterload: referred to as *pulmonary* vascular resistance.

Agonist Drug with a certain affinity for a receptor to produce a predictable response. EXAMPLE: morphine sulfate (Astramorph).

Air-lock Small amount of air, 0.2 to 0.5 cc, added to the syringe after the medication is accurately measured; it enables the clearing of all of the drug from the needle after the medication is injected.

Alopecia Partial or complete lack or loss of hair.

Amphetamines A group of nervous system stimulants that are subject to abuse. Street names and routes: black beauties, lidpoppers, and pep pills, all taken by mouth; speed, an injectable form; and ice, a crystalline form of methamphetamine that is smoked.

Anabolic steroid Any one of several compounds derived from testosterone or prepared synthetically to promote general body growth, to oppose the effects of endogenous estrogen, or to promote masculinizing effects. All such compounds cause a mixed androgenic-anabolic effect.

Analeptics   Also called CNS stimulants. Substances that quicken the activity of the CNS by increasing the rate of neuronal discharge or by blocking an inhibitory neurotransmitter, such as caffeine and amphetamines.

Analgesic   A drug that relieves pain.

Anasarca   Severe, generalized massive edema that often occurs with renal disease when fluid is retained for an extended period.

Angioedema   An acute, painless dermal, subcutaneous, or submucosal swelling of short duration. It involves the face, neck, lips, larynx, hands, feet, genitalia or viscera. It may result from food or drug allergy, infection, or emotional stress.

Anorexiant   A drug or other agent that suppresses the appetite.

Antabuse   A trade name for the alcohol abuse deterrent, disulfiram.

Antagonists   A drug that exerts the opposite action to that of another or competes for the same receptor site.

Antiadrenergic   Pertaining to the blocking effects of impulses transmitted by the adrenergic fibers of the sympathetic system. EXAMPLES: alpha-adrenergic and beta-adrenergic blocker agents.

Anticoagulant   A substance that prevents or delays coagulation of the blood, such as heparin. Heparin interferes with: (1) the formation of thromboplastin, (2) the conversion of prothrombin to thrombin and (3) the formation of fibrin from fibrinogen.

Anticonvulsant   A substance that prevents, reduces, or stops the severity of epileptic or other convulsive seizures.

Antidysrhythmics   Drugs that prevent, alleviate, or correct an abnormal cardiac rhythm.

Antihistamine   Any substance capable of reducing the physiologic and pharmacologic effects of histamine.

Antilipidemics   Agents that reduce the amount of lipids in blood.

Antiparasitic   A substance that kills parasites or inhibits their growth or reproduction, such as amebicides, anthelmintics, and antimalarials.

Antispasmodics   A drug or other agent, such as belladonna and dicyclomine hydrochloride (Antispas), that prevents smooth muscle spasms, as in the uterus, digestive system, or urinary tract.

Antiseptic   A substance that inhibits the growth and reproduction of microorganisms.

Antitoxins   A subgroup of antiserum, such as botulism, tetanus, and diphtheria antitoxins, conferring passive immunity when injected.

Antitussive   Any of a large group of narcotic and nonnarcotic drugs that act on the CNS and peripheral nervous system to suppress the cough reflex. EXAMPLES: codeine and hydrocodone, which are potent narcotic antitussives.

Antivenin   A suspension of venom-neutralizing antibodies that confers passive immunity and is given as part of emergency first aid for various snake and insect bites.

Astringent   A substance that causes contraction of tissues upon application, usually locally or in a bath, such as alum or tannic acid.

Attenuated vaccine A vaccine made from a strain of virus whose virulence has been lowered by a physical or chemical process. It is used to prevent tuberculosis, small pox, measles, mumps, rubella, polio, and yellow fever.

Automaticity A property of a specialized excitable tissue that allows self-activation through spontaneous development of an action potential, as in most of the cells called pacemaker cells in the heart.

Bone marrow depression A suppression of the manufacture and maturation of red blood cells.

Brand or trade name Proprietary name assigned by the manufacturing company. EXAMPLE: Tylenol.

Carcinogen Substance that causes or accelerates the development of cancer.

Cardiac terminology Clinically discussed in terms of positive, meaning a faster or stronger response, and negative, meaning a slower or weaker response. Chronotropic: The act or process of affecting the rate of the heart. Dromotropic: The act or process of affecting the conduction through the heart. Inotropic: The act or process of affecting the contractility of the heart.

Cathartic Also called laxative, a substance that promotes bowel evacuation by stimulating peristalsis, increasing the fluidity or bulk of intestinal contents, softening the stool, or lubricating the intestinal wall.

Cell-cycle nonspecific The action of an agent without regard to the stage of cell division.

Cell-cycle specific The action of an agent at a specified stage of cell division.

Central nervous system (CNS) One of the two main divisions of the nervous system, consisting of the brain and spinal cord. The other main division is the peripheral nervous system.

Ceruminolytic Pertaining to a drug or other agent that loosens or dissolves cerumen (earwax) to allow for removal.

Chemical name The chemical nomenclature. EXAMPLE: N-acetyl-para-aminopenol.

Chemotherapeutic agent The treatment of infections and other diseases with chemical agents. In modern usage, it usually refers to the use of chemicals to destroy cancer cells on a selective basis; not to kill the cells but to impair their ability to replicate. Agents are termed cytotoxic.

Cholinergic-blocking, anticholinergic Pertaining to a substance that blocks the acetylcholine receptors or competes with acetylcholine for its receptor sites.

Cholinergic response Pertaining to a substance that produces effects similar to those from the stimulation of the cholinergic system.

Cholinergic or sympathomimetic Pertaining to the nerve fibers that elaborate acetylcholine at the myoneural junctions; maintains normal, day-to-day functions of the body.

CNS depressant Any drug or substance that decreases the function of the CNS, such as alcohol, barbiturates, and hypnotics. Such drugs can produce tolerance, physical dependence, and compulsive drug use.

Controlled substance Drugs that have the potential for physical or psychological dependence.

Corticotropin   Also called adrenocorticotropic hormone (ACTH); secreted from the anterior pituitary gland, which in turn stimulates the adrenal cortex to secrete other hormones, such as cortisol, in times of stress, fever, or acute hypoglycemia.

CRF   Chronic renal failure.

Cycloplegic   An agent that causes paralysis with relaxation of the ciliary or ocular muscles of accommodation.

Dawn phenomenon   Hyperglycemia only in the early morning, without prior hypoglycemia, resulting from an increased plasma glucose concentration (and related to the growth hormone); treated with an extra dose of insulin.

Decongestant   A substance that eliminates or reduces congestion or swelling, especially in the mucous membranes.

Debriding agent   A substance that removes damaged tissue or cellular debris from a wound to prevent infection and promote healing.

Dependence   Total psychophysical state of one addicted to drugs or alcohol who must receive an increasing amount of the substance to prevent the onset of withdrawal symptoms.

Dependent authority   Prescriptive authority defined by the State Board of Nursing as an activity within the scope of nursing practice for a nurse practitioner requiring physician collaboration or supervision.

Digitalis toxicity   A result of the cumulative effect of digitalis preparations; earliest findings are typically nausea, vomiting, and anorexia; poor feeding in infants

Disinfectant   A chemical that can be applied to objects to destroy microorganisms.

Diuretic   A drug that promotes diuresis, the formation and excretion of urine.

Dysthymia   A chronic depression that tends to occur in elderly persons with debilitating physical disorders, multiple personal losses, or chronic marital difficulties.

Dysthymic disorder   A mood disorder in which the essential feature is a chronic depression of at least 2 years. It is not disabling nor does it prevent the client from normal daily functioning.

Edema   The abnormal accumulation of fluid in interstitial spaces of tissues.
   Pitting edema—most common bilaterally in the feet and ankles from right-sided heart failure or unilaterally from venous congestion or blockage of lymphatic vessels from malignant diseases.
   Anasarca—a generalized, massive edema often observed with renal disease or low serum albumin levels when fluid retention continues for an extended period of time.
   Periorbital edema—edema located in the area surrounding the socket of the eye, and is most commonly an initial sign in children with nephrosis, also called nephrotic syndrome.

Emetic   A substance, such as syrup of ipecac, that causes vomiting, used in the emergency treatment of overdose or in certain cases of poisoning; it can be cardiotoxic if absorbed and not vomited.

Emollient   A substance that softens tissue, particularly the skin and mucous membranes.

End-of-dose deterioration   Return of symptoms before the next dose.

Enteral route   By way of the gastrointestinal (GI) tract.

Epidural   Administration of a drug into the epidural space.

Ergotism   An acute or chronic disease caused by excessive dosages of medications containing ergot: cerebrospinal symptoms, such as spasms, cramps, and dry gangrene.

Expectorant   An agent that promotes expectoration by reducing the viscosity of pulmonary secretions or by decreasing the tenacity with which exudates adhere to the lower respiratory tract.

Extrapyramidal   Exhibiting movement disorders, especially postural, supporting, static, and locomotor mechanisms, similar to those of Parkinson's disease. EXAMPLES: dystonia (impaired muscle tone), akathisia (restlessness, agitation, inability to sit still), and akinesia (hypoactivity or nonmovement as in muscular paralysis).

Extravasation or infiltration   The process whereby a fluid or drug passes into the tissues with findings of pain, swelling, coolness, and a pale color at the infiltration site.

Fetal antiepileptic drug syndrome   A pattern of congenital abnormalities characterized by prenatal and postnatal growth deficiencies, microencephaly, developmental delay, and several congenital defects.

Follicle-stimulating hormone (FSH)   Also called menotropin—a gonadotropin that stimulates the growth and maturation of the follicles in the ovaries in females and promotes spermatogenesis in males.

Gamma-aminobutyric acid (GABA)   An amino acid with neurotransmitter activity found in the brain, heart, lungs, and kidneys.

Generic name   The nonproprietary name assigned by the United States Adopted Names (USAN) Council. EXAMPLE: acetaminophen.

Half-life   Amount of time required to reduce the plasma drug concentration to one-half of the dose.

Hepatitis B vaccine   A genetically engineered vaccine produced in yeast cells by recombinant DNA technology to develop active immunity against hepatitis B.

Hematuria   The abnormal presence of blood in the urine, which may occur with overdoses of anticoagulants.

Hemophilia   A group of hereditary bleeding disorders in which there is a deficiency in one of the factors necessary for coagulation of blood. Hemophilia A (classic) is a deficiency or absence of clotting factor VIII; hemophilia B (Christmas disease) is a deficiency of the thromboplastin component.

Hemorrhage   Loss of a large amount of blood in a short period of time, either internal or external, and from arterial, venous, or capillary sites.

Hemostatic   Pertaining to a procedure or substance that arrests the flow of blood.

Hib (*Haemophilus influenzae*) **type b vaccine**   A vaccine given to children at 24 months to prevent infection by a gram-negative bacterium found in the throats of 30% of normal, healthy people; the organism can cause bacterial meningitis, pneumonia, joint or bone infections, and throat inflammations in children through age 5 and older adults.

Histamine   A compound found in cells and released in allergic, inflammatory reactions with resultant dilation of capillaries, decreased BP, increased gastric secretions and constriction of the smooth muscles of the bronchi and uterus. Anaphylactic shock may result when massive amounts are released.

HTN   Hypertension.

Hyperfunction of the endocrine system   Thyrotoxicosis, hyperglycemia, hyperthyroidism (also called Grave's disease), hyperparathyroidism.

Hyperkalemia   Serum potassium levels > 5.0 mEq/L; a major threat in renal failure or with the diuretic, aldactone, which inhibits the function of aldosterone to reabsorb sodium in the distal renal tubule. Consequently, sodium is lost into the urine and potassium is reabsorbed into the bloodstream.

Hypnotics   A class of drugs often used as sedatives.

Hypochloremic alkalosis   A metabolic disorder resulting from increased blood bicarbonate secondary to the loss of chloride from the body; not uncommon in diuretic therapy with furosemide (Lasix) or bumetanide (Bumex).

Hypofunction of the endocrine system   Addison's disease, cretinism, hypoparathyroidism, hypoglycemia, hypothyroidism.

Hypokalemia   A serum potassium level < 3.5 mEq/L.

Hypomagnesemia   A serum magnesium level < 1.5 mEq/L; both low potassium and magnesium are major threats with thiazide diuretics, hydrochlorothiazide (Hydrodiuril), or loop diuretics, furosemide (Lasix), bumetanide (Bumex); if client is hypomagnesemic, hypokalemic, and on digoxin, an increased risk of digoxin toxicity occurs.

Iatrogenic effect   Caused by treatment or diagnostic procedures.

Idiosyncracy   An individual sensitivity to effects of a drug caused by inherited or other bodily constitution factors.

Immune globulin   Also called immune gamma globulin—passive immunizing agents obtained from pooled human plasma.

Immunity   The quality of being insusceptible to or unaffected by a particular disease or condition.

Immunosuppressive   A substance or procedure that lessens or prevents an immune response.

Independent authority   Prescriptive authority defined by the State Board of Nursing as practice within the scope of a nurse practitioner, which does not require physician collaboration or supervision.

Infertility   Inability to produce offspring.

Infiltration   The process whereby a fluid passes into the tissues.

Inflammation   A protective response of the tissues of the body to irritation or injury. It may be acute or chronic. Cardinal findings are redness (rubor), heat (calor), swelling (tumor), and pain (dolor), accompanied by loss of function.

Inhalation route   By way of the respiratory tract with inspired air.

International normalizing ratio (INR)   An international standardized test for monitoring the prothrombin time when a client has been stabilized on warfarin therapy. Therapeutic range is 2 to 3 with Coumadin therapy.

Intraarticular   Administration of medication into the synovial cavity of a joint.

Intraosseous   Administration of medication into the bone marrow.

Intraperitoneal   Administration of medication into the peritoneal cavity, usually at the site of a tumor.

Intrapleural   Administration of medication into pleural cavity, usually at the site of a tumor.

Intrathecal   Administration of medication by injecting directly into the subarachnoid space of the spine.

Iodism   A condition produced from excessive amounts of iodine in the body, with findings of lacrimation, salivation, rhinitis, weakness, and a typical skin eruption.

Keratolytics   A substance that loosens or causes shedding of the outer layer of skin.

Lennox-Gastaut syndrome   Childhood form of epilepsy manifested by complex, poorly controlled seizures (often of multiple types) and mental retardation.

Liniments   A preparation, usually containing an alcoholic, oily, or soapy vehicle, that is rubbed into the skin as a counterirritant.

Loading dose   Dose that may be required to obtain a therapeutic blood level.

Luteinizing hormone (LH)   A glycoprotein. In women, LH works together with FSH to stimulate the ovaries to secrete estrogen in which high concentrations stimulate the release of a surge of LH, which stimulates ovulation. In men, it induces the secretion of testosterone, which together with FSH stimulates the production of sperm.

Maintenance dose   Daily dose to maintain a therapeutic blood level.

Miotic   An agent such as pilocarpine that causes constriction of the pupil; used to treat glaucoma.

Monoamine oxidase (MAO)   An enzyme that catalyzes the oxidation of amines. The inhibition of this enzyme by MAO inhibitors is used in the treatment of depression. MAO inhibitors interact with foodstuffs and drugs, such as ephedrine, a common ingredient in common cold remedies.

Mucolytic   Any agent, such as acetylsysteine (Mucomyst), that dissolves or destroys mucus.

Mutagenic   Substance or drug that causes genetic mutation.

Mydriatic   An agent that causes dilatation of the pupil from the contraction dilator muscle of the iris. Such drugs as atropine, homatropine, and scopolamine are both mydriatics and cycloplegics.

Myxedema   The severest form of hypothyroidism, characterized by swelling of the hands, face, feet, and the periorbital tissues, at which stage coma may result.

Narcotic analgesics   Acts on the CNS to alter the client's perception of pain; used for severe pain.

Nonnarcotic analgesics   Acts at the site of the pain; does not produce tolerance or dependence or alter the client's perception; used for mild to moderate pain.

Nonvesicant   A drug incapable of causing tissue necrosis when extravasated.

NSAIDs   Nonsteroidal anti-inflammatory drugs—a classification of drugs that decreases prostaglandin synthesis. They are used to treat mild to moderate pain, osteoarthritis and rheumatoid arthritis, and dysmenorrhea (pain associated with menstruation).

On-off phenomenon   Alteration in the control of symptoms from day to day or within each day.

Ototoxicity   Having a harmful effect on the eighth cranial nerve or the organs of hearing or balance from such drugs as aminoglycoside antibiotics, aspirin, furosemide, and quinine. Damage may reverse when the drug is stopped.

PABA   Paraaminobenzoic acid, a topical sunscreen.

Parenteral route   By way of any route other than in or through the digestive tract.

Partial thromboplastin time (PTT)   A test to assess the intrinsic system and the common pathway of clot formation, evaluates clotting factors I, II, V, VIII, IX, X, XI, and XII. Used to monitor heparin.

Peak level   Test obtained to establish the peak, the highest concentration of a drug, may be measured immediately after the drug has been administered.

Peripheral   The motor and sensory nerves and ganglia outside the brain and spinal cord.

Pheochromocytoma   A tumor of the sympathoadrenal system that is usually benign and accompanied by hypertension.

Phlebitis or thrombosis   Inflammation of a vein, often accompanied by a clot, with findings of pain, swelling, redness, and warmth along the inflamed vein.

Photosensitivity   A skin reaction requiring the presence of a sensitizing agent, typically a medication such as tetracycline, and exposure to sunlight or its equivalent.

Preload   The stretch of the myocardial fiber at end diastole, which is related to filling volume.

Premenstrual syndrome (PMS)   A syndrome of nervous tension, irritability, weight gain, edema, headache, mastalgia, dysphoria, and lack of coordination that occurs during the last few days of the menstrual cycle before the onset of menstruation.

Prescriptive authority   Limited authority to prescribe certain medications using established protocol.

Prothrombin time (PT)   A test for detecting plasma coagulation defects caused by a deficiency of clotting factors V, VII, and X.

Psychotropic agents   Substances that affect the mind or modify mental activity.

PVR   Peripheral vascular resistance.

Rapid eye movement (REM) sleep   Sleep periods lasting from a few minutes to 30 minutes that alternate with nonrapid eye movement (NREM) periods. NREM sleep, with its four stages, represents three-fourths of a period of typical sleep; REM represents one-fourth of that total time. Dreaming occurs during REM time. Infants tend to begin a sleep period with REM sleep, whereas adults usually begin with the four stages of NREM sleep before entering REM sleep.

Raynaud's disease   Intermittent episodes of pallor, then cyanosis, then redness to the extremities. The color changes return to normal; usually occurs as a result of exposure to cold, vasoconstriction, or extreme emotional distress.

Rebound insomnia   The inability to sleep worsens after treatment.

Renal failure   Inability of the kidneys to excrete wastes, concentrate urine, and conserve electrolytes. The diagnostic test is an elevated serum creatinine level.

Resistance   A situation when an organism is not affected or only minimally affected by antimicrobial drugs.

Rotavirus   An organism that causes acute gastroenteritis with diarrhea, particularly in infants. This tends to peak during the winter months.

Respiratory syncytial virus (RSV)   A common cause of epidemics of acute bronchitis, bronchopneumonia, the common cold in young children and the sporadic acute bronchitis and mild upper respiratory tract infections in adults. Symptoms include fever, cough, and severe malaise.

Sedative   An agent that decreases functional activity, diminishes irritability, and allays excitement.

Sensitivity   A situation in which an organism is affected by low concentrations of antimicrobial drugs.

Serotonin   Acts as a neurotransmitter in the CNS; found in platelets and the cells of the brain and the intestines. If released in the blood vessels, it is a potent vasoconstrictor; if in the intestines, it stimulates smooth muscles to contract.

Side effect   Also called adverse effect—an undesirable or unintended effect of a drug.

Somogyi effect   Hypoglycemia in the evening results in a rebound hyperglycemia in the early morning. The low blood glucose level measured around 3 AM usually pinpoints the problem.

Status epilepticus   A medical emergency characterized by continual, uninterrupted seizures; commonly treated with IV diazepam (Valium).

Stevens-Johnson syndrome   A systemic erythema manifested by fever, lesions of mouth and eye, and a rash.

Stomatitis   Any inflammatory condition in the mouth.

Superinfection   An infection occurring during antimicrobial treatment for another infection.

Thyroxine (T_3)   Thyroid hormone that influences metabolism.

Triiodothyronine (T_4)   Thyroid hormone produced mainly from the metabolism of thyroxine in the peripheral tissues, but also made by and stored in the thyroid gland. It helps regulate growth and development, control metabolism and body temperature, and, by negative-feedback loop, inhibit the secretion of thyrotropin, a thyroid-stimulating hormone (TSH), by the pituitary gland.

Teratogenic   Substance or drug that causes fetal defects.

Therapeutic dose   Dose that may be required to produce a desired effect.

Therapeutic level   Having a serum blood level that is within normal limits.

Thrombophlebitis   Inflammation of a vein, often accompanied by formation of a clot.

Thyroid storm or thyrotoxic crisis or thyrotoxicosis   A life-threatening situation in uncontrolled hyperthyroidism with characteristic findings: fever as high as 106° F, sweating, tachycardia, extreme nervous excitability, and acute respiratory distress.

Tinnitus   A subjective noise sensation heard in one or both ears. It may occur for no apparent reason; commonly described as "ringing in the ears"; classic finding with too much aspirin or severe lithium toxicity.

Tissue necrosis   Localized tissue death that occurs in groups of cells in response to disease or injury; for example, from an infiltrated, highly caustic, or vasoconstrictive drug, such as norepinephrine (Levophed).

Topical route   By way of a body surface part, such as the skin, mucous membranes, or cornea.

Torsades de pointes   A very rapid ventricular tachycardia with gradual changing QRS complexes. May be self-limiting or turn into ventricular fibrillation. If the QT interval lengthens and the client has PVCs; the drug therapy is *not* Lidocaine, but rather magnesium IV, isuprel, or overdrive pacing.

Toxic effect   Undesirable or unintended effect of a drug when blood levels are above the therapeutic range. EXAMPLES: lanoxin toxicity: serum levels > 2.0 ng/ml; lithium toxicity: serum levels > 1.5 or 2.0 mEq/L; theophylline toxicity: serum levels > 20 mg/ml.

Toxicity   Blood level above the therapeutic range.

Trough   The lowest concentration of a drug, may be measured immediately before the drug is administered.

Tyramine   An amino acid synthesized in the body from the essential acid tyrosine. Tyramine stimulates the release of catecholamines, epinephrine and norepinephrine. Clients on MAO inhibitors must avoid foods with tyramine, particularly aged cheeses and meats, bananas, yeast-containing products, and alcoholic beverages. If restrictions are not followed, severe hypertensive crisis may result.

Vaccines   A suspension of attenuated or killed microorganisms administered PO, IM, IV, or ID to induce active immunity to infectious diseases.

Vesicant   A drug capable of causing tissue necrosis when extravasated.

Xanthine derivative   Any of the closely related alkaloids, caffeine, theobromine, and theophylline. Their pharmacologic properties stimulate the CNS, produce diuresis, relax smooth muscle; most importantly they dilate the bronchioles.

Z-track   Technique for injecting preparations into the muscle without tracking residual medication through sensitive tissue.

Bibliography

Baer C and Williams B: *Clinical pharmacology & nursing,* ed 2, Springhouse, 1992, Springhouse Corp.

Beare P and Myers J: *Principles and practice of adult health nursing,* ed 3, St Louis, 1998, Mosby.

Behrman RE and Kliegman R: *Nelson essentials of pediatrics,* Philadelphia, 1990, WB Saunders.

Clark J, Queener S, and Karb V: *Pharmacologic basis of nursing practice,* ed 6, St Louis, 2000, Mosby.

Deglin J and Vallerand A: *Davis's drug guide for nurses,* ed 6, Philadelphia, 1999, FA Davis Co.

Gahart B. and Nazareno A: *2000 IV Medications,* ed 16, St Louis, 2000, Mosby

Kuhn M: *Pharmacotherapeutics: A nursing process approach,* ed 4, Philadelphia, 1998, FA Davis Co.

Lehne R, Moore A, Crosby L, and Hamilton D: *Pharmacology for nursing care,* ed 3, Philadelphia, 1998, Saunders.

Lilly L. and Aucker R: *Pharmacology and the nursing process,* ed 2, St Louis, 1999, Mosby.

McKenry L. and Salerno E: *Pharmacology in nursing,* ed 20, St Louis, 1998, Mosby.

Mosby's medical, nursing, & allied health dictionary, ed 5, St Louis, 1998, Mosby.

Pagana K and Pagana T: *Mosby's diagnostic and laboratory test reference,* ed 4, St Louis, 1999, Mosby.

PDR: Nurse's handbook, Montvale, NJ, 1999, Medical Economics Company.

Potter P and Perry A: *Nursing interventions and clinical skills,* ed 2, St Louis, 1999, Mosby.

Perry A and Potter P: *Fundamentals of nursing,* ed 4, St Louis, 1997, Mosby.

Reiss B and Evans M: *Pharmacological aspects of nursing care,* ed 5, Albany, 1996, Delmar.

Richardson JK and Richardson L: *The mathematics of drugs and solutions,* ed 5, St Louis, 1994, Mosby.

Rollant P: *Acing multiple choice tests, AJN Career Guide for 1994,* pp. 18-21, 36, Jan 1994.

Rollant P: *Soar to success: Do your best on nursing tests,* St Louis, 1999, Mosby.

Skidmore-Roth L: *Mosby's drug guide for nurses,* ed 3, St Louis, 1999, Mosby.

Skidmore-Roth L: *Mosby's nursing drug reference,* St Louis, 2000, Mosby.

Spratto G and Woods AL: *Nurse's drug reference,* Albany, 1994, Delmar.

Vallerand A: *Nursing pharmacology,* ed 2, Springhouse, 1993, Springhouse Corp.

Wallace L and Wardel S: *Nursing pharmacology,* ed 2, Boston, 1992, Jones & Bartlett Publishers.

Wilson B, Shannon M, and Stang C: *Nurse's drug guide 2000,* Norwalk, 2000, Appleton & Lange.

Wilson B, Shannon M, and Stang C: *Health Professionals nurse's drug guide 2000,* Norwalk, 2000, Appleton & Lange.

Index

Nonnarcotic analgesics
  actions of, 126
  common drugs, 127-128
  nursing implications for, 127
  uses and side effects of, 126-127
Nonnucleoside reverse transcriptase
    inhibitors, 206
Nonsteroidal antiallergy agents
  common drugs, 235
  uses and side effects of, 234
Nonsteroidal antiinflammatory drugs,
    128
Nucleoside inhibitors
  actions of, 205
  common drugs, 206
  uses and side effects of, 205-206
Nurse practitioners, prescriptive authority
    for, 9
Nurses, medication administration rules
    for, 7-9

O

Ophthalmic drops and ointments,
    medication administration through,
    44
Oral anticoagulants
  actions of, 184
  common drugs, 186
  nursing implications for, 185-186
  uses and side effects of, 184-185
Oral contraceptives (birth control pills)
  actions of, 322
  common drugs, 324t-326t
  uses and side effects of, 322
Oral route for medication administration,
    39-40
Osmotics
  actions of, 176
  common drugs, 177, 311
  uses and side effects of, 177
Otic drops, medication administration
    through, 44
Ovulation stimulants, uses and side
    effects of, 327
Oxazolidinediones, uses and side effects
    of, 333
Oxytocics
  ergot alkaloids, 214-215
  oxytocin, 214

P

Pain
  mixed narcotic agonist-antagonist
      agents for treating, 125
  narcotic antagonists for treating,
      126
  narcotics for treating, 124-125
  nonnarcotic analgesics for treating,
      126-128
  nonsteroidal antiinflammatory drugs for
      treating, 128
Parathyroid hormone
  actions of, 216
  common drugs, 217
  uses and side effects of, 216
Parenteral anticoagulants
  actions of, 186
  common drugs, 188
  nursing implications for, 187
  uses and side effects of, 186-187
Parenteral route
  effects on absorption process, 21t
  for medication administration, 11
Parkinson's disease, defined, 75
Penicillins
  actions of, 259
  drug categories, 260
  substitutes, 266-267
  uses and side effects of, 259-260
Peptic ulcer disease
  antacids for treating, 292-293
  anticholinergic agents for treating,
      294-295
  antimicrobials for treating, 295
  H_2 histamine receptor antagonists and
      gastric protectants for treating,
      293-294
  proton (acid) pump inhibitors for
      treating, 294
Peripherally acting antiadrenergic agents,
    160
Pharmacodynamics phase of drug therapy,
    23-24
Pharmacokinetics phase
  absorption, 20-21
  distribution, 22
  excretion, 23
  metabolism, 22